Introduction to
to
DIAGNOSTIC
IMAGING

ISADORE MESCHAN, M.D.
Professor of Radiology

and

DAVID J. OTT, M.D.
Associate Professor of Radiology,

Bowman Gray School of Medicine,
Wake Forest University,
Winston-Salem, North Carolina

1984
W.B. Saunders Company
Philadelphia / London / Toronto / Mexico City / Rio de Janeiro / Sydney / Tokyo

W. B. Saunders Company: West Washington Square
Philadelphia, PA 19105

1 St. Anne's Road
Eastbourne, East Sussex BN21 3UN, England

1 Goldthorne Avenue
Toronto, Ontario M8Z 5T9, Canada

Apartado 26370—Cedro 512
Mexico 4, D.F., Mexico

Rua Coronel Cabrita, 8
Sao Cristovao Caixa Postal 21176
Rio de Janeiro, Brazil

9 Waltham Street
Artarmon, N.S.W. 2064, Australia

Ichibancho, Central Bldg., 22-1 Ichibancho
Chiyoda-Ku, Tokyo 102, Japan

Library of Congress Cataloging in Publication Data

Meschan, Isadore.

Introduction to diagnostic imaging.

1. Diagnosis, Radioscopic.   2. Imaging systems in
   medicine.   I. Ott, David J. (David James), 1946–   .
   II. Title.   III. Title: Diagnostic imaging. [DNLM: 1. Radiography. WN 200 M578i]

RC78.M386 1984   616.07'57   83–4643

ISBN 0–7216–6277–3 (pbk.)

Introduction to Diagnostic Imaging   ISBN   0-7216-6277-3

Last digit is the print number: 9   8   7   6   5   4   3   2   1

DEDICATION
To our families

Preface

The goal of this text is to teach the fundamentals of diagnostic imaging to the advanced medical student and to the family practitioner who has been caught in the great avalanche of imaging techniques that have become available in the last decade.

In most medical curricula, the medical student is taught an introduction to radiographic anatomy; somewhat later the student is usually exposed to a didactic course of limited hours in the fundamentals of diagnostic imaging, nuclear medicine, and radiation therapy; he or she then reviews with the preceptor the films on those patients assigned during the clinical clerkship.

In many curricula there is no obligated time for the teaching of diagnostic imaging in an organized fashion beyond this point, although in many medical schools an elective is provided for this purpose.

This text has been designed primarily for that group of students who have been given the opportunity to elect radiology at this point in their medical training, and for students who are denied the opportunity of such an elective in diagnostic radiology.

Thus this text is divided into the following basic parts:

1. In every section, we have introduced an area of diagnostic imaging with preliminary didactic material. In this area, we have tried to outline, as briefly as space would permit, a "methodology" for the approach to diagnostic imaging, even as the student has learned a "methodology" in the courses in physical diagnosis.

2. Once this methodology has been mastered, we present certain basic roentgen signs of abnormality that we have learned through the years are most frequently encountered in general practice.

3. Thereafter, we have utilized the "quiz case" approach to see whether the student has grasped the fundamentals. The "questions" in these cases are of the type utilized on National Board Examinations. The discussion following each quiz case is divided into three parts: (a) the roentgen signs that should have been observed by the student; (b) the differential diagnosis derived from the integration of the "given" clinical data and these roentgen signs; and (c) a discussion of the clinical entity illustrated, particularly in relation to similar entities, with points of difference illustrated wherever feasible. In this manner it is our hope that the student may grasp a concept of the entire process of integration of the clinical, laboratory, and diagnostic imaging techniques.

Although the number of pages consumed by this text seems great at first glance, it will be noted that much of the text is devoted to illustrative material. We believe that the entire text is not too expansive for a "four-week" curriculum in which we have tried to adapt our own thinking to help those who might use this text material for an equivalent amount of time in study.

ISADORE MESCHAN, M.D.
DAVID J. OTT, M.D.

Acknowledgements

For a number of years, one of us (I.M.) had taught medical students at an advanced level from his book *Synopsis of the Analysis of Roentgen Signs* (2nd edition, 1976). We now use this text as an overview for first year residents in diagnostic radiology.

It was Dr. Joseph E. Whitley who pointed out to us (1) that this didactic text experience was too vast for the senior medical student; and (2) that there was little time left to teach the student from a personal experience approach. We owe Dr. Whitley a debt of gratitude for altering these earlier errors of judgment to what we now feel is a better approach after several years of development by one of us (D.J.O.).

Our colleagues have been very generous in leading us to examples for "quiz cases" as well as to illustrations for discussion. We hope there has been appropriate acknowledgement in every instance.

The basic text for this presentation was originally written by one of us (I.M.) for presentation as a chapter in Dr. Robert E. Taylor's *Family Practice: Principles and Practice* (2nd edition, New York, Springer Verlag, 1983) by personal copyright, so that we could retain those parts most relevant to this presentation, in which the other of us (D.J.O.) could make an optimum contribution. There is obviously some resemblance between the two presentations in didactic (non-exercise) materials. In all other respects, this latter text is entirely different and significantly amplified. To Dr. Taylor we owe a debt of gratitude for his earlier critical comments and editorial assistance, especially since the family practitioner is an important segment of our audience.

To our secretaries, Mrs. Nadeene Temple, Mrs. Edna Snow, and Mrs. Carolyn Ezzell, theirs has been a "labor of academia." Mrs. Snow has helped one of us (I.M.) through several textbooks, and this is Mrs. Temple's second. Good secretaries are essential to the process of writing; producing the text would have been impossible without their assistance.

Our Department of Audiovisual Resources, under the direction of Mr. George Lynch, has been extremely helpful, as he has been in all our publications.

Last but not least, our deep appreciation goes to our publishers, W. B. Saunders Company, who have helped inestimably in the organization of the material as it is being presented and who have provided the editorial guidance that has allowed us to achieve the definitive "chapter approach."

In the ultimate, the authors must take full responsibility, with the hope that, as Dante has said, "give light and people will find their way."

I.M.
D.J.O.

Contents

1

The Scope of Diagnostic Imaging

Diagnostic radiology (including ultrasonography) has undergone tremendous strides in the past decade, particularly since the introduction of computerization techniques, and it has become increasingly difficult for the non-radiologist to acquire a sufficient overview of the field to utilize its many component parts to the best advantage of his patient.

The direct photographic effects of ionizing radiation were applied very quickly. Thereafter, image intensification with the use of intensifying screens contained within cassettes, the utilization of extremely small focal spots in x-ray tubes, and the development of vacuum tubes, the rotating anode to facilitate cooling, and the utilization of full wave rectification denoted great progress toward a rapid image with minimal exposure to ionizing radiation. The high resolution was enhanced with the introduction of the Potter-Bucky diaphragm, which helped eliminate scattered radiation.

The introduction of the image intensifier tube allowed the fluoroscopist to use the cone vision of his retina, instead of rods in complete darkness, and television viewing and video tape recording have become readily available.

Alongside these great discoveries was the increased mechanization of the development and fixation process of the film itself, which allows high resolution and excellent contrast, with film interposed for development after exposure of the latent image, and the viewing of a completely dry image of excellent quality in 90 seconds.

The transverse axial computerized image, with its algorithmic reconstruction to other planes, will be described subsequently. Other developments of the more recent past include ultrasonography, emission tomography, tremendous advances in nuclear medicine, and the application of nuclear magnetic resonance.

DIAGNOSTIC IMAGING IN MANAGEMENT OF CLINICAL PROBLEMS

After a physician has obtained his clinical history, and performed a thorough physical examination, he defines for himself certain pathophysiological disturbances in his patient.

In sorting these out, he virtually makes an outline to approach a definitive diagnosis. In so doing, he evolves a plan for action—sometimes referred to as an algorithm—in which a decision tree is formed.

Some aspects of this format involve clinical pathology or other similar tests, whereas in over one half of his patients he will most likely decide to resort to one or another method of diagnostic imaging, usually employing the consultative services of a radiologist. It will be our purpose in this text to provide an overview of diagnostic imaging in its many ramifications.

Radiology, more broadly conceived in this text as diagnostic imaging, since more is involved than ionizing radiation, begins therefore with an understanding of the clinical problem at hand for which a certain methodology is chosen. Having obtained the end results of these methodologies, the radiologist analyzes each in a careful, systematic fashion, eliciting signs of abnormality. He then refers back to the patient, perhaps for a different or more accurate elucidation of these objective findings, so that he may narrow the clinical problem down. Some have called this "triangulation" in which the

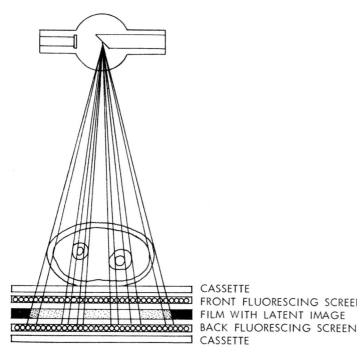

CASSETTE
FRONT FLUORESCING SCREEN
FILM WITH LATENT IMAGE
BACK FLUORESCING SCREEN
CASSETTE

Figure 1–1. Diagram illustrating x-rays from the target of an x-ray tube striking the forearm and passing through a cassette containing film. The remnant radiation passes through the forearm, producing a latent image on the film. (From Meschan, I.: Synopsis of Analysis of Roentgen Signs in General Radiology. Philadelphia, W. B. Saunders Co., 1976.)

"signs of abnormality in the diagnostic image" are integrated with the "clinical and laboratory studies" to render a "differential diagnosis opinion."

Very often this opinion will be a "statistical one" dealing with entities that are "most likely" as against those that are "least likely." Noninvasive procedures are chosen first in preference to "invasive" ones, which carry an element of risk. However, there is a place, as we shall note, for interventional techniques when appropriate in the course of the ultimate study.

Diagnostic imaging basically involves three technologies: (1) The transmission of ionizing radiation through an organ or anatomic part—and a record made of the beam emitted on film, a cathode ray oscilloscope, or a television apparatus (Fig. 1–1). (2) The emission of ionizing radiation from the patient after he has had an injection of an appropriate pharmaceutical. The emitted image is recorded on a special camera device (with or without a computer in the circuit) and a photograph is rendered by this camera (nuclear medicine). (3) The passage of a sound beam through the body or anatomic part, with a recording of the reflected echo (ultrasonography). These technologies will be more thoroughly discussed in their appropriate sections.

METHODOLOGIES

Plain Film Studies

Plain films, without the introduction of contrast studies or other special techniques in diagnostic radiology, compose the great bulk of diagnostic imaging. For example, over half the workload of the average x-ray department involves plain films of the chest. In other areas of the body, plain films compose the baseline for comparison of all contrast studies. The first consideration, therefore, in respect to diagnostic imaging should be in this area.

Contrast Studies

Contrast studies involve the introduction of a suitable agent that is opaque to x-rays into an organ or vascular lumen. Contrast enhancement of the organ or vascular lumen will be shown to be basic to most diagnostic imaging with ionizing radiation.

Angiology and Cardiovascular Imaging by Special Catheterization Techniques

This modality requires that a catheter be introduced into a remote blood vessel and passed through the vascular system under fluoroscopic control to the appropriate blood vessel or cardiac chamber desired. A suitable water-soluble contrast agent is injected, either manually or by special mechanical devices, for contrast enhancement of the appropriate vascular system or cardiovascular chambers.

This technique is considered invasive, and is indicated where a visualization of the blood supply of an organ or body part is necessary to make a definitive diagnosis. There are some rare complications that involve bleeding from the blood vessel puncture site, and *very rarely* there are problems of embolism, catheter breakage, and direct trauma to the vessels from the catheter or its guide wire. The technique is, therefore, carefully selected for certain clinical problems only. "Digital subtraction" overcomes many of these problems, is utilized wherever possible, and will be described subsequently.

Interventional Radiology

There is an increasing involvement of radiologists in both diagnostic and therapeutic interventional procedures. Many interventional diagnostic procedures involve both selective and nonselective arterial examinations: e.g., aortography; visceral angiography; renal arteriography; coronary arteriography; neuroangiography; many venous examinations involving the lower extremity and the superior and inferior vena cava; renal venography; pulmonary angiography; adrenal venography; and epidural venography. Other interventional special procedures include musculoskeletal arthrography for visualization of joints particularly; myelography; transhepatic cholangiography; splenoportography; sialography; bronchography; hysterosalpingography; and lymphangiography. Some of these interventional techniques involve percutaneous biopsies of the breast, lung, liver, or kidney. At times, when the diagnostic image is adequate for the purpose, a transcatheter therapeutic embolization is carried out to obliterate the blood supply to a malignancy. This measure and such interventional techniques as the nonoperative extraction of retained biliary calculi fall more properly into the therapeutic realm. Transluminal angioplasty is likewise a therapeutic procedure for opening up major blood vessels responsible for ischemia of organs such as the kidney, but is undertaken

only after the diagnostic imaging is appropriately accomplished.

Computed Tomography of the Transmission Type

In this newly developed technology, at first a fine pencil-like beam was employed which was transmitted through the body to cover a cross-sectional slice approximately 1 cm. in thickness. The remnant radiation following this transmission was received by an appropriate phosphorescent solid or liquid material. The pencil beam was moved at one-degree intervals, and the receptor device recording the remnant radiation backtracked its information to a computer, "informing" the computer of the number of photons absorbed in the transmission (Fig. 1–2). In this technology, the cross-section traversed in this manner at one-degree intervals was divided into thousands of small volume elements (called voxels) measuring approximately $1.3 \times 1.3 \times 0.5$ cm. By the application of an appropriate algorithm to the computer, the computer was enabled to record within the voxel the number of photons absorbed during the transmission by each volume element. This information was thereafter electronically translated to a cathode ray oscilloscope or television monitor and an image re-created in respect to the photon absorption by each volume element. In this fashion, the anatomy of the cross-section was virtually recreated. The original computed tomography of the transmission type has undergone many stages of development utilizing a fan beam (Fig. 1–3) instead of the pencil-like beam, and utilizing much more sophisticated computer technology. It is now possible to re-create a television image of the cross-section in as little as one second.

Computed Tomography of the Emission Type

In emission type tomography the photons being recorded in the volume elements are those obtained from the body itself, after an appropriate radionuclide has been introduced into the body. This technology has not at this writing achieved the high resolution of transmission type computed tomography, but may well have applications in the future, particularly in the recording of important physiologic changes. Emission tomo-

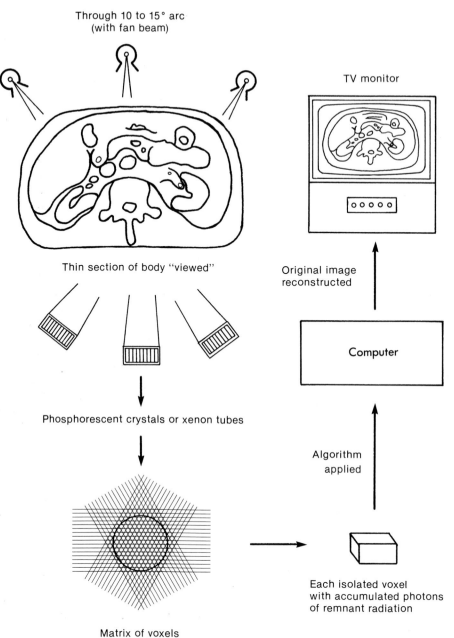

Figure 1–2. Line diagram illustrating the basic theory of operation of computed axial tomography.

graphs are used very little at this time and will be given only brief mention in this text.

Nuclear Medicine

The peaceful uses of nuclear medicine have involved the development of appropriate radiopharmaceuticals. In this technology the radionuclide is administered usually intravenously, but occasionally orally, and is especially applicable for visualization of the brain, skeleton, liver, spleen, bone marrow, lungs, heart, thyroid, tumors and abscesses, and the kidney. This technology is useful not only for the morphology but also for information regarding physiologic function and disturbances in the body, and these methods will be appropriately described.

Clinical Ultrasonography

Diagnostic clinical ultrasonography involves the utilization of sound waves, which are propagated through the body, by a

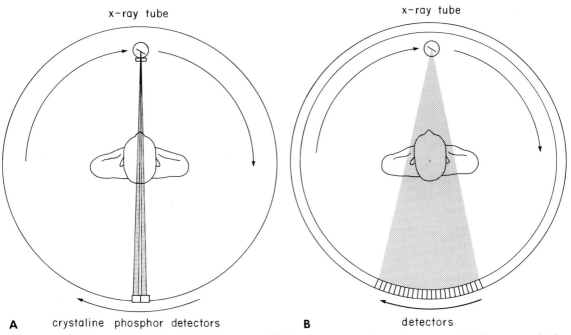

Figure 1–3. *A,* Movement of tube and detectors: 180 degrees at one degree increments. *B,* Movement of tube and detectors: 180 degrees in 10 degree arc increments. Detectors are crystalline phosphors or xenon gas tubes. There have been further developments beyond this "fan beam" to involve a complete circle of detectors and even multiple x-ray tubes. (From Bo, W. J., Meschan, I., and Kreuger, W. A.: Basic Atlas of Cross-Sectional Anatomy. Philadelphia, W. B. Saunders Co., 1980, p. xiii.)

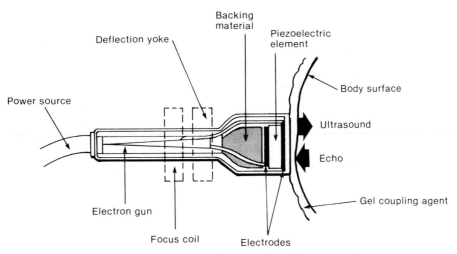

Figure 1–4. Diagram of a transducer used in ultrasonography.

"transducer" mechanism. Sound waves have different velocities in common biologic materials, although, with the exception of air, bone, fat, water, and the lens of the eye, most biologic tissues transmit sound with an average of 1540 meters per second. The sound intensities encountered in medical imaging vary over a wide range. The sound wave may be depicted as striking an object and then being partially reflected backward toward the transducer, with some of the sound energy entering the object itself where it is again possibly reflected. Thus, separate echoes from various portions of the objects struck excite the very same transducer that originally emitted the sound wave. This pulse-echo mode is the basis for ultrasonic medical imaging. The transducer (Fig. 1–4) receiving the echo processes this signal, passes it along to an electronic memory, and thereafter to an appropriate monitor display mechanism. Variations and applications of clinical ultrasonography will be described.

Xeroradiography

A xeroradiograph is the photographic image of a thin layer of selenium on a rigid aluminum support on which a uniform electrostatic charge has been "disturbed" by the remnant radiation passing through an anatomic part. The electrostatic image so produced is made visible by spraying a charged image powder onto the rearranged selenium particles. This powdered image is transferred to a charged paper, and thereafter it is fused to the paper by heat. The peculiar attributes of "edge-enhancement" of this technology and its particular usefulness in mammography, bone radiology, and cadaveric study will be discussed in greater detail.

Thermography

Photographs obtained with an infrared camera of different parts of the human body, discerning different temperatures in tissues, is called *thermography*. This technology has been used as a screening technique in breast cancer and also in investigations for peripheral vascular disease. It is not widely represented in radiology departments in this country at this time.

Specialized Subtraction Techniques Utilizing Computers (Digital Radiography)

Digital radiography and fluoroscopy, which are rapidly coming to the fore at this writing, involve the simple intravenous injection of a contrast agent and computerized subtraction of all surrounding tissues. It is conceivable that this technology will replace some catheterization techniques. This method is still developmental and is being rapidly and successfully achieved.

Nuclear Magnetic Resonance

When a body or organ (as well as a chemical) is placed in a strong magnetic field, and radiofrequency waves allowed to pass through that field, there is a primary and secondary movement of the hydrogen ions particularly of protons in that field. This movement is recorded with the aid of a detector and computer device and ultimately visualized on a monitor in much the same way as computed tomography. This modality of imaging has the great advantage over ionizing radiation in that no deleterious effects have thus far been reported from either the magnetic field or the radiofrequency waves employed. It is still in a developmental phase, but augurs well for the future. The images produced resemble those obtained with transmission type computed tomography to some extent, but since the modality of producing the image is entirely different, a new set of normals will be required. Images resembling those obtained with computed tomography are already of excellent quality in the case of the head.

2

Basic Radiologic Physical Principles

Since ionizing radiation is basic to most of the modalities described in Chapter 1, certain basic physical and interpretive radiologic principles must be discussed, and the hazards of ionizing radiation understood.

In direct radiography, the x-ray beam passes through the body part and is attenuated variably, depending on the density of the portions of anatomy traversed. This results in five basic densities (Fig. 2–1) on a film: air appears black; fat appears dark gray; soft tissues, which are near unit density, appear a lighter gray; bone appears moderately white; and metallic densities appear very white. Until recently these were the main densities recorded on x-ray film. With the advent of computed tomography, many additional orders of density, based upon the "absorption of x-ray photons in tissues of differing densities and composition" ("absorption coefficient"), are now possible. In deference to the inventor of this apparatus, these absorption coefficients are now referred to as "Hounsfield units," or "H." Graphs such as the one demonstrated in Figure 2–2

have been devised but, unfortunately, these numbers vary not only from manufacturer to manufacturer but also in the same models of machines made by one manufacturer. The graph presented does demonstrate the tremendous capabilities of computed tomography in expanding the five basic densities illustrated in Figure 2–2.

When the x-ray beam itself is used to photosensitize the silver halide emulsion on the film, the film is described as a "no-screen film." Usually, however, the x-ray film is interposed between two intensifying screens in an *x-ray cassette*. The x-ray cassette is a lightproof housing, and contains both a front intensifying screen and a backscreen, coated with a phosphorescent material, which is somewhat thicker. The phosphorescent material so employed on intensifying screens varies, and almost invariably, the x-ray beam, when it strikes the phosphorescent material, is converted to ultraviolet light. It is the ultraviolet light image that photosensitizes the x-ray film emulsion. Many screens so employed are highly sensitive to the x-ray

VERY RADIOLUCENT	MODERATELY RADIOLUCENT	INTERMEDIATE	MODERATELY RADIOPAQUE	VERY RADIOPAQUE
Gas	Fatty tissue	Connective tissue Muscle tissue Blood Cartilage Epithelium Cholesterol stones Uric acid stones	Bone Calcium salts	Heavy metals

Figure 2–1. Classification of tissues and other substances with medical application in accordance with five general categories of radiopacity and radiolucency. This tabulation relates to conventional, but not computerized, tomographic radiography. An entirely different scale of densities will be shown for computed tomography (formerly called "computerized" tomography).

7

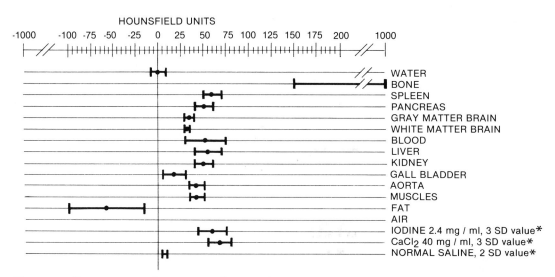

Figure 2–2. Representative absorption coefficients of different tissues expressed as Hounsfield units. These are known to vary from machine to machine and even from the same manufacturer, but are representative of the greater latitude in differentiating tissues that computed tomography offers. (Modified from Zatz, L. M.: in Ter-Pogossian, M. (ed.): Workshop on Reconstruction Tomography in Diagnostic Radiology and Nuclear Medicine (Proceedings). Baltimore, University Park Press, 1977.)

beam, but in most instances the greater the sensitivity the less is the resolution. Some sacrifice is made for "speed" of exposure as against "detail" or resolution of the image. The *rare earth* screens that have recently become available allow a considerable reduction in the amount of ionizing radiation necessary to produce a high resolution image. These screens are as yet very expensive and are not routinely employed. Their use reduces x-ray exposure by a factor of two, sometimes three.

Fortunately many organs of the body are encased in an envelope of fat (the so-called tela subserosa), and as a result the black x-ray depiction of the fat provides contrast and permits visualization of the contour of the organ. This is particularly true of such organs as the kidney and many of the muscles—especially those of the retroperitoneum.

Another format in which diagnostic imaging is produced conventionally by ionizing radiation is fluoroscopy. All modern fluoroscopes are equipped with image intensifier tubes. This type of image amplification allows the viewer to see the diagnostic image with the cones of his retina, rather than with the rods, as by older techniques. In addition to the markedly increased resolution and detail it affords, this type of image amplification has obviated light adaptation prior to fluoroscopy. The great advantage of fluoroscopy in diagnostic imaging is that the organ

or organ part is viewed in rapid sequence, recording its physiologic motor activity and slight changes in respect to time.

Diagnostic imaging may be obtained by films exposed in rapid sequence, as is often done in the permanent recording of a contrast-enhanced blood stream through various parts of the body—producing the so-called "angiogram." This technique is applied successfully in studies of the brain, heart, lungs, kidneys, viscera, and extremities.

INTERPRETIVE ASPECTS OF DIAGNOSTIC IMAGING

Basic Positions and Views in Diagnostic Imaging with Ionizing Radiation

Basic positions, such as anteroposterior, lateral, and oblique, compose most standard radiologic examinations. A projection is named by virtue of the portion of the body that is entered first by the ionizing beam of radiation. Thus, a *posteroanterior projection* of the chest is one in which the patient stands in front of the film-bearing cassette so that the ionizing beam will enter the posterior aspect of the patient first, traverse the patient, and exit through the anterior aspect thereafter. Radiation that remains after traversing the patient, not having been absorbed in the patient, is called "remnant radiation." As previously indicated, this strikes the film, producing the photosensitization of the silver halide emulsion on the film, either by the direct effect of the ionizing radiation or by the phosphorescence on the crystals of the intensifying screen. The accompanying illustration (Fig. 2–3) demonstrates the positions and projections commonly employed.

Anyone who would undertake the interpretation of roentgenograms must not only familiarize himself with these various positions and projections but must also learn in great detail the anatomy so depicted. This anatomy, of course, is correlated with the dissected anatomy learned in prior exercise. However, the degradation of the ionizing radiation, its "scattering," its "resolution," and artefacts that might be obtrusive in the way of the ionizing beam are understood thoroughly, so that the ultimate interpretation may be accomplished in three dimensions.

Routinization of Study of the Radiograph

When the radiograph is obtained and viewed it is studied in a routine fashion, so that even the most minute abnormalities can be detected. Just as physicians adhere to a standard routine for obtaining a detailed history and performing a physical examination so that nothing of importance is overlooked, so is the radiograph viewed. Certain of these routines will be demonstrated in appropriate sections.

Nine Basic Roentgen Signs

Just as the pathologist has organized his thinking in terms of basic processes that may occur anywhere in the human body (general pathology), such as hyperemia, inflammation, neoplasia, hyperplasia, hamartoma, and the like, the radiologist has formulated a *radiologic pathology* that is particularly suited to any roentgenogram of any organ system. We have subdivided these generally into nine basic roentgen signs, which may be tabulated as follows:

1. Alterations in *size* of the organ or part of the organ ●
2. Alterations in *number* ●
3. Changes in *density* with respect to the ionizing radiation ●
4. Changes in *shape* from the normal ●
5. Changes in *position* from the normal ●
6. Changes in *architecture*, both internal and external ●
7. Alterations in *function* of the organ or a part of an organ system ●
8. *Changes with respect to time* when one views radiographs in sequence ●
9. Changes with respect to *treatment* ●

Each of these nine basic roentgen signs requires that the observer learn the normal and its variations as they relate to the patient's age, sex, and even racial characteristics. The normal *size* and *number* of organs and systems are well understood. Duplications of some single organs may occur (esophagus, stomach, and other portions of the gastrointestinal tract). As indicated earlier, *density* was originally thought to have five basic presentations (see Fig. 2–1). With the advent of computed tomography, this concept has been significantly altered, and tissues may now be classified according to the number of photons of ionizing radiation absorbed by them (see Fig. 2–2). Although this concept continues to change with each new development in this instrumentation, one can readily note that in the brain, the gray matter may be differentiated from the white, and the cerebrospinal fluid can be clearly visualized as separate from the brain. In the spinal canal, the leptomeninges can be clearly differentiated from the spinal cord. In the abdomen, the liver is considerably denser than other organs of the abdomen and can be clearly differentiated from such other abdominal viscera as the pancreas, the aorta, the inferior vena cava, and many of the major arterial and venous branches. In the muscles, the facial planes can often be clearly differentiated and individual muscles identified. In the bones, trabeculae can be seen in great detail and dense compact bone clearly differentiated from that which is medullary. (With regard to metallic density, the metal must be of a subdued variety because scattering occurs readily from metal and reduces the accuracy of computed tomography.) Contrast substances, when utilized in moderate dilution, have a wide applicability in computed tomography, and this applicability is spoken of as "contrast enhancement."

Alterations in *contour* or *shape* require

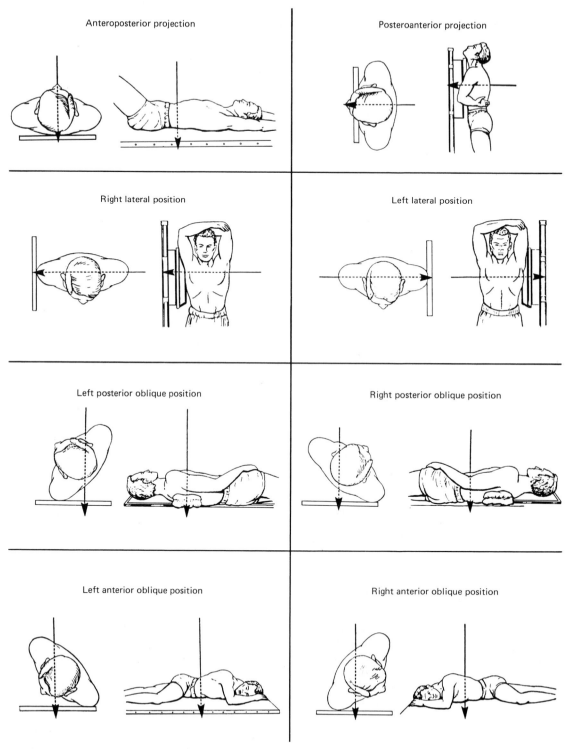

Figure 2–3. The commonly employed positions and projections of an anatomic part in diagnostic imaging with ionizing radiation. (From Standard Terminology for Positioning and Projection. American Registry of Radiologic Technologists, Minneapolis, Minnesota.)

that the observer know the normal from the abnormal. As examples, the slightest alteration in the contour of the kidney may have great significance: an outpouching may signify the presence of a tumor, whereas an indentation may be caused by a scar from infarction or pyelonephritis. The shape of the stomach, even though highly variable because of peristalsis, may sometimes indicate the presence of a rigid tumor as in linitis plastica, ulcer, or cancer. The shape of a bone may indicate whether the epiphyses, metaphyses, or diaphyses have developed normally, findings that are highly significant in the diagnosis of certain diseases and syndromes. Shape must be studied in three dimensions, not just from a single planar view. With ordinary radiography, this is accomplished by the multiplicity of projections. With computed tomography, computerized isometric reconstruction may be accomplished with appropriate algorithms.

The *position* of an organ or part may be the most important abnormality. For example, kidneys may be ectopic, giving rise to a condition known as "crossed ectopia." The stomach may be displaced on the basis of a vector principle when a mass lesion is adjoining it. The visceral pleura surrounding the lung may be displaced from its normal position by inflammation or tumor. The heart or mediastinum may be displaced from a normal position by atelectasis or by a solid lesion.

The intricate *architecture* of an organ or organ part consists primarily of two parts: the *outer boundary* and the *inner structure*. The outer boundary may or may not be capsular. The capsule, if present, may be discontinuous and either thin or thick. Each of these characteristics has a separate pathologic connotation. The inner architecture of an organ or an organ part also is significant. Familiarity with the architecture of the kidney, for example, is essential. The cortex of the kidney has a finite thickness. The pyramids of the kidney have finite thickness as well as shape. The calyces and collecting system of the kidney have a very specific internal architectural pattern. The colon, too, when filled with double contrast media, lends itself to architectural analysis. By filling the colon appropriately with high-density barium and air, it is possible to see changes in internal architecture that approach 5 mm. in size, indicating polypoid masses or even neoplasia.

The *function* of many organs can be ana-

lyzed radiologically. For example, we can cite the gallbladder. When certain contrast agents are introduced orally, they interact with bile in the upper gastrointestinal tract, are absorbed into the blood stream, and when traversing the liver react with glucuronidase to form a complex. This in turn is absorbed by the liver parenchyma and secreted into the biliary system. As this passes through the biliary system and gallbladder, it remains in the gallbladder long enough to become concentrated normally. When this does not occur, particularly after two doses conventionally utilized in this examination, a diseased gallbladder may be diagnosed, if the gallbladder is present, with an accuracy exceeding 95%.

The function of the kidney is another case in point. Most of the contrast agents employed for visualization of the collecting system of the kidney measure the ability of the kidney in terms of glomerular filtration. Some agents, such as Hippuran, measure tubular function primarily, but these are seldom used when filtration fraction may be calculated. The motor function of the gastrointestinal tract lends itself readily to fluoroscopic study. The presence or absence of appropriate peristalsis in the esophagus, when the patient is in the recumbent position, may determine the diagnosis of scleroderma. Peristalsis in the stomach may not occur when the stomach is rigid as the result of an infiltrative process by a neoplasm (linitis plastica). The heart may be visualized as functioning abnormally fluoroscopically when its pulsatile activity is aberrant. The detection of *alterations in respect to time* require that at least two films of the patient be available for study on two separate occasions. These "serial film studies" permit differentiation between acute and chronic illness. This differentiation has an important bearing on etiology and pathologic significance.

Alterations with respect to treatment must be known by the physician before analysis of the radiograph is feasible. For example, a patient originally may have had considerable lymphadenopathy of the mediastinum, which virtually disappears when treated with an appropriate quantity of x-rays. If the patient is seen after treatment, the diagnosis may not be made. Surgery almost invariably alters many of the normal roentgen signs. Not only may an organ be absent, but it may be altered in size, shape, position, or contour by surgery.

These nine basic roentgen signs are applicable not only to the organ as a whole but to each part as it is studied in sequence radiographically.

Amalgamation of Roentgen Signs with History and Physical Examination

After the basic roentgen signs are elucidated, the patient's history and physical examination are once again carefully reviewed. These are integrated with the roentgen signs to achieve differential diagnosis. It must be presumed that the original examination ordered is based on an appropriate evaluation of the history and physical findings. Once the differential diagnosis is achieved, other examinations may be indicated—both by diagnostic imaging and by clinical pathology. For example, jaundice is an obvious indication for a serum bilirubin test. The usual findings in blood analysis will bring some diagnoses to the fore and suppress others. An elevated globulin, for example, also differentiates certain diseases.

Having achieved this more finite differential diagnosis, the physician is now prepared to separate the *more likely* entities from those that *are very likely.* The practice of medicine has been likened to the field of statistics. The physician draws heavily on statistical methods when correlating roentgen findings with the information obtained through history, physical diagnosis, and laboratory findings. When a patient is referred for radiologic study, the radiologist should be apprised of these elements.

HAZARDS OF RADIOLOGY

Radiation, as it traverses the anatomic part, introduces ionization. Ionization in tissues is undesirable, but experience has shown that within certain limits it is "tolerable." It is expressly important that the physician understand certain physical principles that are fundamental to ionizing radiation.

Radiation has been quantified by employing the term "roentgen," which is a measurement in reference to *ionization in air.* This can be understood readily if one visualizes a cubic centimeter of air under standard conditions of pressure and temperature, and realizes that one roentgen is measured when the ions produced in this cubic centi-

meter by radiation produce one electrostatic unit of electricity.

Radiobiologists have realized for some years that ionization in air is not the best reference point for the use of ionizing radiation in human beings. As a result the term "rad" was devised, which is a *measurement of absorbed dose.* Fortunately, in the diagnostic range of the kilovoltages and milliamperages utilized in diagnostic imaging, the roentgen and rad are very similar to one another, and such differences as exist are of primary importance to the radiotherapist rather than to those who employ ionizing radiation for diagnostic techniques.

It is difficult to assess the harmfulness of ionizing radiation to the biologic mechanism in those doses used in diagnostic imaging, but certain truisms can be enumerated:

1. In diagnostic radiology, exposure of the anatomic part is more appropriately measured in thousandths of rads, or *millirads,* than in rads.

2. Exposure of the neonate or infant is many times more "harmful" than exposure of the adult, the fetal and infantile tissues having greater sensitivity than those of the adult.

3. No one can accurately define the so-called "minimum tolerable dose" for a patient who is being studied for a disease process. However, as a point of reference, those who are occupationally exposed are required to stay within standards that do not allow exposures in excess of 5 rads per year beyond the age of 18. The usual allowance, then, is in the order of 50 to 60 rads per lifetime. The main hazard in those who are occupationally exposed is the *genetic* hazard. However, if they receive repeated and excessive exposure, the carcinogenic and leukemogenic effect of radiation may take hold, and either cancer or a reduction in life span may result. It is generally estimated that those who are not occupationally exposed and who are not patients should not receive more than 0.5 rads per year after the age of 18. This begins to approach the environmental exposure to ionizing radiation in the atmosphere. If one follows these general guidelines, it is believed that the genetic pool of man will not be impaired. For an understanding of the exposure of skin and gonads during the most common examinations performed, the reader is referred to Table 2–1. Exposure in the region of the gonads, which obviously requires the greatest caution, is most likely to occur

Table 2–1 RADIATION DOSE RECEIVED BY SKIN AND GONADS FOR COMMONLY EMPLOYED RADIOLOGICAL STUDIES

Examination Site	kvp.	mas.	Focus Film Distance (in.)	Added Filtration (mm. Al)	Skin Dose (mrad)	Gonadal Dose (mrad) Male	Female
Skull (5 views)	74–90	20	36	3.0	635.6	2.32	.72
Paranasal sinuses (3 views)	66–86	20	36	3.0	327.2	<0.03	<0.03
Hand and wrist (3 views)	54	5	40	2.5	—	<0.01	<0.01
Chest, PA	100	5	72	2.5	9.21	0.02	0.04
Chest, lat.	110	15	72	2.5	37	0.03	0.08
Chest, obl.	100	10	72	2.5	17	0.02	0.04
Thoracic spine, AP	100	30	40	2.5	249	0.19	0.26
Thoracic spine, lat.	110	60	40	2.5	707	0.17	0.54
Lumbar spine, AP	100	30	40	2.5	221	14.7	70.4
Lumbar spine, lat.	120	60	40	2.5	820	9.77	61.5
Lumbar spine, obl.	120	40	40	2.5	290 (× 2)	20 (× 2)	94 (× 2)
Lumbosacral spine, lat.	120	70	40	2.5	1100	55	82
Pelvis, AP	100	30	40	2.5	219	83.0	79.0
Abdomen, AP	100	20	40	2.5	159	11.6	51.1
Upper GI series							
Fluoroscopy	90	—	—	3.0	328/min.	.348/min.	12.8/min.
Spot film	90	PHT	—	3.0	101/film	.07/film	2.68/film
4 routine films	100–120	20–40	40	2.5	1237	25.99	138.5
Barium enema							
Fluoroscopy	90	—	—	3.0	480/min.	11/min.	140/min.
Spot film	90	PHT	—	3.0	110/film	3.20/film	28.0/film
Gallbladder series							
Fluoroscopy	90	—	—	3.0	400/min.	0.1/min.	0.6/min.
3 views	90–120	20–30	36–40	2.5–3.0	684	17.39	82.59
Spot film	90	PHT	—	3.0	173/film	1.0/film	7.1/film
IVP, AP abdomen	120	30	40	2.5	675/film	60.2/film	132/film
IVP, bladder, AP	120	30	40	2.5	659/film	181/film	105/film
IVP, Tomo, Kidneys	120	20	40	2.5	450/film	12/film	80/film
Arm, AP and lat.	70	5	40	2.5	—	<0.01	<0.01
Thigh, AP and lat.	100	20	40	2.5	328	124.7	73.9
Fluoroscopy, chest	90	—	—	3.0	150/min.	.03/min.	0.38/min.
Myelogram							
Fluoroscopy	90	—	—	3.0	360/min.	3.0/min.	45/min.
Spot films	90	PHT	—	3.0	820/film	16/film	94/film

From Antoku Shigetoshi, and Walter J. Russell: Dose to the active bone marrow, gonads, and skin from roentgenography and fluoroscopy. Radiology *101*:669–678, 1971. (The kilovoltage for gallbladder studies is more frequently 60 to 70 and IVP's 80 to 85, which would increase the gonadal dose slightly.)

during examinations of the pelvis or lumbosacral spine and examinations that require fluoroscopy and filming in the course of examination, as in studies of the gastrointestinal tract and in hysterosalpingograms.

4. Even in patients, one must realize that there is probably a cumulative effect, and very little repair occurs in the course of a lifetime. When one considers the genetically significant dose to the population as a whole, recent surveys have demonstrated that although medical diagnostic x-rays are by far the biggest source of man-made radiation, the genetically significant dose for medical x-rays is still much less than the average dose from natural background radiation. Thus, although the av- erage annual genetically significant dose in millirems for natural background is considered to be 90, by a 1970 estimate the similar average annual genetically significant dose from diagnostic radiology was considered to be 20. Needless to say, gonadal shielding should be used wherever feasible and appropriate. Physicians themselves should always wear lead aprons in fluoroscopy rooms and lead gloves if they help to maintain a correct position and posture of a patient. Even those protective barriers, equivalent to 0.5 mm of lead in most instances, are only designed to protect against *scattered radiation* and not the direct x-ray beam itself.

5. In a female in the childbearing years, radiation should be avoided unless abso-

lutely necessary, or confined if possible to a "safe" period when an impregnated ovum may not be involved.

6. In the child, ionizing radiation should be avoided unless the "risk-to-benefit" ratio is carefully evaluated.

Apart from the hazards of ionizing radiation there are certain hazards in the use of contrast media, especially those that are soluble and injected intravenously directly into arteries via catheterization. The exact cause of these hazards is not completely understood. An accurate incidence is not known, but contrast media are believed to cause outright death in 1:20,000 or up to 1:100,000 examinations. Short of such severe sequelae, other major effects include "allergic swelling," convulsions, pulmonary edema, respiratory failure, and cardiac arrest. It is impossible to anticipate by any testing modality at this time which patients will or will not react. Those who would employ contrast media of this type must be well prepared to employ every type of treatment necessary in the event a reaction occurs—including cardiopulmonary resuscitation if necessary.

3

The Chest

Routine diagnostic imaging of the chest consists primarily of posteroanterior and lateral views taken at a sufficiently long target-to-film distance to avoid magnification (6 to 10 feet). Oblique or special views are thereafter obtained for clarification as required. The posteroanterior view of the chest is preferred to the anteroposterior to avoid obscuration of the upper lungs by the scapulae.

There is no set way in which to study the plain films of the chest, but we have adopted a routine that has served us well (Figs. 3–1 and 3–2).

The observer begins with the costophrenic angles, noting the sharpness therein and the level of the diaphragm. A quick survey is made of the area beneath the diaphragm, noting areas where air is normally contained: underneath the left hemidiaphragm, particularly in the gas bubble of the stomach, and perhaps even in the splenic flexure of the colon.

Thereafter the chest wall is considered in its entirety, including its various soft tissues and bony components. In the female the breast shadows are carefully examined.

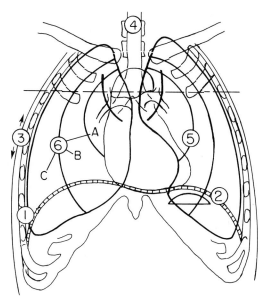

1. Costophren. Sinuses
2. Diaphragm level (and gas bubble)
3. Chest wall (axillas, pect. mm. breast)
4. Neck and trachea
5. Mediastinum and heart and major vessels and azygos
6. 3 zones of lung

Figure 3–1. Routine for study of posteroanterior film of the chest.

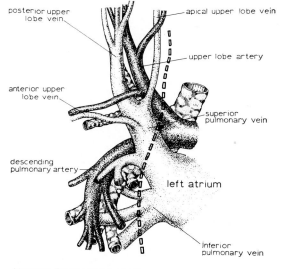

posterior upper
lobe vein

apical upper lobe vein

upper lobe artery

anterior upper
lobe vein

superior
pulmonary vein

descending
pulmonary artery

left atrium

inferior
pulmonary vein

Normal Right Hilar Anatomy

B.J. Bensam, M.D.

Figure 3–2. Diagrammatic representation of vasculature of right lung. Note the concave hilar angle formed by the intersection of the superior pulmonary vein and the descending pulmonary artery. Note also the relationship of the posterior upper lobe vein and artery. (Courtesy Doppman, J. L., Lavender, J. P.: Radiology *80*:931–936, 1963.)

Each rib of the thoracic cage is traced out individually and observed for the nine basic roentgen signs described previously. Interspaces are compared to ascertain symmetry; asymmetry could signify disease.

Once the chest wall and the supraclavicular area have been carefully examined, the position of the trachea and the mediastinal structures is observed. In the posteroanterior view, the trachea is seen in the midline up to the thoracic inlet, which can be readily identified by noting the symmetry of the manubrioclavicular joints on either side of the thoracic spine. Minimal deviation of the trachea is encountered in children because of slight redundancy, but otherwise the midline position of the trachea should be clear. The obtuse angulation of the right mainstem bronchus with respect to the trachea is noted.

Cradled between the trachea and the right mainstem bronchus is a curvilinear shadow spoken of as the "azygous node" or "azygous arch," depending on whether it consists of lymph node tissue or of the distal end of the azygous arch just prior to its entry into the superior vena cava.

We next observe the position of the heart, and consider the nine basic roentgen signs as they apply to the heart and pericardial shadows. These will be described later. The aortic knob is to the left, and the anatomic structures represented by the border structures of the cardiopericardial silhouette in each of the major projections of the heart are demonstrated (Figs. 3–3 to 3–6).

Thereafter the relative positions of the pulmonary arteries are noted. The left pulmonary artery is slightly elevated with respect to the right, since it lies *above* the left mainstem bronchus whereas the right pulmonary artery lies *below* the right bronchus. A reversal of this relationship is an immediate indication of abnormality. Normally, the pulmonary artery and pulmonary veins do not exceed 2 cm in diameter at their first bifurcation visible on the frontal view of the chest. If they do exceed this dimension, abnormality must be suspected and an explanation given.

Continuing the examination of the frontal view, the lung fields are studied and divided into three zones, spoken of as the inner or A zone; the middle or B zone; and the outer or C zone (see Fig. 3–1). The A zone, as indicated earlier, contains structures that seldom exceed 2 cm. in diameter and can be related specifically to elements of pulmonary anatomy. The B zone likewise contains branches of the pulmonary artery and pulmonary veins, and its structures seldom exceed 5 mm, in diameter. The outermost, or C zone, contains structures that seldom exceed 1 mm in diameter normally. Early recognition of abnormality in any of these three zones gives one an immediate lead to the abnormality of the chest.

Text continued on page 21

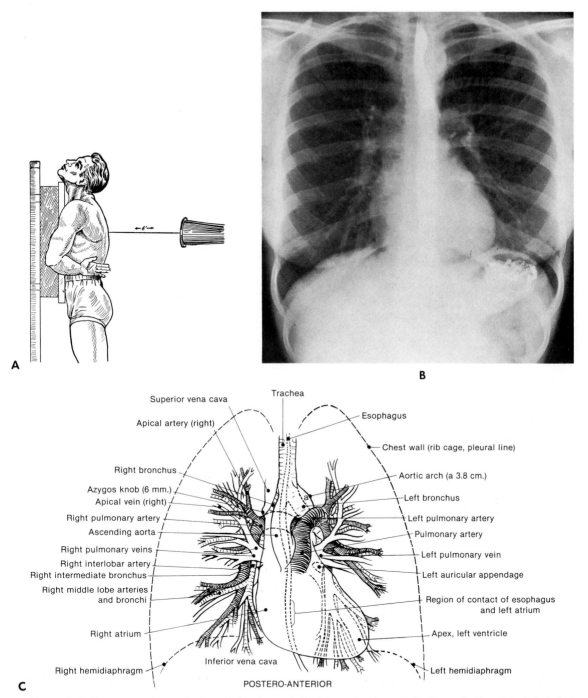

Figure 3–3. Posteroanterior projection of the chest. *A,* Position of patient. *B,* Radiograph (female). *C,* Labeled representation of chest.

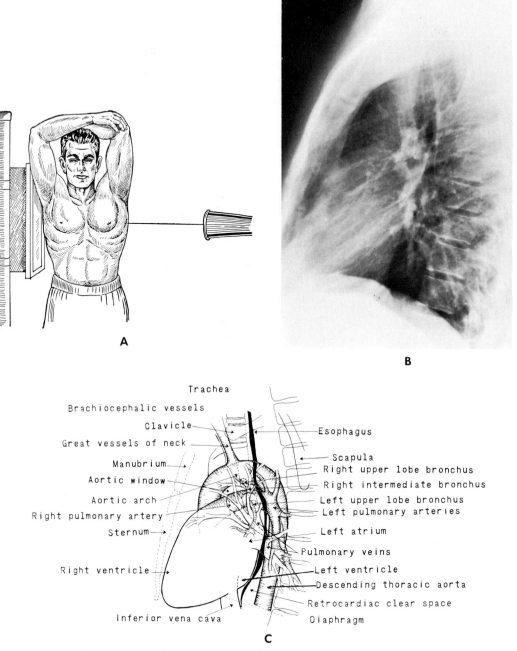

Figure 3–4. Lateral projection of chest. *A,* Position of patient. *B,* Radiograph. *C,* Lateral view of chest with anatomic parts labeled.

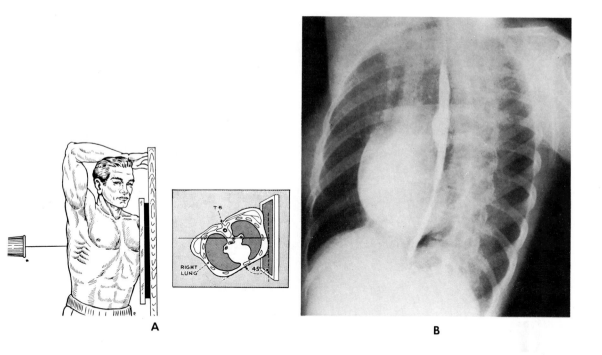

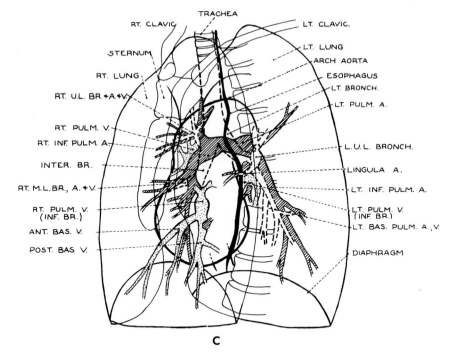

Figure 3–5. Left posteroanterior oblique projection of chest. *A*, Position of patient. *B*, Radiograph. *C*, Labeled tracing of *B*.

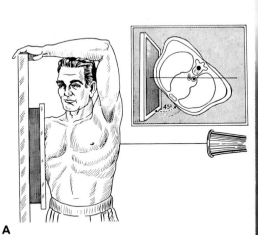

A

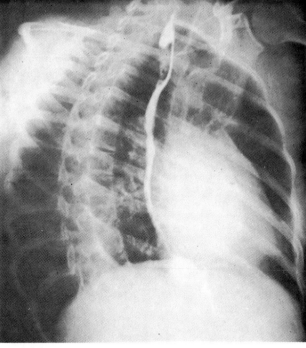

B

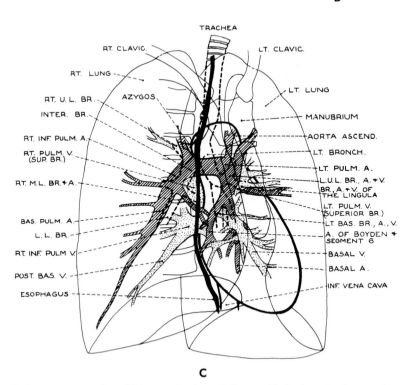

C

Figure 3–6. Right posteroanterior oblique projection of chest with barium in the esophagus. *A*, Position of patient. *B*, Radiograph. *C*, Labeled tracing of *B*.

It is difficult to differentiate arteries from veins on the radiograph. However, in the upper lung zones veins can frequently be traced beyond the appropriate pulmonary artery toward a venous communication, whereas the artery can be identified as a pulmonary artery branch. Medially, in respect to the apical branches, the artery is usually medial to the vein, with a bronchus intervening (Fig. 3–2). Since the blood flow in the chest, with the patient erect, is three times greater in the dependent portion of the chest than it is in the upper zone of the lung, normally the vein and artery juxtaposed on either side of the apical bronchus seldom exceed 1 or 2 mm in diameter. If the vein is 5 mm in diameter or greater, or if the artery begins as a structure that is 5 mm in diameter and tapers rapidly, one suspects hypertension of either the venous or arterial side, as the case may be. Venous hypertension or "cephalization of flow" is the earliest indicator of (1) cardiac failure with passive (venous) hyperemia, (2) mitral backup from a mitral stenosis into the venous structures of the lung, and (3) arterial-venous malformations of congenital heart disease. Interstitial edema, which is easier to recognize, often accompanies these early manifestations of cardiac failure and helps to reinforce the diagnosis.

The lateral view of the chest may be approached similarly. After examining the dome of the diaphragm and the costophrenic sinuses, the chest wall is examined carefully.

The sternum and manubrium are clearly identified, and the space between the sternum and the soft tissue lining the inferior aspect of the sternum on a good lateral view should not exceed 2 or 3 mm in width. There is a slight normal scalloping of these structures reflecting the pleura lining the chest wall at rib indentations. If this scalloping is exaggerated, or if the thickness of the pleura is greater than that indicated, such abnormalities as lymph node enlargement of the internal mammary chain, pleural effusion, or encasement of the lung by pleural fibrosis should be suspected. The thoracic cage is further examined in the lateral view by noting especially the degree of angulation and structure of the thoracic spine and its vertebral components. In the lateral view, the tracheobronchial tree is once again identified, and the hilar structures immediately adjoining the carina of the trachea are clearly outlined. The heart forms a considerable portion of the silhouette, and the right and left ventricles, anteriorly and posteriorly respectively, are clearly defined. The curvilinear relationship of the right ventricle to the sternum is carefully noted, as is the clear space between it and the sternum, which should be no greater than 3 cm normally. Obliteration of this clear space becomes one of the earliest indicators of anterior mediastinal or cardiac disease. The curvature of the arch of the aorta is clearly identified as it blends with the shadow of the descending thoracic aorta, and it may or may not be clearly defined,

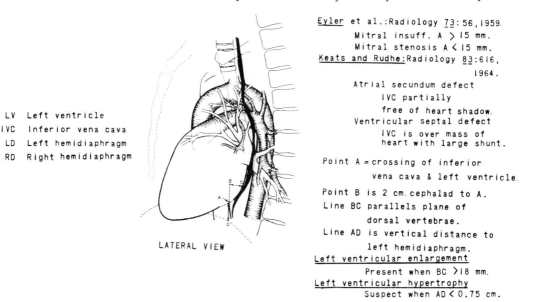

LV   Left ventricle
IVC Inferior vena cava
LD   Left hemidiaphragm
RD   Right hemidiaphragm

LATERAL VIEW

Eyler et al.:Radiology 73:56,1959.
   Mitral insuff. A > 15 mm.
   Mitral stenosis A < 15 mm.
Keats and Rudhe:Radiology 83:616,
                              1964.
   Atrial secundum defect
        IVC partially
        free of heart shadow.
   Ventricular septal defect
        IVC is over mass of
        heart with large shunt.

Point A = crossing of inferior
          vena cava & left ventricle.
Point B is 2 cm.cephalad to A.
Line BC parallels plane of
        dorsal vertebrae.
Line AD is vertical distance to
        left hemidiaphragm.
Left ventricular enlargement
        Present when BC >18 mm.
Left ventricular hypertrophy
        Suspect when AD < 0.75 cm.

Figure 3–7. Diagram of chest in its lateral projection for definition of the heart and left ventricle, particularly with respect to the inferior vena cava, to define normalcy or enlargement of left ventricle.

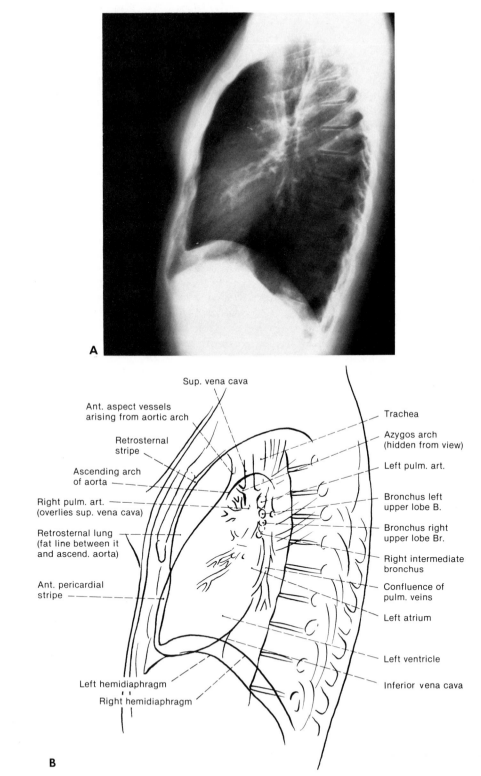

Figure 3–8. *A,* Lateral radiograph of the chest. *B,* Tracing of radiograph, labeled to show some of the more detailed anatomic features.

depending upon the presence or absence of atherosclerosis. On close examination, calcium may be seen in its arterial wall. The exact relationship of the left ventricle to the shadow of the inferior vena cava as it penetrates the right hemidiaphragm is carefully noted. Normal size of the left ventricle is gauged by measuring from a point 2 cm above the point of penetration of the diaphragm by the inferior vena cava to the posterior margin of the left ventricle. This distance should not exceed 18 mm (Figs. 3–7 and 3–8). Generally, the esophagus is not delineated with barium in routine filming of the chest unless it is clearly understood that no abdominal studies are entertained in the immediate future, since the barium in the abdomen will interfere with plain film studies of the abdomen. However, the demonstration of the esophagus with barium at the time of study of the chest is ideal from the standpoint of better understanding of the heart and mediastinum.

In addition to posteroanterior and lateral views of the chest, oblique studies are also obtained. For study of the lung fields, these may be rotated under fluoroscopic control for the ideal position of an abnormality and visualization of its contour. On the other hand, standard positions in the oblique usually require approximately a 45-degree angulation and are named as indicated in Figures 3–5 and 3–6.

In addition to these basic views, there are certain special plain views of the chest, each with its particular purpose.

1. The *apical lordotic* view is obtained with the patient leaning in the anteroposterior projection backward toward the film, so that the clavicles are projected above the lung apices and the apices may therefore be more clearly identified.
2. At times *inspiration and expiration* views are obtained. Although inspiration views are required for best visualization of the lung in full ventilation, at times it is the expiration view that shows air entrapment or a pneumothorax to best advantage. It is particularly advantageous in suspected foreign body inhalation, when a swaying mediastinum may be demonstrated.
3. *Decubitus views* with the patient lying on one side or the other are likewise employed, so that fluid can be more clearly identified and the lung substance above it more clearly seen.
4. If rib disease or abnormality is suspected,

special views of the ribs are required, usually in three different obliquities, with an opaque marker placed over the area of maximal pain, to alert the physician to the possible location of abnormalities. These are usually rib fractures, but they may represent areas of infiltration due to pneumonia or pleurisy, or other pathologic rib processes.

CLASSIFICATION OF ABNORMALITIES SEEN IN THE LUNG PARENCHYMA

Although a 5-mm abnormality is about the smallest that can be detected on the chest radiograph, particularly in the middle and outer zones, it is important to understand the more minute structure of the lung at the histopathologic level to recognize disease processes radiographically. The primary lobule of the lung, as orginally conceived by Miller (Fig. 3–9), is of considerable historic interest because it demonstrates a terminal bronchiole entering into a series of atria, and surrounding each atrium are the alveoli. Capillaries surround the alveoli, and the original primary lobule was envisaged as containing nerves and lymphatic and venous structures. The value of this historic histopathologic concept is the parallel that can be drawn to the radiograph when one realizes that the "primary lobular structure" may be filled with a transudate, an exudate, hemorrhagic constituents such as red cells, or cellular constituents of either neoplastic or non-neoplastic origin (Table 3–1). Obviously, shadows that occupy the primary lobule are much too small to be seen, but when clustered in a sufficiently large number and involving the portion of the lung parenchyma that is distal to a terminal bronchiole, called the "acinus," they form the smallest roentgenographic appearance visualized. The primary lobule of the lung may be considered as highly theoretical, but in viualizing the acinus it consists of all the respiratory bronchioles, alveolar ducts, and alveoli supplied by this terminal bronchiole and measures approximately 5 to 7 mm in diameter. Theoretically, it may contain as many as 18 of the last-order respiratory bronchioles considered by Miller. The acinus, as visualized radiographically, is ill-defined, of increased density, and typically is near unit density. Acini may be conglomerated further, involving whole segments of

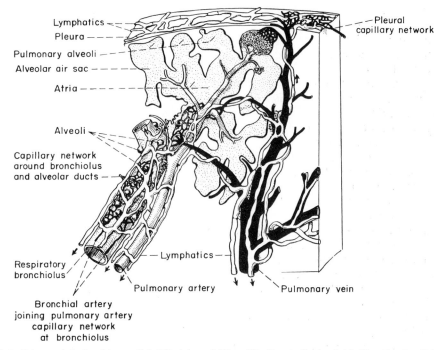

Lymphatics
Pleura
Pulmonary alveoli
Alveolar air sac
Atria
Alveoli
Capillary network
around bronchiolus
and alveolar ducts
Respiratory
bronchiolus
Lymphatics
Pulmonary artery
Bronchial artery
joining pulmonary artery
capillary network
at bronchiolus
Pleural
capillary network
Pulmonary vein

Figure 3–9. Primary lobule of lung. (Modified from Miller, The Lung. Springfield, Ill., Charles C Thomas, 1950. Courtesy of Charles C Thomas, Publisher.)

lung or lobes, and may produce a shadow in the lung as a lobe or even the entire lung itself as containing the ill-defined, homogeneous shadow characteristic of this structure.

In consideration of the alveolus it is also important histopathologically to recognize the following:

1. The lining cells of the alveolus are identified as flat epithelial cells, known as pneumocytes I, and cuboidal cells, known as pneumocytes II (Fig. 3–10).
2. The alveolus is a complex structure in which air exchange occurs predominantly on one side. The cellular constituents of the greater connective tissue support structures on the other side are lined with a composite surfactant-hypophasic compound that maintains a low surface tension so that the alveoli remain distended.
3. The surfactant-hypophasic compounds are approximately 90% dipalmitoyl lecithin and 10% mucopolysaccharides, manufactured by the cuboidal cells known as the pneumocytes II.
4. Macrophages reside within the alveolus and the interstitium to act as scavengers to remove debris from the alveolus cephalad from the alveoli.
5. Capillaries, connective tissue, lymphatics,

and other blood constituent cells—as well as nerve tissues—may also be found surrounding the alveolus.

6. *Pores of Kohn* are small perforations in the alveolus that allow an "air drift" between alveoli—just as the *canals of Lambert* allow an air drift between the acini.
7. The canals of Lambert reside in the distal portions of the bronchiolar tree; they are lined by epithelium and provide an accessory route for the passage of air directly between acini and even segments of the lung. The *pores of Kohn* are pores in the alveoli measuring about 10 to 15 microns in diameter. These permit the transfer of gases, fluids, or particulate matter between alveoli. They become particularly important if bronchial occlusion exists and ventilation continues through these collateral channels. This is known as "collateral air drift."

In addition to the tracheobronchial airways, other important structural components of the lungs are the main and branching pulmonary arteries, capillaries, pulmonary veins, bronchial arteries and veins, and lymphatics of the lungs including those of the bronchi, arteries, veins, and pleura, and ultimately the mediastinal lymph nodes.

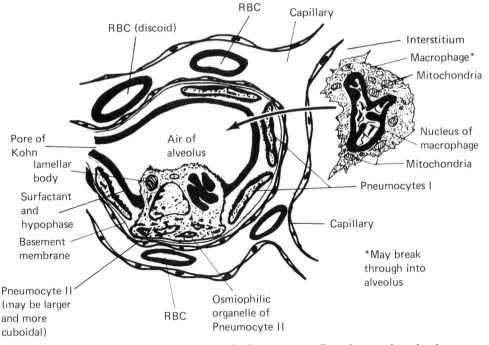

RBC (discoid)

RBC

Capillary

Interstitium

Macrophage*

Mitochondria

Nucleus of macrophage

Mitochondria

Pneumocytes I

Pore of Kohn

Air of alveolus

lamellar body

Surfactant and hypophase

Basement membrane

Capillary

Pneumocyte II (may be larger and more cuboidal)

RBC

Osmiophilic organelle of Pneumocyte II

*May break through into alveolus

Figure 3–10. Diagrammatic anatomic sketch of constituent cells and parts of an alveolus.

Important component parts of the thoracic cage that may be visualized radiographically are (1) the soft tissue structures of the thoracic wall, such as the skin, breasts, and muscular tissues, (2) the bony structures of the thoracic cage, consisting chiefly of ribs, costal cartilage, sternum, and thoracic spine, (3) the pleura, both visceral and parietal, and (4) the diaphragm. For further elucidation of these basic anatomic concepts the reader is referred to Meschan's *Atlas of Anatomy Basic to Radiology.*

In the various patterns in lung disease, we note five variations in density:

1. Ill-defined homogeneous shadows consisting primarily of transudates, exudates, hemorrhage, or cellular constituents
2. Nodular densities of miliary size or larger, possibly even cavitary; and those that contain calcifications
3. Linear densities that have a rather reticular and nodular component as well as the linear
4. Increased lucencies of lung that may either be localized, consist of large cavities, or even involve an entire lung, as in widespread pulmonary emphysema
5. Abnormalities of the pleura and lymphad-

enopathies are included in this tabular reference, although they more literally apply to the chest wall in the case of pleural effusion; and to mediastinal structures in the case of the lymphadenopathies.

Close correlation with the clinical history, physical findings, and other laboratory findings is essential in differentiating the ultimate morphologic pathology represented by these radiologic appearances.

With regard to pulmonary nodules, computed tomography is coming to the fore. The density of a nodule is closely related to its histology—and the latter, its Hounsfield computed tomograph number. This, in essence, is the average number of photons of x-rays absorbed within a given voxel. Generally, it is believed that benign lesions have average numbers greater than 164 H (Hounsfield units). No malignant lesions were recorded by Siegelman* having more than 175 H. There are, of course, "indeterminate" nodules which cannot be specifically identified in this manner.

_____

*Siegelman S. S., Zerhouni, E. A., Leo, F. P., et al.: CT of the solitary pulmonary nodule. AJR *135*:1–13, 1980.

Table 3–1 VARIOUS PATTERNS IN LUNG DISEASE

Ill-Defined Homogeneous
Alveolar Water or Unit Density

Transudate
- Pulmonary edema (Example 1)
- Aspiration drowning
- Pulmonary alveolar proteinosis
- Inhalation of fumes
- Congestive heart failure

Exudate
- Pneumonia (Example 2)
- Tuberculosis
- Fungi
- Systemic bacterial infection
- Parasite
- Viral pneumonia
- Mucoid impactions

Hemorrhage
- Infarction
- Hemosiderosis
- Chest contusion
- Hemorrhagic diathesis
- Goodpasture's syndrome

Cellular
- Non-neoplastic
  - Sarcoid
  - Tuberculosis
  - Fungi
  - Respiratory distress syndrome
  - Cytotoxic agents
  - Drugs (surfactant disease)
  - Eosinophilic granuloma
  - Allergies and collagen arteritides
- Neoplastic (Example 3)
  - Bronchiolar-alveolar carcinoma
  - Lymphomas
  - Histiocytosis(?)
  - Bronchogenic carcinoma
  - Adenomas
- Atelectasis

Nodular Densities
Miliary
- Tuberculosis
- Sarcoid
- Hemosiderosis
- Lymphomas
- Histiocytosis X
- Histoplasmosis
- Viral pneumonia

Slightly Larger Nodules and Cavities
- Bronchogenic carcinoma (Example 4)
- Metastatic carcinoma
- Malignant lymphomas
- Sarcoid
- Tuberculosis and fungal granulomas
- Parasitic
- Collagen disease (rheumatoid, polyarteritis nodosa, Wegener's necrotizing granuloma)
- Neurofibromatosis
- Arteriovenous fistula
- Pneumoconiosis (silicosis)
- Pulmonary infarction
- Embolic phenomena

Linear Densities—Diffuse Bilateral
(Includes Reticulonodular) (Example 5)
- Progressive system sclerosis
- Rheumatoid arthritis
- Dermatomyositis
- Progressive usual interstitial pneumonitis
- Desquamative interstitial pneumonitis
- Tuberculosis
- Lymphangitis carcinoma
- Malignant lymphomas
- Mucoviscidosis
- Amyloidosis
- Interstitial edema
- Post-irradiation pneumonitis
- Tuberous sclerosis
- Asbestosis
- Histiocytosis (honeycombing)
- Congestive heart failure and active hyperemias

Increased Lucencies
(Indiscriminate or General)
- Honeycombing of reticuloendotheliosis
- Collagen honeycombing
- Cavities and abscesses (Example 6)
- Cysts
- Emphysema (Example 7)
- Cystic bronchiectasis
- Lipoid pneumonias

Larger Cavities
- Tuberculosis, granulomas, carcinoma and malignancies
- Fungi, malignant lymphoma, sarcoid rarely
- Systemic embolic infections
- Pulmonary thromboembolism and infarction

*   *   *

Calcifications
- Tuberculosis, fungi
- Progressive systemic sclerosis
- Hyperparathyroidism
- Hypervitaminosis D.
- Milk-alkali syndrome
- Destructive bone disease with bone formation
- Calcinosis
- Varicella pneumonia
- Pulmonary alveolar microlithiasis
- Amyloidosis
- Occasional tumor metastases

Pleural Effusions
- Systemic lupus and other collagen diseases
- Tuberculosis
- Fungi (actinomycosis, nocardiosis, coccidiodomycosis)
- Malignant lymphomas
- Pulmonary infarction
- Myxedema
- Liver cirrhosis
- Pancreatitis
- Meig's syndrome
- Congestive heart failure
- Chest injury

Lymphadenopathies
- Tuberculosis
- Sarcoid
- Histoplasmosis and other fungi or mycoses
- Mucormycosis
- Varicella and infantile exanthemata
- Bronchogenic carcinoma
- Metastatic carcinoma
- Malignant lymphomas
- Silicosis
- Farmer's lung
- Collagen disease
- Histiocytosis X
- Mucoviscidosis
- Infectious mononucleosis
- Thalassemia major

Table 3–1 *Continued*

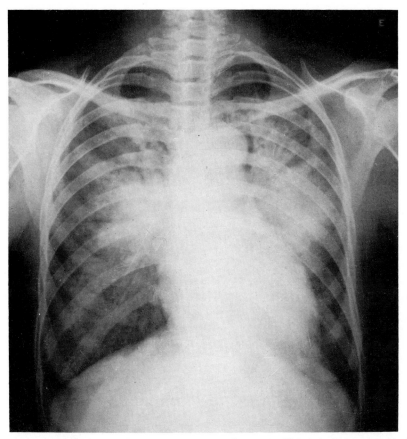

Example 1. Edematous infiltrate occurring in association with uremia. This is indistinguishable from pulmonary edema from other causes and is described as the "bat-wing" appearance.

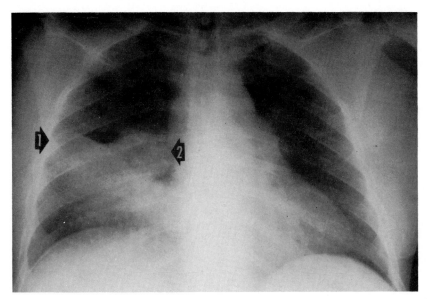

Example 2. Confluent pneumonia involving the right middle lobe (1) and the right lower lobe (2).

Table continued on following page

Table 3–1 *Continued*

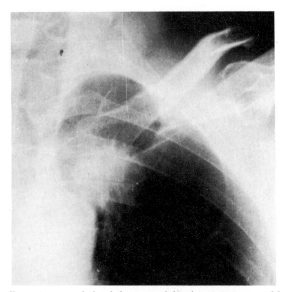

Example 3. Squamous cell carcinoma of the left upper lobe forming in an old scar and hence called "scar carcinoma."

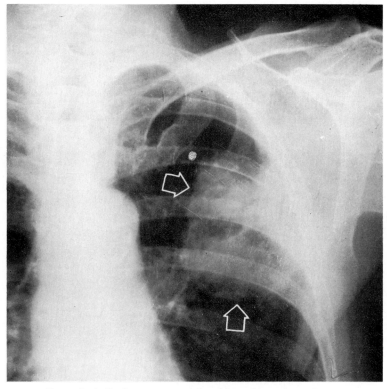

Example 4. Cavitary type peripheral bronchogenic carcinoma.

Table continued on opposite page

Table 3–1 *Continued*

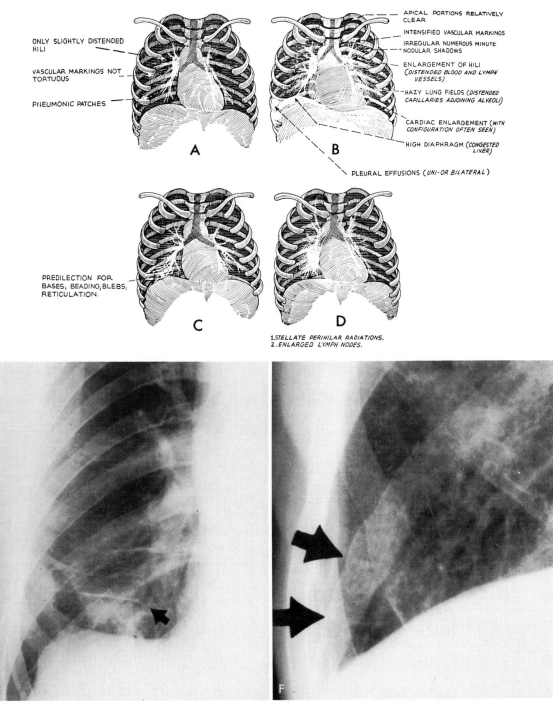

Example 5. *A*, Active hyperemia. *B*, Chronic passive hyperemia. *C*, Peribronchial fibrosis. *D*, Lymphangitic accentuation. *E*, Platelike (segmental) atelectasis. *F*, Kerley's "B" lines.

Table continued on following page

Table 3–1 *Continued*

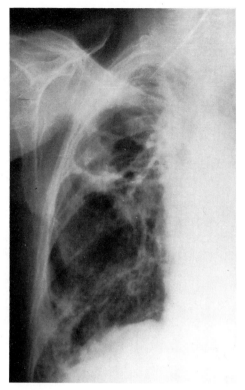

Example 6. Cavitation throughout the right lung in far advanced pulmonary tuberculosis.

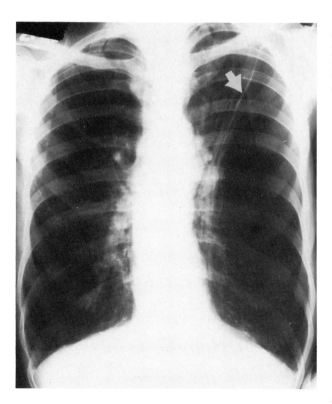

Example 7. Bullous emphysema of the chest. The lower two thirds of the chest is virtually one large bullous emphysematous area with no demonstrable lung substance contained within. Very often such findings are progressive in the course of time, and hence the term "vanishing lung disease."

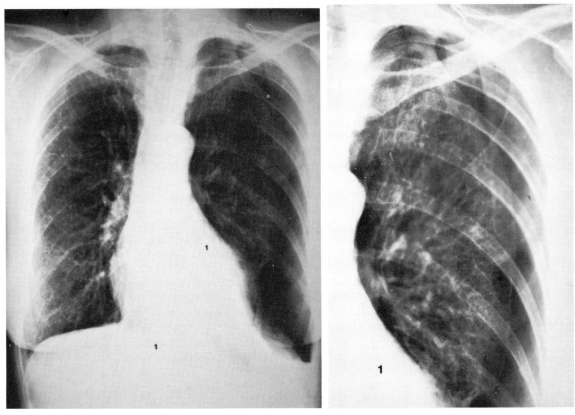

A   B

Figure E–1.

CLINICAL FINDINGS

You are shown first the posteroanterior chest film (Fig. E–1) of a young female, 24 years old, who came into the Emergency Room after experiencing an acute exacerbation of left chest pain. The two films shown are *A,* the PA film of the chest as it was first obtained, and *B,* a coned-down view of the left hemithorax.

Question

    1–1. The MOST likely diagnosis is

    A. Pulmonary infarction.

    B. Bronchopneumonia.

    C. Pleural effusion with an acute exacerbation of pleurisy.

    D. Spontaneous pneumothorax.

    E. A fractured rib.

Radiologic Findings. On these two views of the chest the most outstanding feature is the demonstration of a clear space between the parietal and visceral pleura. The left lung is partially collapsed and on the full film of the chest *(A)* there is a small amount of fluid in the left costophrenic sinus. On the coned-down film of the left hemithorax *(B)* there is an increased clarity between the parietal and visceral pleura as well as the pericardium and the visceral pleura medially. There are no associated homogeneous shadows of increased density and there is no indication of a fractured rib.

Differential Diagnosis. The most likely diagnosis in this instance is **pneumothorax** (actually **hydropneumothorax**, since there is a small amount of fluid in the left costophrenic sinus). The fact that there are no ill-defined homogeneous shadows in the lung fields proper would exclude a phenomenon which might be related to transudate, exudative processes, hemorrhagic phenomena such as pulmonary infarction, and any cellular infiltrative or consolidative process such as might be related to either a non-neoplastic, neoplastic, or atelectatic process.

The appearance of increased linearity through the visualized lung is due to the diminished expansion of the lung, with the blood vessels appearing closer together than would normally be obtained in a fully expanded lung. These linear densities are therefore a secondary phenomenon and not related to a disease process proper.

The left pulmonary artery is difficult to distinguish because the pneumothorax surrounds the entire left lung medially, producing an air space overlying the left pulmonary artery and depressing it caudad slightly. This is all due to the pneumothorax. The appearance of the right pulmonary artery and right lung are completely normal. There is no indication of lymphadenopathy.

Although *multiple views are considered necessary to exclude conclusively the possibility of a fractured rib*, there is no indication on the films obtained that such views might be necessary and all of the ribs and bony structures of the thoracic cage appear intact.

Exercise 2: Middle-aged Female with Progressive Shortness of Breath and Hemoptysis

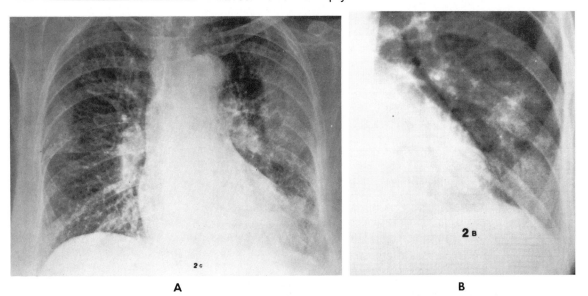

A

B

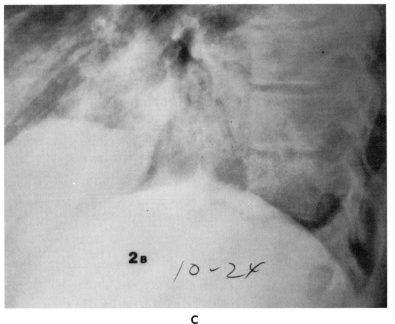

C

Figure E–2.

CLINICAL FINDINGS (Fig. E–2)

This patient is a 49-year-old female who had been experiencing considerable short-ness of breath for a period of several months. Throughout this period she had been coughing somewhat and occasionally bringing up clear, frothy sputum. She came in to the hospital on this occasion having experienced multiple episodes of considerable chest pain, both right and left, and the sputum began to contain considerable blood.

Question

2–1. The MOST likely diagnosis is
A. Bronchopneumonia.
B. Lobar pneumonia of a confluent type.
C. Pleural effusion.
D. Metastatic carcinomatosis.
E. Multiple pulmonary infarcts.

Radiologic Findings. In Figures E–2 *A, B,* and *C* there are multiple ill-defined areas of increased density throughout the lung parenchyma on both sides. The left costophrenic sinus is partially obscured whereas the right is clear. The cardiopericardial silhouette is enlarged chiefly in the region of the left ventricle. The pulmonary arteries are moderately prominent but in normal relationship. A careful study of the vascular pattern of the lungs, especially in the right upper lobe, will reveal a redistribution of blood flow strongly suggestive of "cephalization." The lung fields show an increased linearity of both arteries and veins. The areas of increased density are pleural based for the most part. They are not extremely sharply circumscribed apart from the normal geographic positions of the fissures but moderately so. The areas of homogeneous density on the left side are considerably more numerous than those on the right, which would appear to occupy the basilar portion of the right upper lobe resting upon the minor fissure.

Discussion. The most likely diagnosis in this patient is **cardiac hypertrophy and dilatation of the left ventricular type with chronic passive hyperemia of the lungs and numerous areas of pulmonary infarction** (E).

Against the diagnosis of bronchopneumonia on an objective basis is the fact that the ill-defined areas of increased density are predominantly pleural based and associated with a large heart in failure with chronic passive hyperemia of the lungs. It is true that bronchopneumonia may coexist with pulmonary infarction and cardiac failure, but this illustration is so typical of the one diagnosis that the diagnostician would be less likely to consider both at this time *unless this patient were highly febrile.* In bronchopneumonia, the areas of ill-defined increased density of a homogeneous type extend in patchy fashion throughout the lungs. These are not associated with evidence of an enlarged left ventricle or passive hyperemia of the lungs. Although there are occasional cases with pulmonary emboli presenting with a radiographic picture of this type, these are distinctly in the minority and *approximately two thirds of patients with pulmonary infarction will have evidence of cardiac failure* and chronic passive hyperemia of the lungs.

Lobar pneumonia (Fig. E–3 *A* and *B*) is not a very likely diagnosis, since the areas of ill-defined homogeneous density are not predominantly confined to lobes or even segments of lung. There is a confluent segmental involvement of the left lower lobe obscuring the left hemidiaphragm but not obscuring the left costophrenic sinus. It is important to emphasize that the costophrenic sinus would be the last area of involvement with lobar consolidation, whereas with pleural effusion,

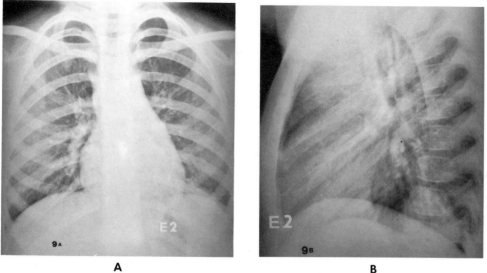

A   B

Figure E–3. *A* and *B*, Pneumonia, left lower lobe.

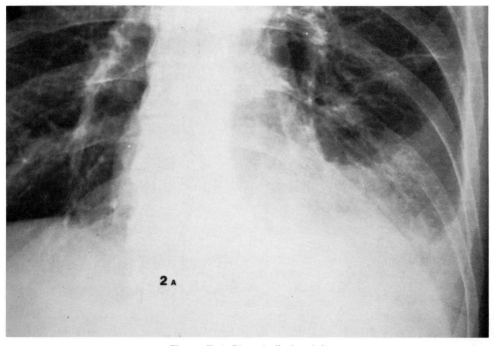

Figure E–4. Pleural effusion, left.

shown in Figure E–4, the costophrenic sinus is the first area to be obliterated. Note also that with pleural effusion there is a curvilinear upward margin which is highest laterally and most caudad medially. If this patient were to be fluoroscoped, this curvilinear ill-defined margin would move upward as the lung expands and caudad as the patient exhaled. This distinction of a pleural effusion occupying the costophrenic sinus first and having a curvilinear upper ill-defined margin, particularly before organization sets in, is a most important differentiation between pleural effusion and other areas of ill-defined homogeneous density. Incidentally, it is very likely that there is a small amount of fluid in the left costophrenic sinus in our primary patient with the cardiac failure and multiple pulmonary infarcts, but this would not be unusual in view of the pleurisy that accompanies pulmonary infarction.

Figure E–5 shows a patient with highly irregular carcinomatous metastases to the lung whose primary lesion was in the pancreas. Here, the areas of ill-defined increased density are profusely distributed throughout the lower two thirds of the lung in highly scattered fashion with no definite pattern identifiable. At times there is a tendency toward sharp circumscription of some of these shadows, suggesting minimal nodulation. Metastatic tumors of the lung have a highly variable appearance, as indicated in Figure E–6, A through F. At times these are of the miliary or lymphangitic type, and on other occasions they appear highly spherical with multiple nodules in both lungs or even coarsely nodular, with an intermixture of ill-defined homogeneous shadows. At times, metastatic tumors in the lung may be characterized only by a pleural effusion, which may become rather massive. And lastly, as shown in F, they may be peribronchial, nodular, or even pneumonic in type. It is probable that approximately 15 per cent of the pulmonary metastases will be no more clearly identifiable than indicated in Figure E–5, and hence, the differential diagnosis will depend to a great extent upon (1) a knowledge of the patient's history and physical findings to suggest the patient has a primary malignancy elsewhere; (2) the chronicity of the illness; (3) no indication (as was present in our patient) of cardiac failure, and chronic passive hyperemia of the lungs. There are, of course, other diagnoses indicated

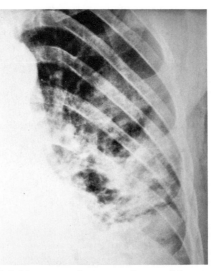

Figure E–5. Metastases from a carcinoma of the pancreas.

METASTATIC TUMORS OF THE LUNG

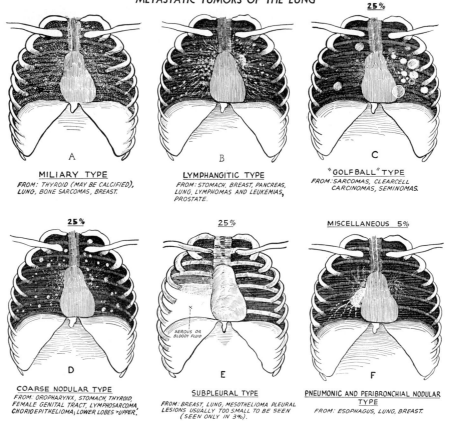

A

MILIARY TYPE
*FROM: THYROID (MAY BE CALCIFIED),
LUNG, BONE SARCOMAS, BREAST.*

B

LYMPHANGITIC TYPE
*FROM: STOMACH, BREAST, PANCREAS,
LUNG, LYMPHOMAS AND LEUKEMIAS,
PROSTATE.*

C
25%

"GOLFBALL" TYPE
*FROM: SARCOMAS, CLEARCELL
CARCINOMAS, SEMINOMAS.*

D
25%

COARSE NODULAR TYPE
*FROM: OROPHARYNX, STOMACH, THYROID,
FEMALE GENITAL TRACT, LYMPHOSARCOMA
CHORIOEPITHELIOMA; LOWER LOBES >UPPER.*

E
25%

SUBPLEURAL TYPE
*SEROUS OR
BLOODY FLUID*
*FROM: BREAST, LUNG, MESOTHELIOMA PLEURAL
LESIONS USUALLY TOO SMALL TO BE SEEN
(SEEN ONLY IN 3%).*

F
MISCELLANEOUS 5%

**PNEUMONIC AND PERIBRONCHIAL NODULAR
TYPE**
FROM: ESOPHAGUS, LUNG, BREAST.

Figure E–6. *A* through *F,* Diagrams illustrating the various roentgen appearance of metastatic tumors of the lung.

in a patient with hemoptysis, such as (1) hemosiderosis, (2) chest contusion, (3) hemorrhagic diathesis, or (4) Goodpasture's syndrome. With hemosiderosis there is often a fine nodularity and weblike linearity in the lung accompanying long-standing cardiac failure. In Goodpasture's syndrome there would be an indication of renal disease. With a chest contusion or a hemorrhagic diathesis, the history and other physical findings would be highly indicative and important in differentiation.

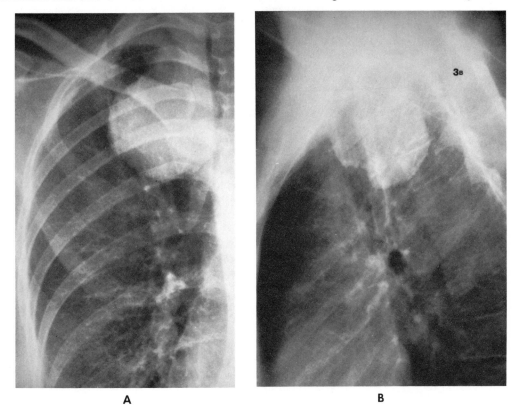

A   B

Figure E–7.

CLINICAL FINDINGS (Fig. E–7)

This patient is a 55-year-old male who was taken to the Emergency Room after a car accident in which he had sustained considerable skin bruising over many parts of his body. He was otherwise relatively asymptomatic. In carefully eliciting this patient's history, it was found that for several months he had been experiencing increased fatigability, some loss of weight, and a chronic cough.

Question

3–1. The MOST likely diagnosis in this patient is
A. Neurofibroma.
B. Hematoma of the lung.
C. Squamous cell carcinoma of the lung.
D. Lipid granuloma of the lung.
E. Oat cell carcinoma of the lung.

Radiologic Findings. The posteroanterior and lateral views of the chest in this patient reveal a sharply circumscribed mass lesion that measured approximately 6 × 7 cm projected in the right subapical region extending to the trachea in frontal perspective but posterior to the trachea in the lateral view. The mass lesion was sharply circumscribed but in the lateral view contained a notch at approximately "seven to eight o'clock." The mass lesion was homogeneous, contained no calcification, and was unassociated with cavitation. There were no associated rib abnormalities or vertebral body erosions. There was no evidence of fracture in association with the injury described. There was a minimal thickening of the pleura, producing a "pleural cap" overlying the right lung apex. There was no deflection of or encroachment upon the tracheobronchial tree.

Discussion. Of the five entities given as potential diagnoses the most likely is **squamous cell carcinoma of the lung.**

To discuss each of the other possibilities in order: A neurofibroma is usually a posterior mediastinal mass lesion that is also sharply circumscribed but is primarily mediastinal in origin and is paraspinous in its usual location. It is very often associated with either rib erosion or erosion of the intervertebral foramina or margins of an adjoining vertebral body (Fig. E–8, A and B).

A squamous cell carcinoma of the lung is often sharply circumscribed, as is the case in this patient, peripherally situated in the lung although it may be centrally situated, and is a mass lesion without calcification. Some distinguishing features of solitary lung lesions in this respect are shown in Table E–1. The two most frequent peripherally situated histologic carcinomas of the lung are the squamous cell carcinoma, sharply circumscribed as is this one, and the adenocarcinoma, which has a stellate, highly irregular margination (Fig. E–9).

A bronchogenic squamous cell carcinoma of the lung may also occur centrally in the immediate vicinity of the carina, as does the oat cell or undifferentiated bronchogenic carcinoma (Fig. E–10).

Since the lesion of the patient in question is peripheral, the most likely histologic carcinoma types are the squamous cell or the adeno-, with the squamous cell being sharply circumscribed and the adeno- being much more stellate in its peripheral margin.

A lipid granuloma can very closely simulate a bronchogenic carcinoma. In general, however, there are three types: (1) that which accompanies generalized systemic lipid disease; (2) alteration in the lung following longstanding atelectasis; (3) granuloma formation following aspiration of lipid material. Usually the lipid granuloma (Fig. E–11) is more easily confused with an adenocarcinoma of the lung, in view of the irregular margination, and a history to correlate with either aspiration or generalized systemic disease may often be evolved. With aspiration, cavitation may occur if gastric contents are aspirated simultaneously, especially if these contain highly acid material. Although lipid granuloma might enter into the differential possibilities in this patient, it would not be considered most likely.

A pulmonary hematoma may appear as a large nodule or mass lesion in the lung (Fig. E–12 A, B, C, and D). Usually this nodular appearance is related to hemorrhage in the lung having a lesser density than that contained in the patient in question, and if one were to follow such a hemorrhagic process for several days, it might well cavitate when the patient coughs up the hemorrhagic material contained within the hematoma.

Very often a hematoma of the lung will be accompanied by bony injury to the thoracic cage or a hemothorax—with both of these entities lacking in this instance.

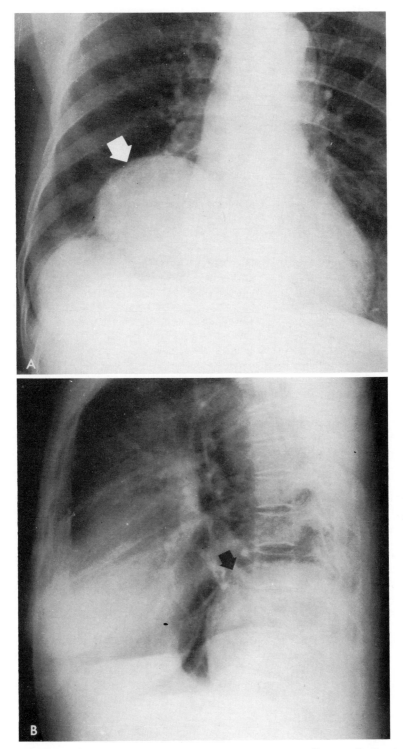

Figure E–8. *A* and *B,* PA and lateral films of the chest demonstrating a neurofibroma affecting the posterior inferior mediastinum. Although these films were not obtained for bone detail, the erosion of the intervertebral foramina in the lower thoracic region is readily demonstrated.

Table E–1.   DISTINGUISHING FEATURES OF SOLITARY PULMONARY LESIONS

Characteristic	Favors Benign Lesion	Favors Malignant Lesion
Roentgenologic findings:		
Size	Less than 1 cm.	More than 4 cm.
Shape	Regular	Irregular
Margin	Smooth and round	Notched or indefinite — Rigler's notch sign
Calcification		
"Popcorn" type	Hamartoma probable	Absent
Laminated type	Granuloma probable	Absent
Central type	Granuloma probable	Absent
Marginal flaky type	May be granuloma	May be malignancy
Cavitation		
Smooth internally	Benign abscess or cyst	Usually absent
Rough internally	Less likely to be benign	Eccentric, usually present
Incidence	Granulomas — approximately 40 per cent Adenomas — 2 to 4 per cent Hamartomas — 7 per cent	Approximately 30 per cent

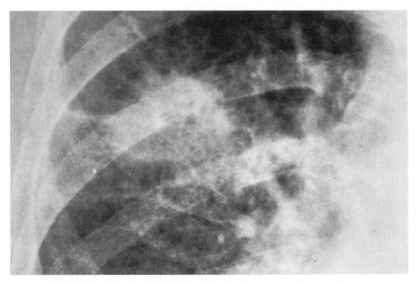

Figure E–9. Bronchogenic adenocarcinoma demonstrating stellate margin.

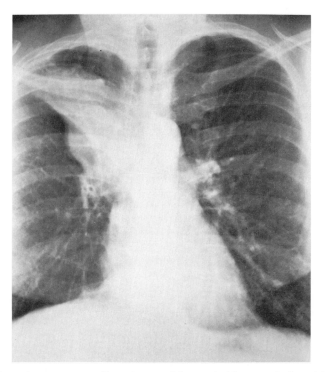

Figure E–10. Bronchogenic squamous cell carcinoma of the central type producing atelectasis in the right upper lobe and Morton's "S" curve in conjunction with the elevated minor fissure.

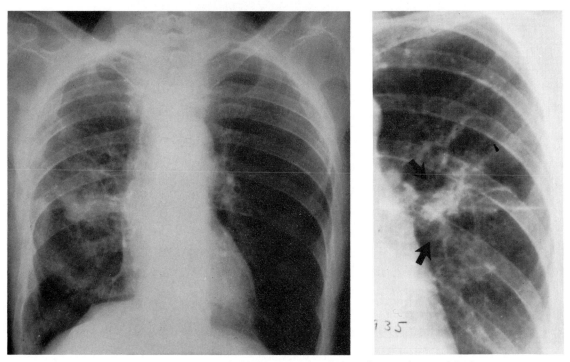

Figure E–11. Lipid granuloma simulating a peripheral type adenocarcinoma of the lung.

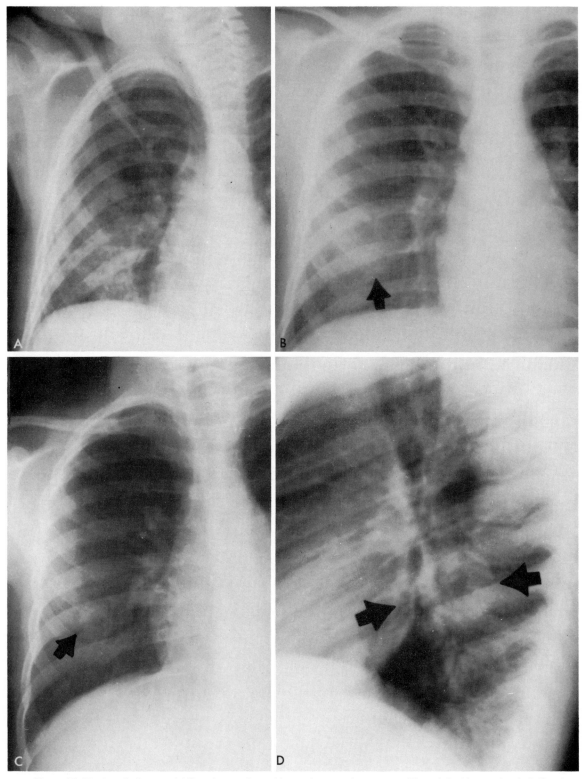

Figure E–12. *A* to *D,* Sequential films in a patient with a pulmonary hematoma. The original hemorrhagic infiltration as a result of trauma became cavitary in a period of 6 days (*C* and *D*).

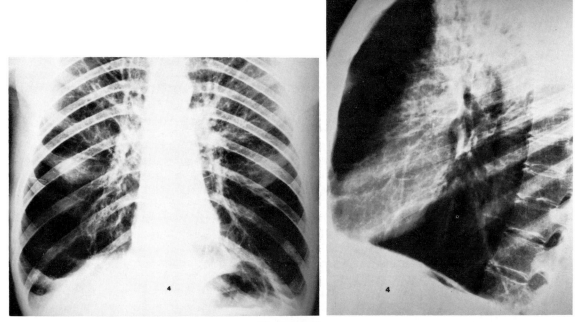

Figure E–13.

CLINICAL FINDINGS (Fig. E–13)

This patient is a 62-year-old male who has been smoking a minimum of two packages of cigarettes per day for approximately 35 years. He is now experiencing some shortness of breath and wheezing and recently has had occasional bouts of coughing of a frothy sputum and febrile episodes lasting as long as 24 hours.

Question

4–1. The MOST likely diagnosis is

A. Idiopathic hyperlucent lung, of the Swyer-James type.
B. Pulmonary cryptococcosis.
C. Chronic obstructive pulmonary disease.
D. Intravenous drug abuse, chronic.
E. Acute bronchiolitis.

EXERCISE

Radiologic Findings. The posteroanterior and lateral films of the chest (Fig. E–13 *A* and *B*) show considerable hyperlucency of both lung fields with an accentuated linear pattern in their upper thirds.

The diaphragm is flattened bilaterally and the costophrenic sinuses are obtuse. The anterior mediastinal clear space on the lateral view is considerably widened due to a marked hyperlucency. The aorta can be clearly defined, as can the branches derived from the aorta and the superior vena cava. There is anterior bowing of the sternum centered just below the manubriosternal junction. The ribs tend to flare, and there is a narrowness of the cardiopericardial silhouette, so that it appears suspended within the chest. The pulmonary arteries are prominent and, where visualized in the upper lobes, appear to taper rapidly bilaterally.

Discussion. The correct diagnosis is **chronic obstructive pulmonary disease.** The cardinal signs can be listed as follows: (1) overinflation with hyperlucency of the lungs; (2) increased vascular markings and interstitial shadows; (3) marked increase in the anterior mediastinal clear space which measures considerably in excess of 3.0 cm; (4) the pulmonary arteries as seen in the upper lobes taper suggesting pulmonary artery hypertension; (5) there is flaring of the ribs and flattening of the diaphragm; (6) where bronchi are identified in the lateral view, the walls appear considerably thickened ("tram-line" sign of chronic bronchitis).

The other diagnoses mentioned among the list of "distractors" are untenable for the following reasons:

With *acute bronchiolitis* in infants and adults there is an associated bronchial asthma, especially in the adult. Although there is general overinflation of the lungs, usually widespread, fine miliary nodulations can be identified and the process is accompanied by *acute* systemic illness. The patient shown has been chronically ill.

Idiopathic hyperlucent lung (Fig. E–14, *A* to *D*) is usually unilateral and is often called the Swyer-James or MacLeod's syndrome. Its etiology is unknown but it may be related to a childhood infection or pneumonia with bronchiolitis obliterans, bronchiectasis, and distal air-space distention and destruction very early in life. This in turn results in marked hyperlucency of one lung, which also has a diminutive pulmonary vasculature. Although the hilar vasculature is present, vessels on the affected side are very small. Air is trapped during expiration with a swing of the mediastinum toward the normal side in exhalation always present. Bronchography and angiography may be used to establish the diagnosis. With bronchography the terminal bronchioles appear bronchiectatic (Fig. E–14 *C* and *D*) and end abruptly in the vicinity of the fifth or sixth divisions. There is also an obstructive emphysema suggested, but no obstructing lesion is seen in the lobar or central bronchus. Angiography is probably not necessary but will usually demonstrate the diminutive partially obliterated pulmonary artery.

Pulmonary cryptococcosis is a granulomatous disease that is fungal in origin. The yeast cell can usually be identified in sputum when the latter is mixed with a drop of India ink and examined wet under a cover slip. It probably occurs just as frequently in the lungs as in the central nervous system but may spread anywhere in the body. The granulomatous lesion in the lung usually has a caseous necrotic center. Unlike the case in question the commonest form of pulmonary manifestation is a fairly well circumscribed mass 2 to 8 cm or more in diameter. These are usually peripheral and based near the pleura. In most instances the disease is confined to one lobe, with a lower lobe predominance. There is usually *no concomitant hyperlucency of the lung* as is found in the case in question, and patients with this disease are usually asymptomatic, or they may have a mild cough, chest pain, and low-grade fever at times. Very often they are neurologically abnormal, suggesting an expanding intracranial lesion or a psychiatric problem.

With intravenous drug abuse, especially Methadone, there are two distinct patterns: (1) widespread micronodulation without loss of lung volume; (2) both

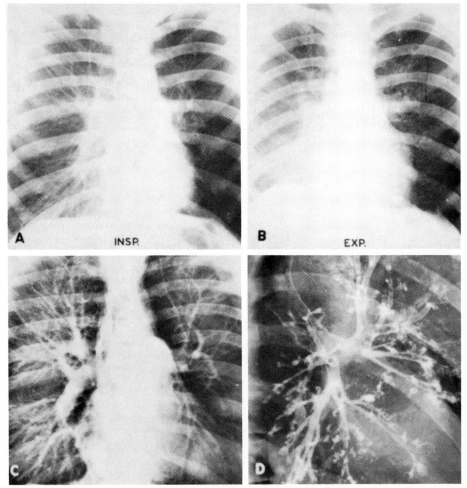

Figure E–14. Idiopathic unilateral hyperlucent lung with small left hilus. *A* and *B*, Inspiration and expiration films. There is hyperlucency of the left lung that persists on expiration. The heart shifts toward the left on inspiration, and the left hemidiaphragm shows poor excursion. *C*, The pulmonary angiogram shows marked decrease in the size of the left main pulmonary artery and its branches, with compensatory increase on the right. *D*, The bronchogram shows a peculiar diffuse form of bronchiectasis with absence of "alveolar" filling. This suggests the presence of a peripheral form of obstructive emphysema. (From Margolin, H. N., Rosenberg, L. S., Felson, B., and Baum, G.: Amer. J. Roentgenol., 82:63, 1959.)

general and local loss of volume with a nodular pattern consisting of multiple discrete opacities in the range of about 1 ml. Changes in the upper lung zones may indeed resemble progressive massive fibrosis such as occurs with pneumoconiosis.

It is thus apparent that chronic obstructive pulmonary disease may generally be diagnosed readily radiologically, when the indicated roentgen signs are present. It is interesting to correlate the roentgen signs with morphologic and clinical diagnoses. The radiologic diagnosis is accurate in nearly all moderate to severe cases and may be made on this morphologic basis even when the condition is not suspected clinically. Indeed, *the clinical correlation is based primarily upon pulmonary function studies.* Such tests as timed vital capacity, the expirogram, maximum breathing capacity, measure of breathing reserve, compliance, forced expiratory vital capacity, and dyspnea index provide a ready measure of the extent of obstruction or restriction produced by the pulmonary disease. Arterial blood assays for oxygen saturation and carbon dioxide content provide a further indication of the efficiency of alveolar ventilation. *Despite these extensive function studies, however, when correlation with the histologic appearance is made, the radiologic correlation is found in some 85% of cases, with only 65 or 70% correlation in the clinical group alone.* One must, however, not underestimate the appearance of the clinical evaluation despite the greater morphologic accuracy of the radiologic assessment. The pulmonary physiologist evaluates not only the mechanical factors in ventilation, the lung volume, oxygen and carbon dioxide diffusion, pulmonary capillary blood flow, and lung compliance but also the distribution of air ventilating alveoli, whereas the radiologist evaluates these various factors to a limited extent only and certainly does not evaluate the distribution of the air-ventilating alveoli.

EXERCISE

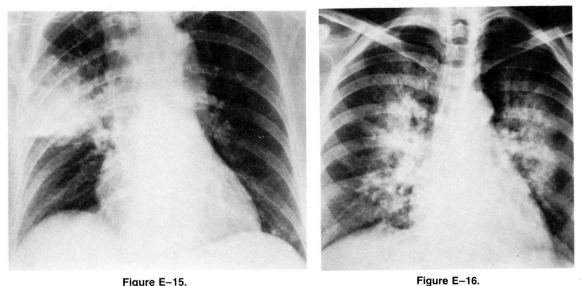

Figure E–15.   Figure E–16.

CLINICAL FINDINGS

You are shown the posteroanterior chest films of four adult patients.

Case 5–1 (Fig. E–15). This patient was admitted to the emergency room acutely ill, febrile, and coughing up blood-streaked sputum.

Case 5–2 (Fig. E–16). This patient, who was known to have chronic renal disease, began to cough up a frothy sputum but was afebrile.

Questions

5–1. The MOST likely diagnosis in Case 5–1 (Fig. E–15) is
A. Pulmonary infarction.
B. Nonspecific bronchopneumonia.
C. Bronchogenic carcinoma.
D. Pulmonary tuberculosis.
E. Lobar pneumonia.

5–2. The MOST likely diagnosis in Case 5–2 (Fig. E–16) is
A. Bronchopneumonia, nonspecific.
B. Disseminated lupus erythematosus.
C. Hodgkin's disease.
D. Pulmonary edema.
E. Bronchomoniliasis.

Exercise 5: Differentiation of Parenchymal Shadows in the Lung *Continued*

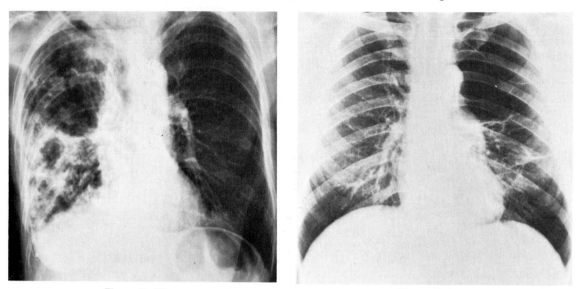

Figure E–17.   **Figure E–18.**

Case 5–3 (Fig. E–17). This patient was a chronic alcoholic who was brought to the emergency room after an inebriated state which apparently had lasted several days. It was indicated by his family that he would habitually lie on his right side.

Case 5–4 (Fig. E–18). This adult patient had suffered all his life from what he described as "asthmatic attacks" with occasional bouts of outright pneumonia.

5–3. The MOST likely diagnosis in Case 5–3 (Fig. E–17) is
A. Wegener's granulomatosis.
B. Aspiration pneumonitis.
C. Bronchogenic carcinoma.
D. Pulmonary tuberculosis.
E. Cavitary pulmonary infarction.

5–4. The MOST likely diagnosis in Case 5–4 (Fig. E–18) is
A. Bronchiectasis.
B. Chronic lung abscess.
C. Mucoviscidosis.
D. Bullous emphysema of the lung.
E. Tuberculosis, reactivated.

Radiographic Findings. In Figure E–15, Case 5–1, there is a homogeneous shadow of increased density that extends cephalad to the minor fissure of the lung and out to the pleura and lung periphery. The upper half of the right upper lobe does not appear to be significantly involved. There are no other radiographic findings of note in other portions of the chest, although the right hemidiaphragm is slightly elevated.

In Figure E–16, Case 5–2, there is a "butterfly" pattern to the parenchymal involvement that is both linear and to some extent acinar in the ill-defined, homogeneous category. There is no scalloping or margination of the butterfly pattern to suggest that the major involvement is that of bronchopulmonary lymph nodes. The cardiopericardial silhouette is normal.

In Figure E–17, Case 5–3, the major pathologic findings are at the right lung base, where there are scattered areas of infiltration surrounding areas of increased lucency representing probable cavitation. There is an elevation of the right hemidiaphragm. The process extends throughout the right lung base into the right costophrenic sinus. There is a slight shift of the mediastinum toward the right, and the left lung is clear.

In Figure E–18, Case 5–4, there is complete lucency in the upper half of the left lung, and the lower half is occupied by horizontal linear shadows interspersed with some areas of lucency. There are scattered foci of ill-defined homogeneous density, but these are minimal, extending out below the linear areas of increased density. In the right lung there are more linear areas of increased density and some increased lucency, especially at the lung base, but there are no circumscribed areas of lucency. The walls surrounding the lucent areas are extremely thin. The pulmonary sector of the cardiopulmonary silhouette is very prominent, especially on the left side.

Discussion. The answer to Case 5–1 (Fig. E–15) is **pneumococcus or lobar pneumonia** (E). Generally, nonspecific bronchopneumonia appears in scattered foci throughout both lung fields, and even histologically the alveoli are not completely or solidly occupied by exudative materials. It is rarely confluent, as is the shadow of Figure E–15. Bronchogenic carcinoma, when peripheral, is usually of the squamous cell variety or adenocarcinoma. When it is of the squamous cell carcinoma type, the lesion is nodular, quite often very large, with rather sharp circumscription. When the bronchogenic carcinoma is of the adeno-type, its margination is more stellate and irregular but it would still appear to be rather nodular. It may appear cavitary. It is not necessarily confined by a fissure, when it is near a fissure. Occasional cases of bronchogenic carcinoma simulate pneumonia, but in these cases there is chronicity that leads one to the adage that "any patient with a pneumonia lasting 8 weeks or longer should be considered a carcinoma suspect until proven otherwise by every available means." This patient, however, was acutely ill and did not conform to this history.

With regard to pulmonary tuberculosis, there are occasional cases of the pneumonic type but these are rare. In the adult reactivated tuberculosis, the lesion is usually initially subapical and somewhat nodular, with fanning of a linear type toward the hilus. As time goes on, cavitation may supervene and ultimately the process becomes fibronodular when healing occurs. This certainly would not conform to the present description.

With regard to Case 5–2 (Fig. E–16), the most likely diagnosis is **pulmonary edema.** Although certain types of bronchopneumonia, such as tularemia, may at times be of this central type, there is no indication in this history that this patient had been hunting or had been infected in the hands with axillary lymph node involvement such as occurs in this disorder. With disseminated lupus erythematosus, there is often a pleural as well as pericardial effusion and the process tends to be basilar with a linearity extending toward the cardiopericardial silhouette. With Hodgkin's disease, the process is primarily lymph nodal, involving paratracheal and bronchopulmonary lymph nodes in asymmetrical fashion. The fact that lymph nodes are involved would give some sharp circumscription usually to the areas of involvement, suggesting that they are not parenchymal in origin. The shadows shown in this case would definitely appear to be parenchymal.

In bronchomoniliasis or candidiasis, the disease usually occurs when the host is rendered vulnerable to disease by immunosuppression. It is often preceded by buccal membrane involvement with mucocutaneous infection. It may occur in other organs such as the esophagus and lung but is usually associated by evidence of other disease which had required immunosuppression, such as cancer, leukemia, lymphoma, etc. At times it occurs in patients who have been treated with broad-spectrum antibiotics, which apparently have eradicated the normal bacterial flora and permitted an unchecked growth of the fungi. In the lung it may simulate tuberculosis but the other aspects of the history would certainly strongly suggest the diagnosis.

In Case 5–3 (Fig. E–17) the most likely diagnosis is **aspiration pneumonitis.** Wegener's granulomatosis is an acute necrotizing vasculitis with granuloma formation that often affects the upper respiratory tract, lungs, and kidneys. Associated with the lesion in the lung there is often a necrotizing process in the nasopharynx, especially with necrosis of the bony nasal septum. The appearance radiologically can simulate that shown in Figure E–17. The fact that this patient was alcoholic and habitually lay on his right side would suggest that he had aspirated during the course of his inebriated state and subjected his lung to digestive action from gastric juices in the lung, giving rise to the appearance of cavitation. This is particularly true by the gravitational effect of habitually lying on his right side. In general, aspiration pneumonitis is a gravitational phenomenon and in the erect posture is most likely to occur in the lung bases.

Although bronchogenic carcinoma can simulate any cavitary process in the lung such as this one, the very considerable associated adjoining pulmonary disease of a linear and ill-defined homogeneous, as well as nodular type, without evidence of nodulation within the cavity proper, would militate somewhat against this diagnosis. The history, of course, is most important in differentiating a bronchogenic carcinoma from aspiration pneumonitis in an alcoholic.

Pulmonary tuberculosis can simulate many diseases in the lung, is often cavitary, but is usually primarily subapical in origin in the reinfection type. Cavitation occurs most frequently in the upper thirds of the lungs rather than in the lung bases. There is a tendency for pulmonary tuberculosis to gravitate diagonally to the opposite lung base when the subapical portion is involved first. With the history given, pulmonary tuberculosis would be less likely than aspiration pneumonitis. With regard to cavitary pulmonary infarction, one must postulate that the patient had an infarct primarily, which had become cavitary in the course of time. Pulmonary infarction of this type can occur particularly in patients with cardiac failure, and two thirds of the patients with pulmonary infarction are in cardiac failure at the time. There is no indication of cardiac failure in this patient's history, which would certainly militate against this diagnosis.

In Case 5–4 (Fig. E–18), the most likely diagnosis is **bullous emphysema of the lung.** The term bullous emphysema refers to any form of emphysema that produces large subpleural blebs or bullae. The bullae are large emphysematous spaces, and in this case, occupy the upper half of the left lung. Bullous emphysema occurs most frequently near the apex and is subpleural. It may occur in relation to old tuberculous scarring. It results from progressive destruction of septal walls encompassing many contiguous pulmonary acini. The insufficient lung substance produces an increased resistance to air flow as well as increased pulmonary arterial pressure, and pulmonary hypertension may also be associated.

Bronchiectasis is a far less likely probability in this instance, since bronchiectasis is usually a bibasilar process that on plain films of the chest is characterized by a peribronchial fibrotic linearity, bleblike alterations in the lung bases due to sacculations, and interspersed areas of platelike atelectasis. With regard to chronic lung abscess, there is usually a significant reactive zone around the area of lucency, much like that seen in Figure E–17, to indicate the presence of an infective reaction surrounding the zone of lucency, with the lucency representing necrosis, and suppuration. There is no such appearance in this instance.

In patients who survive to adulthood with mucoviscidosis, there is evidence of a widespread and diffuse increased linearity to indicate that the presence has been subject to frequent bouts of pneumonia with a fibrosing alveolitis and chronic fibrotic changes throughout both lungs. Mucous plugging is related to abnormal bronchial secretions, and these in turn result in the frequent episodes of pneumonia. In this instance, there is no such indication of the fibrotic changes of mucoviscidosis characteristic in the adult. The problem of reactivated tuberculosis comes into consideration, in that bullous emphysema is sometimes associated with old tuberculous scarring, but the appearance here is certainly not that of the usual cavitary tuberculosis one encounters. With cavitary tuberculosis, as with chronic lung abscess, there is usually a reactive zone around the zone of lucency to indicate reactive changes in the lung surrounding the area of infection. There very frequently is associated fibronodular disease of a much more severe type than is present in this instance.

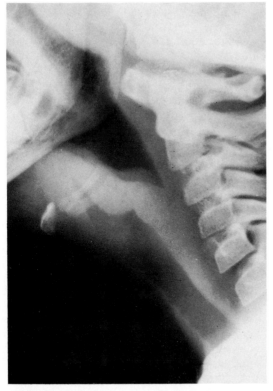

Figure E–19. Illustration courtesy of Dr. J. S. Dunbar.

CLINICAL HISTORY (Fig. E–19)

You are shown a lateral film of the neck of a 7-year-old patient who experienced sudden pain in the throat, difficulty in swallowing, and respiratory distress with considerable stridor.

Question

6–1. The MOST likely diagnosis is

A. Hypertrophied tonsils and adenoids due to a fulminating infection.

B. Acute epiglottitis and aryepiglottis.

C. Tracheomalacia.

D. Croup.

E. Retropharyngeal abscess.

Radiologic Findings. A careful study of the soft tissue lateral film of the neck in Figure E–19 demonstrates a massively swollen epiglottis and aryepiglottic folds. The trachea appears to be normal in dimension. The tonsillar tissue seen in the uppermost portion of the film beneath the clivus is normal for a 7-year-old child, and the tonsils and adenoids do not appear to be hypertrophied. The retropharyngeal tissues appear not to be swollen by actual measurement and by comparison with the dimensions of the vertebral bodies of the adjoining cervical spine.

Discussion. The most likely diagnosis is **aryepiglottitis** and **epiglottitis.** These structures appear to fill the entire hypopharynx, whereas the subglottic trachea appears clear and there is no particular widening of the pre- or post-tracheal soft tissues. Epiglottitis ordinarily has a very rapid progressive course with a high mortality rate and may be associated with upper respiratory obstruction leading to death. It results most commonly from infection by *Haemophilus influenzae* and although it most frequently occurs between the ages of 2 and 4 it can occur at the age of 7 but rarely is seen after the age of 8. The most common symptoms are those manifested in this case, consisting of pain, difficulty in swallowing and respiratory stridor with distress.

In contrast with epiglottitis, *tracheomalacia* (Fig. E–20A) is caused by a weakness of the tracheal wall and softening of the supporting cartilage with a hypotonia of the muscular and elastic elements of the trachea. The anterior and posterior walls of the trachea begin to approximate one another, producing a diminution in the tracheal lumen. This marked narrowness is particularly apparent during exhalation. There are two recognized types of this disorder—a *primary* tracheomalacia and one that is *secondary.* The primary tracheomalacia is usually congenital and is often associated with other congenital abnormalities involving the larynx, palate, nasopharyngeal choanae, and ear. Ordinarily, if the patient survives, the softening of the trachea corrects itself by the age of one or two, and hence would not be found in a child of 7. Secondary tracheomalacia is acquired and occurs in somewhat older individuals. In this instance, the trachea becomes somewhat wider and longer in inspiration but tends to contract and shorten in exhalation. These changes are somewhat greater in children but may occur in adults. In infants the primary symptoms are those of severe stridor with dyspnea, periods of cyanosis, and *tracheal* obstruction. It is possible to relieve this obstruction readily by passage of a bronchoscope through the narrow area, and the flaccid tracheal wall may thereby be visualized. In both inspiratory as well as expiratory films in the anteroposterior and lateral projections, there is a persistent narrowness or even a collapse of the trachea at the level of the first and second thoracic vertebrae. It is important to note that the persistence of the finding of collapse during the expiratory phase is an important one, since in asymptomatic infants the trachea has been shown to have as small a diameter as 1 to 3 mm under certain circumstances.

In *croup,* the walls of the conus elasticus of the trachea in the subglottic region show a convexity medially instead of a concavity (Fig. E–20B). Above the level of the conus, the true cords appear normal. There may be a secondary collapse of the trachea, particularly during inspiration, but ordinarily this disappears during expiration, unlike tracheomalacia. The hypopharynx with croup very often appears abnormally aerated with increased rather than decreased inspiratory pressure, as would be the case with hypertrophied tonsils and adenoids or a retropharyngeal abscess.

With a *retropharyngeal abscess,* the retropharyngeal soft tissues are markedly widened by comparison with the dimensions of the vertebral bodies of the cervical spine and there is no sharp delineation of the tonsillar or adenoid tissue as would be the case if the soft tissue swelling were associated with hypertrophied tonsils and adenoids. The tonsillar tissues can be identified, superimposed over the other oropharyngeal and retropharyngeal structures, somewhat caudad to the adenoid area. *The posterior margin of the tongue as well as the epiglottis can be well identified and are usually within normal limits under these circumstances.* Hypertrophied tonsils and adenoids are very often related to streptococcal or staphylococcal infections.

There are other lesions in the retropharynx that must come into consideration, such as those that are illustrated and others:

(1) Hemangiofibromas of the nasopharynx;
(2) Chondrosarcomas involving the base of the skull;
(3) Chordomas;
(4) Burkitt's lymphoma;
(5) Tuberculous lymphadenitis; and
(6) Pontine glioma, which erodes the base of the skull into the nasopharynx.

 · **Hemangiofibroma** (Fig. E–20C) of the nasopharynx has a high degree of vascularity (♦), is very dangerous to biopsy because of hemorrhage, and it usually grows anteriorly to erode the bone of the pterygoid pillars. This erosion can be detected by lateral inspection of the pterygoid processes (◊) and by computed tomography by spreading of the pterygoid fossa (so-called "bowing sign" [Fig. E–20C]).

 · **Chondro- or osteosarcomas** involving the base of the skull are very rare primary or secondary tumors arising in the enchondral bone of the clivus.

 · **Chordomas** (Fig. E–20D) are primary tumors that are rare in infants and children, and arise from the primitive notochord. They affect the base of the skull and often destroy the clivus (◊). They also involve the sacrococcygeal area. They tend to be avascular.

 · **Burkitt's lymphoma** in the neck is endemic in South Africa. It is probably caused by a virus. In the United States it is more likely to involve the abdominal region.

 · **Tuberculous lymphadenitis** may involve the cervical lymph nodes and spine, but the cervical spine is least commonly affected. A paraspinal abscess

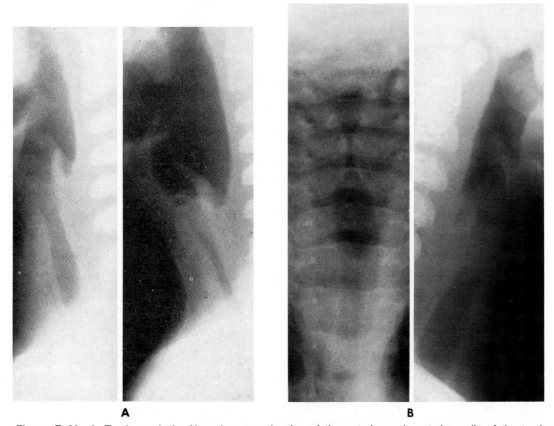

A   B

Figure E–20. *A,* Tracheomalacia. Note the approximation of the anterior and posterior walls of the trachea particularly evident during expiration. (Inspiration *left* and expiration *right*) *B,* Radiographic appearance of croup. The walls of the conus elasticus of the trachea in the subglottic region show convexity medially instead of concavity. A secondary collapse of the trachea may appear, particularly during inspiration, but ordinarily disappears during expiration. (*A* and *B* courtesy of Dr. J. S. Dunbar.)

Illustration continued on following page

with destruction of the bone and adjoining interspaces is characteristic. Usually the chest is also involved. The most frequent location is the thoracic spine.

· A **pontine glioma** (Fig. E–20*E*) is an axial glioma arising in the pons that may destroy the clivus (□) and bulge into the nasopharynx, obliterating the cisterna pontis and displacing the fourth ventricle posteriorly. In angiograms the basilar artery is also displaced.

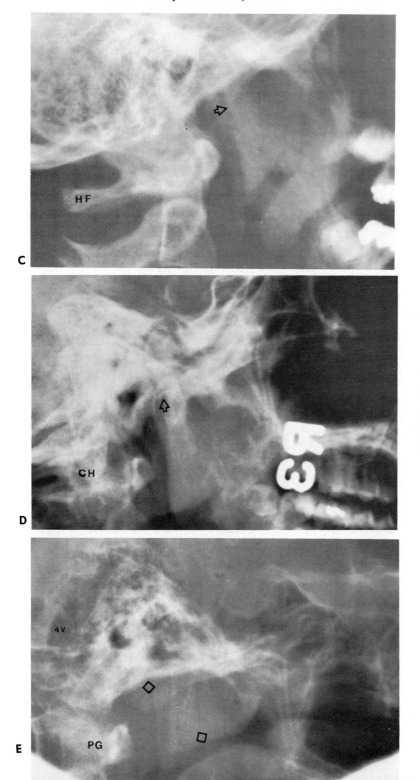

Figure E–20 *Continued. C,* Hemangiofibroma of the nasopharynx in a 14-year-old boy. *D,* Chordoma in an adult. Note the destruction of the clivus (◊). *E,* Pontine glioma with destruction of the clivus and production of a soft tissue mass in the nasopharynx (◇).

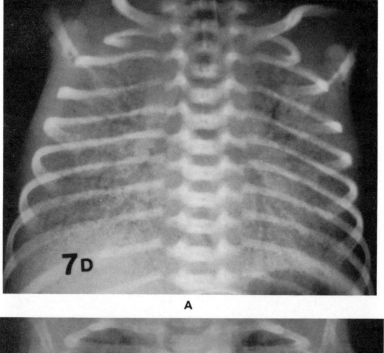

A

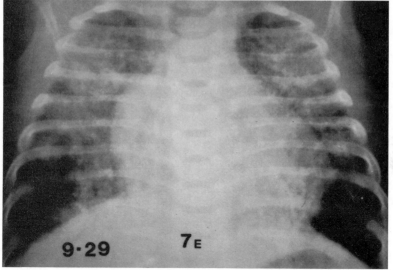

B

Figure E–21.

CLINICAL FINDINGS

This patient is a newborn premature infant who appeared to be in marked respiratory distress from the time of his birth on July 5 (Fig. E–21A), but who apparently had no respiratory stridor. His respiratory distress was severe enough to require tracheal intubation. At first he did not respond to 50% oxygen, but he continued to survive and by August 1 he required 100% oxygen. His respiratory distress continued although he could be maintained in the newborn nursery. However, he died shortly after the film was obtained on September 29 (Fig. E–21B).

Question

7–1. The MOST likely diagnosis is
A. Hyaline membrane disease ultimately leading to bronchopulmonary dysplasia.
B. Mikity-Wilson disease.

C. Tachypnea of the newborn.
D. Streptococcal pneumonia.
E. Staphylococcal pneumonia.

Radiologic Findings. In the series of two films shown on this neonate one notes that at the time of birth on July 5 (Fig. E–21A) there was a fine, discrete nodulation throughout both lung fields with occasional areas of segmental atelectasis. Occasional areas of lucency are seen but the amount of respiratory distress is significantly inordinate in comparison with the *supposed* aeration of the lungs as visualized herein, necessitating intratracheal intubation, as shown. The patient required supplementary oxygen therapy, and on August 1 the lungs were increased in their radiability, but these foci were circumscribed and large.

On the final film of September 29 (Fig. E–21B), obtained shortly before death, the appearance is that of coarse nodulation throughout both lung fields with interspersed large bulla-like shadows especially at the lung bases.

Discussion. The correct diagnosis in this neonate is **hyaline membrane disease of the newborn eventually developing a bronchopulmonary dysplasia** prior to death.

In hyaline membrane disease, approximately 90% of cases are premature and about one half die within the first 24 hours of life. Those who survive proceed to develop various stages of bronchopulmonary dysplasia ending in what Northway has called Stage 4 bronchopulmonary dysplasia, well exemplified by Figure E–21B. The disease is due to a loss or deficiency of surfactant within the lung resulting in a marked proliferation of the pneumocytes II responsible for surfactant production; their destruction; and entry into the alveoli of macrophages, which also undergo destruction, releasing a fibrosing enzyme. There is also a resultant acinar atelectasis. As the result of these changes, the lungs at first appear diffusely granular, with the secondary lobules and acini full of the cellularity described. There are scattered air-filled alveolar ducts giving rise to "bubbles" of air contained within the homogeneous ground-glass and granular appearance. Air bronchograms may also result.

The *bronchopulmonary dysplasia* represents an end stage apparently related to the oxygen toxicity as well as to the surfactant deficiency. There is an indication of coalescence of the emphysema with large bulla formation and focal thickening of capillaries. Although the lung appears "spongy," at autopsy it is significantly heavier than normal—frequently three times normal weight. This heaviness of the lung, coupled with its characteristic purplish hue, is pathognomonic of the diagnosis at autopsy.

It is thought by some that *Mikity-Wilson syndrome* or *pulmonary dysmaturity* is a representation of surfactant deficiency in a *somewhat older* child who does not develop the surfactant deficiency until several months of age. Although a respiratory disturbance may be noted in these patients in the neonatal period, the respiratory embarrassment is most evident several weeks later. Approximately one half of these patients die and the others improve slowly after a period of 6 months to a year. As in the case of hyaline membrane disease, it is characterized by linear and reticular areas of density with interspersed "cystlike" areas of lucency resembling bronchopulmonary dysplasia to some extent. Wilson and Mikity have indicated no residual pathologic or radiologic findings in infants who survive and recover—unlike the bronchopulmonary dysplasia resulting from hyaline membrane disease. In some infants, findings may completely disappear at 4 to 11 months of age. In an intermediate stage the pattern may be coarse with streaks radiating from the hilus, most commonly into the upper lobe, with air trapping and emphysema in the lower lobes.

With *transient tachypnea of the newborn* (Fig. E–22 A and B) there are also miliary densities throughout both lung fields and air bronchograms at birth extending far into the periphery. These patients usually first present with pulmonary overexpansion, and ordinarily the findings radiologically are more likely to be linear and streaky in contrast to the fine stippling characteristic of hyaline membrane disease. Despite this early respiratory distress, these infants may be treated by conservative measures, and the lung fields clear rapidly, even within 24 hours, as illustrated in Figure E–22B.

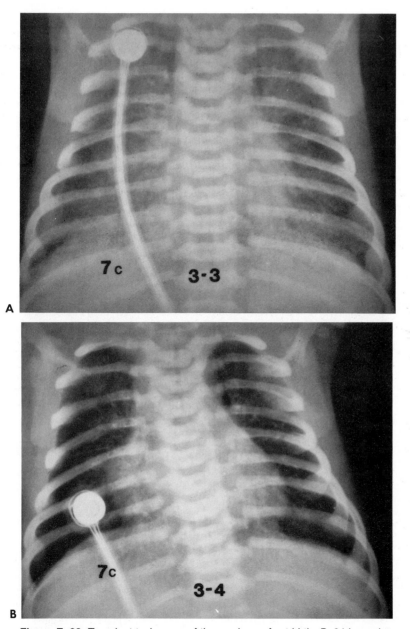

Figure E–22. Transient tachypnea of the newborn. *A,* at birth; *B,* 24 hours later.

In *streptococcal pneumonia,* the beta-hemolytic *Streptococcus* is the organism that may be cultured from sputum or pleural effusion. It may occur as a complication of measles or other childhood exanthemata and occasionally follows streptococcal infections of the pharynx or tonsils. Prior to the advent of antibiotics, it was a very acute fulminating disease wherein the patients frequently died within 36 hours, characterized at autopsy by hemorrhagic edema of the lung parenchyma, particularly of the lower lobes. Considerable alveolar wall necrosis and cavitation developed in those who survived for 4 to 5 days.

In infants it might resemble an acute staphylococcal pneumonia closely, and the radiologic appearances may be indistinguishable. However, the tendency to pneumatocele formation and pyopneumothorax, so characteristic of staphylococcal pneumonia, is usually absent. Clinically, the disease process is characterized by marked shaking chills, fever, and a cough productive of purulent and often blood-tinged sputum. By auscultation, areas of decreased breath sounds may be heard at the lung bases, particularly together with coarse rales and rhonchi. The disease process may occur in either infants or adults. At present, response to appropriate antibiotic therapy is good.

Staphylococcus pneumonia (Fig. E–23) is particularly frequent in infants during the first year of life but not necessarily in neonates. It is highly virulent, and the causative organism is *Staphylococcus aureus,* which is coagulase positive and hemolytic. Radiologically, the disease process extends to the pleura early, rapidly causing a pleural effusion, empyema, pneumothorax, and at times, bronchopleural fistula. Pleural complications are very characteristic, even as are the *pneumatoceles,* which are thin-walled, air-containing, spherical cystlike areas within the lung that may be single or multiple and of any size. The pneumatoceles may rupture and produce a pneumothorax. The pneumatoceles may persist for weeks or months after recovery, and ordinarily do not require surgical intervention despite the very large size they may acquire. Resolution of the staphylococcus pneumonia takes several weeks, even with appropriate antibiotic therapy, and a residual thin wall may remain for a considerable period of time thereafter.

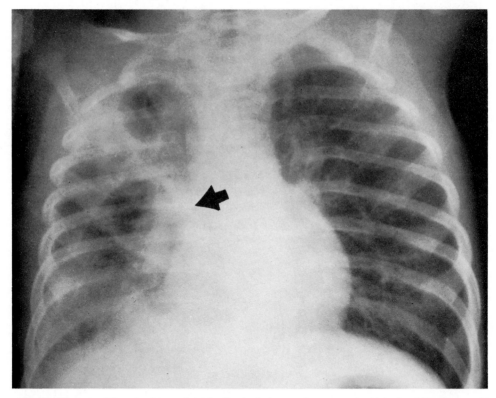

Figure E–23. PA view of the chest in an infant with staphylococcal pneumonia. Note the following combination of findings: (1) Unilaterality; (2) pleural involvement; (3) pulmonary consolidation; (4) pneumatocele formation. The arrow points to a large pneumatocele adjoining the right side of the mediastinum.

Exercise 8: Young Adult Female with "Bat-wing" Enlargement of Bronchopulmonary Lymph Nodes

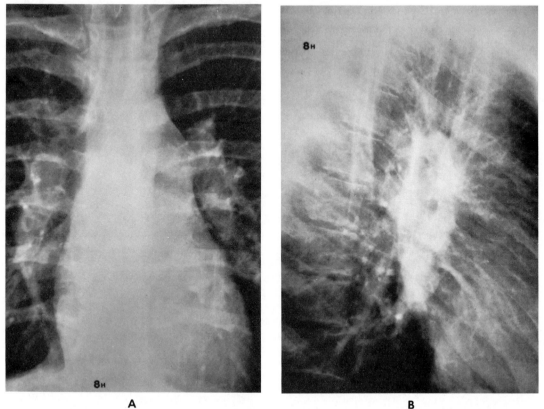

A   B

Figure E–24.

CLINICAL FINDINGS

Figure E–24 *A* and *B* are radiographs of a 27-year-old black female who has relatively few complaints with the exception that she has noted a low grade fever, especially in the afternoon, on several occasions in the last several weeks.

Question

8–1. The MOST likely diagnosis is
A. Hodgkin's disease.
B. Lymphosarcoma of the mediastinum.
C. Histoplasmosis of the mediastinum.
D. Tularemia.
E. Sarcoid of the mediastinum.

Radiologic Findings. In the frontal (Fig. E–24A) and lateral views (Fig. E–24B) of the mediastinum it is noted that there is bilateral and symmetrical enlargement of *bronchopulmonary lymph nodes.* In the lateral view these are midmediastinal, involving carinal nodes and extending somewhat inferiorly from the carina. *There is no paratracheal extension.* There is a clear space identifiable surrounding the entire cardiopericardial silhouette, separable from the enlarged lymph nodes, indicating that the involved nodes are specifically bronchopulmonary rather than paratracheal.

Discussion. With the clinical history given and the radiographic appearance of the mediastinum, **sarcoid of bronchopulmonary lymph nodes** is the most likely diagnosis.

In the differential diagnosis, one should consider the following alternative possibilities: A) Hodgkin's disease; B) lymphosarcoma of mediastinal lymph nodes; C) histoplasmosis or some other infectious lymph nodal or granulomatous process such as even primary tuberculosis.

Hodgkin's disease involves lymphatic tissue, especially with histologic presence of Reed-Sternberg cells and variable proliferation of the lymphocytes and histiocytes. It is usually regarded as neoplastic and related to the malignant lymphomas. Although the most common type of initial involvement is in the cervical lymph node bearing region, dissemination occurs by spread to contiguous lymph node areas such as the mediastinum. It is noteworthy that systemic reactions, particularly fever, are prominent—even more so than with lymphosarcoma and reticulum cell sarcoma, and patients often show symptoms due to debility, pressure from the lymph nodes involved, and infiltration of the lungs peripherally. *The disease process is far more likely to be clinically symptomatic than is sarcoid of the lung or mediastinum,* and mediastinal or even retroperitoneal

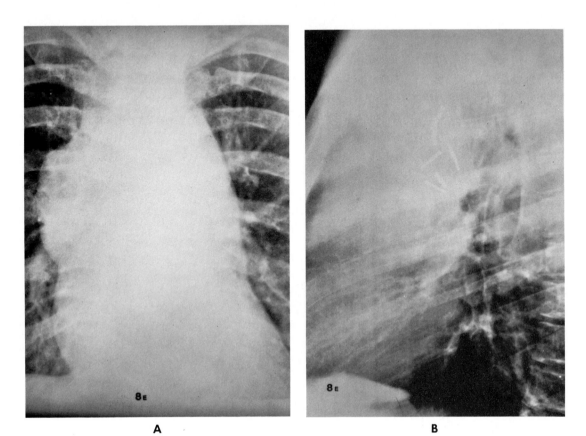

A   B

Figure E–25. Hodgkin's disease.

lymph nodes may be enlarged before those in other areas of the body. Four different types of the disease are recognized: 1) lymphocytic predominance, 2) nodular sclerosis, 3) mixed cellularity, and 4) lymphocytic depletion, but nodular sclerosis accounts for approximately 40% of cases. At times there appears to be a natural evolution of the disease histologically from lymphocytic predominance to mixed cellularity and thereafter to lymphocytic depletion. *The involvement of Hodgkin's disease, as with lymphosarcoma in the mediastinum, is more frequently paratracheal and hilar than bronchopulmonary,* although this itself might not be sufficient to prove the diagnosis, and biopsy with mediastinoscopy is needed.

A case of Hodgkin's disease that obviously has been operated upon, as shown by the metal clips in the lateral view (Fig. E–25 *A* and *B*), is shown.

The radiologic differentiation of Hodgkin's disease of the mediastinum from lymphosarcoma may be virtually impossible. Complete regression of lymph nodes involved by lymphosarcoma following radiation therapy is demonstrated in Figure E–26 *A* and *B*. In the *search for mediastinal disease* it is often desirable—indeed necessary—to obtain *heavier exposure films* than routine studies would afford. Despite the high degree of variability in the appearance of the mediastinum involved by lymphosarcomatous lymph nodes, one would *not* seriously entertain this diagnosis in our patient (Fig. E–24 *A* and *B*) for the following reasons: 1) the symmetrical *bronchopulmonary lymph node involvement* is much more frequent with sarcoid than with lymphosarcoma. In lymphosarcoma, even though the mediastinum or retroperitoneum may be the first site of involvement, there is often associated back pain, considerable patient discomfort, and systemic complaints such as malaise, fever, weight loss, excessive sweating, and pruritis. These latter systemic complaints occur in at least one fifth of the patients. More

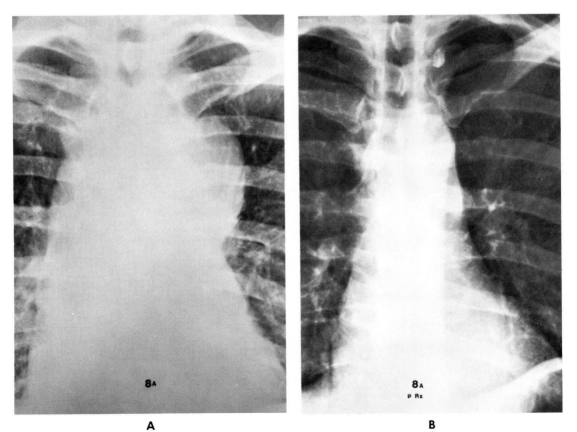

A   B

Figure E–26. *A,* Malignant lymphoma before radiation therapy. *B,* After radiation therapy.

specific symptoms are highly variable, being determined by the organ systems involved. In the chest there is often an associated cough, substernal pain, dysphagia, and even evidence of superior vena caval obstruction or paralysis of the recurrent laryngeal nerve. The diagnosis can be established only by biopsy.

Histoplasmosis is a systemic fungal disease that spreads via the pulmonary lymphatics and blood to mediastinal lymph nodes and elsewhere in the body such as the spleen, liver, gastrointestinal tract, kidneys, skin, central nervous system, and other organs. It has a great variability in its clinical presentation, being at times asymptomatic and benign but at times producing highly significant symptomatology and illness progressing to eventual fatality. Our patient might easily have been diagnosed as having histoplasmosis, although on a preferential basis, the involvement of the bronchopulmonary lymph nodes is much more frequent with sarcoidosis than histoplasmosis. Acute primary histoplasmosis could readily be excluded on the basis that our patient did not have a persistent febrile respiratory disease or widespread parenchymal disease of the lungs. As a general rule, however, differentiation is extremely difficult even from tuberculosis without supporting laboratory and microscopic data.

Most cases of *tularemia* are related to the handling or ingestion of infected animal tissues, to inhalation of infected aerosols or to transmission to humans by insect vectors such as ticks or deer flies. Characteristically, there is an initial focal ulcer at the site of entry of the causative bacilli, and thereafter there is enlargement of regional lymph nodes and a constitutional reaction of severe fever, systemic prostration, muscle aches and pains, and headache. There may be a full-blown pneumonia, occasionally accompanied by pleurisy or a typhoid-like illness. Lung involvement does occur in all forms of tularemia subsequent to the bacteremia. The incubation period varies from 2 to 5 days. There may be parenchymal involvement in the lungs as well as the hilar adenopathy.

Usually these patients are severely ill, and usually with careful history, the mode of entry of the bacillus can be traced. Our patient did not have the severe type of illness nor the portal of entry that would characterize it as a tularemia.

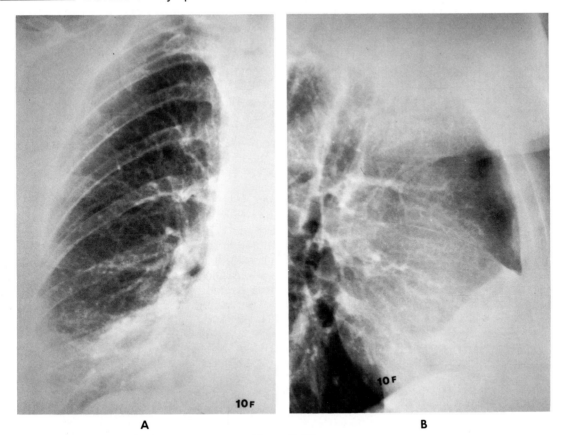

A   B

Figure E–27.

CLINICAL FINDINGS

This patient is a 58-year-old male who had a chest film as part of an executive examination, and as the result of this, posteroanterior (Fig. E–27A) and lateral (Fig. E–27B) films of the chest were obtained. Figure E–27A shows the right half of the thoracic cage, the left half being completely normal. No symptomatology, physical findings, or laboratory abnormalities were recorded.

Question

9–1. The MOST likely diagnosis is
A. Bronchogenic cyst
B. Pericardial lipoma
C. Neurofibroma
D. Thymoma
E. Middle lobe syndrome

Radiologic Findings. On the posteroanterior film of the chest (Fig. E–27 *A*) there is a shadow of increased density which is moderately well circumscribed, having the appearance of a quarter segment of a sphere, in the right cardiophrenic angle anteriorly. Lung substance could be visualized through this shadow, which was posteriorly situated behind it. The margin of the right atrium could be clearly delineated, as were the lower branchings of the right pulmonary artery. On the lateral chest radiograph (Fig. E–27 *B*) the shadow of increased density is anteriorly situated, appearing to occupy a portion of the right middle lobe anteriorly. It blended with the minor fissure anteriorly and the major fissure inferiorly, with a rather sharp line of circumscription between these two fissures. This shadow of increased density was not associated with the hilus, and the anterior clear space was clearly identified above the minor fissure anteriorly. The shadow of the inferior vena cava and the posterior cardiac margin were also clearly defined.

Discussion. The diagnosis in this patient proved to be a **pericardial lipoma.**

The pericardial lipoma and pericardial cyst ordinarily occupy a similar location and are very difficult to differentiate radiologically, except by computed tomography, where the attenuation coefficient is that of fat, whereas with a pericardial cyst it would be that of water. Computed tomography is, therefore, the method of diagnosis, and would probably have made it unnecessary for the patient to have been operated upon. Occasionally, a herniation through the foramen of Morgagni will also produce a shadow of this type, sometimes in association with organoaxial rotation of the stomach and tenting of the mesentery and transverse colon upward through the foramen of Morgagni. This was not the case here.

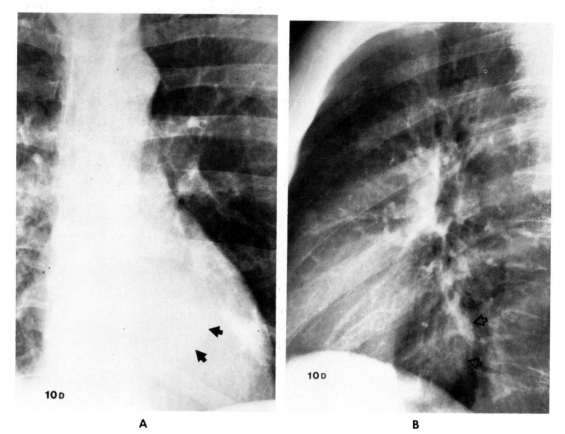

A   **B**

Figure E–28. Bronchogenic cyst: PA and lateral views.

A *bronchogenic cyst* (Fig. E–28 *A* and *B*) does not have this appearance. It usually arises from the tracheobronchial tree near the carina or one of the major bronchial branches and extends posteriorly like a gloved finger or inferiorly and posteriorly from this situation, resembling a "hanging sack." In Figure E–28*B* the hanging "sac" can be seen behind the heart on the left and it blends with the posterior cardiac margin in the posterior mediastinum.

As previously indicated, the *neurogenous tumors* are almost exclusively in the posterior mediastinum, as is indicated in the radiographs, Figure E–29 *A* and *B*. They are sharply circumscribed and are at times associated with erosive changes in the posterior margins of the vertebral bodies or the intervertebral foramina, and they are usually either neurofibromata (as was the case here) or ganglioneuromas.

The *thymoma* is ordinarily an *anterior* mediastinal tumor, usually occupying at least a portion of the *anterior mediastinal clear space,* as seen in Figure E–30 *A* and *B,* but it also may be somewhat more inferiorly situated.

A normal-appearing thymus in an infant sometimes fills the anterior mediastinal clear space in the lateral view and in the posteroanterior projection appears as a "sail"; hence this is referred to as the "thymic sail sign" in the infant.

The *middle lobe syndrome* is caused by blockage of the right middle lobe bronchus. Lymph nodes may be responsible, either inflammatory or neoplastic in origin. Bronchoscopy and computed tomography are very helpful in establishing this diagnosis, although a tissue diagnosis would be necessary to differentiate between an inflammatory or a neoplastic origin.

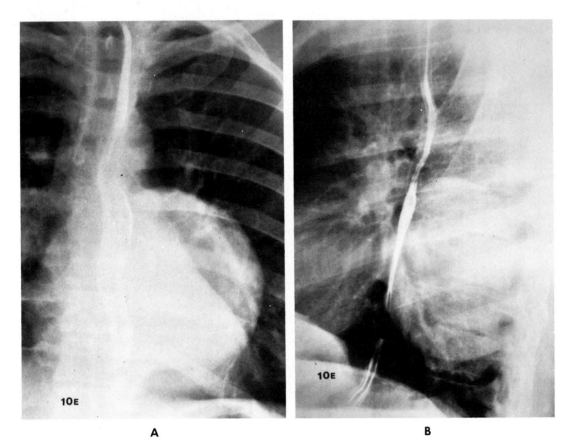

A   B

Figure E–29. Neurofibroma: PA and lateral views.

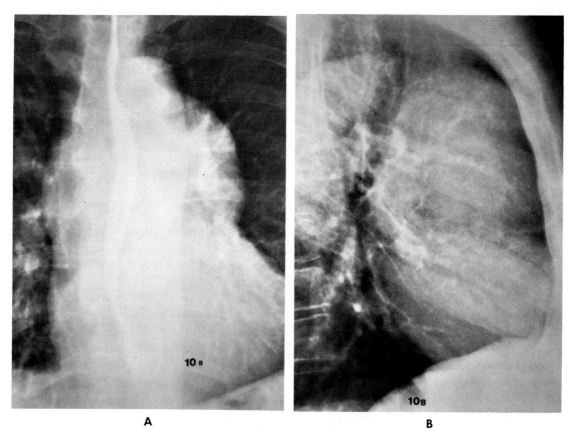

A   **B**

Figure E–30. Thymoma: PA and lateral views.

HEART AND MEDIASTINUM

The study of the complexity of the anatomy of the heart and mediastinum are greatly facilitated by specialized contrast techniques to be described later. By plain film studies in routine positions with barium in the esophagus (combined with fluoroscopy when feasible), the heart and mediastinum generally can be well analyzed. Once a lesion has been localized to the mediastinum from all perspectives, its location in the lateral chest radiograph often *statistically* denotes its probable histology (Figs. 3–11 and 3–12).

Computed tomography offers distinct advantages in the study of the mediastinum if one is familiar with the normal anatomy by this modality. With computed tomography, abnormal or questionable contours of the mediastinum may be evaluated more accurately than by conventional tomography. Morever, the extent of a mediastinal tumor can be estimated and its localization determined, a particular advantage in the appropriate staging of bronchogenic neoplasms prior to undertaking treatment. Also, previously considered "blind spots" in the mediastinum can now be evaluated. These are located especially at the thoracic inlet, the intrapericardial great vessels, the azygoesophageal recess, and the diaphragmatic crura.

Diagnostic roentgen imaging of the heart is possible without added chamber or vessel contrast enhancement when routine views with barium in the esophagus and fluoroscopy are employed. When a diagnosis of cardiac disease is suspected, the following details are noted:

1. The *anatomic configuration* of the heart and its major chambers and outflow tract are delineated.

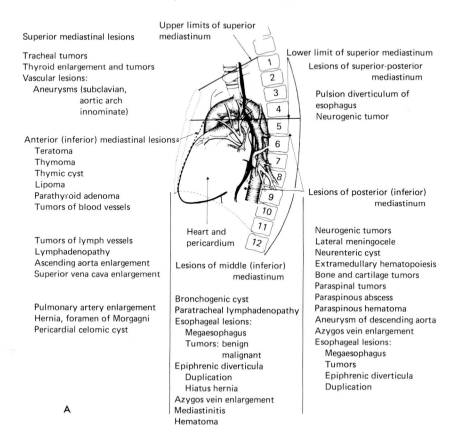

Figure 3–11. *A,* Most frequent sites for mediastinal lesions.

Illustration continued on following page

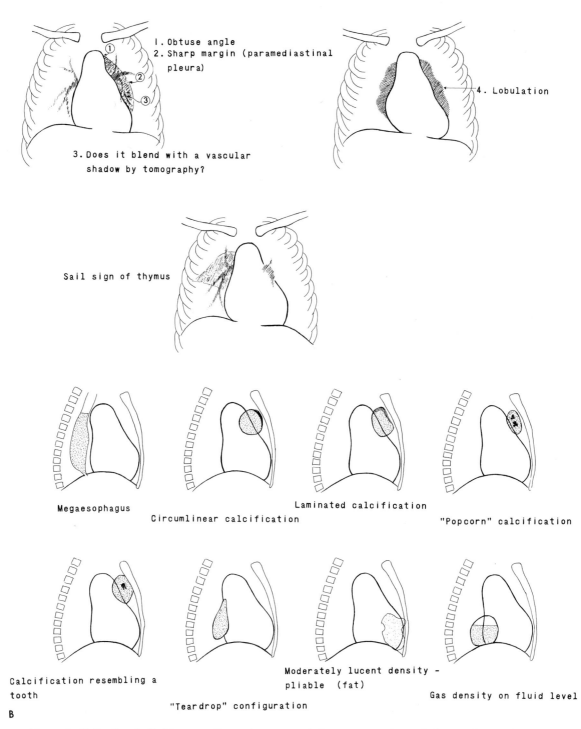

1. Obtuse angle
2. Sharp margin (paramediastinal pleura)
3. Does it blend with a vascular shadow by tomography?

4. Lobulation

Sail sign of thymus

Megaesophagus

Circumlinear calcification

Laminated calcification

"Popcorn" calcification

Calcification resembling a tooth

"Teardrop" configuration

Moderately lucent density — pliable (fat)

Gas density on fluid level

B

Figure 3–11 *Continued. B,* Diagrams illustrating some of the roentgen signs of abnormality with respect to mediastinal lesions. *C* 1 and 2, Diagram at thoracic level 15 and T7-T8 at cut no. 13 showing anatomic parts encountered in these slices. 3, Figure for orientation.

Illustration continued on opposite page

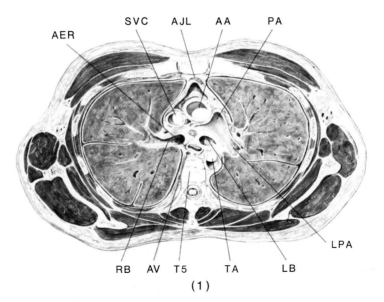

(1)

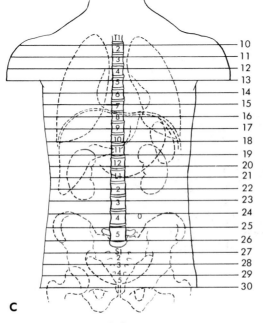

(2)

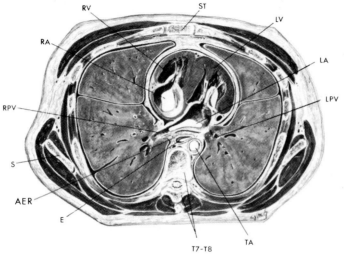

C

(3)

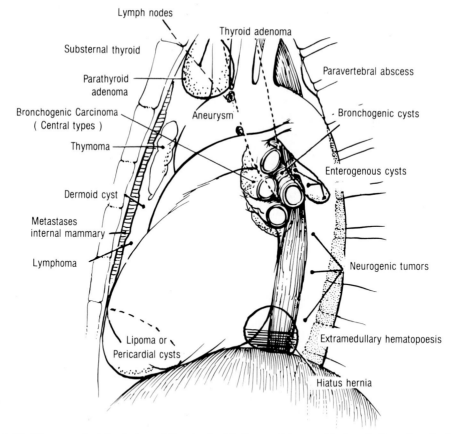

Figure 3–12. Diagram of a lateral view of the chest with the most frequent lesions indicated and where they are most likely to occur in relation to the mediastinum.

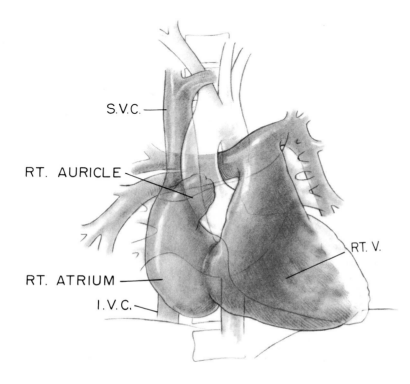

Figure 3–13. Frontal view of the heart showing the relationship of inflow and outflow tracts to the right cardiac chambers. I.V.C. = inferior vena cava; S.V.C. = superior vena cava; RT.V. = right ventricle. (After Schad, N., et al.: Differential Diagnosis of Congenital Heart Disease. New York, Grune & Stratton, 1966. Used with permission of Grune & Stratton.)

2. The *electrical conductive* activity of the heart and its resultant pulsatile activity are evaluated fluoroscopically. Admittedly, electrocardiographs are more accurate in this regard.

3. A determination is made by actual measurement as to *whether the heart is enlarged.*

4. The *presence or absence of cardiac failure* is indicated by "cephalization of flow" on posteroanterior roentgenograms of the chest in the erect position, and interstitial edema or pleural effusion as well as cardiac enlargement are further evaluated.

5. From the analysis of size and shape, assuming that cardiac failure has not supervened, the *etiology of heart disease* often can be ascertained. This is particularly true of rheumatic heart disease with valvular involvement.

6. The presence or absence of pericardial *calcification* can be determined.

7. *Treatment* is planned, whether medical or surgical.

A further elucidation of each of these seven criteria in respect to cardiac disease is now in order.

The *anatomic configuration* of the heart is readily elucidated from reference to Figures 3–13 through 3–15. The external borders of each chamber are readily visualized by frontal, lateral, and oblique perspectives radiologically and fluoroscopically if possible. In some instances, valvular disease of a specific type may be suspected (i.e., mitral, especially).

Cardiac mensuration for possible enlargement of the heart is the best single indicator of cardiac disease. Only the coronary atherosclerotic heart may be small and yet seriously diseased. The most accurate (and only method strongly recommended) for cardiac mensuration requires erect posteroanterior and lateral teleroentgenograms of the chest and the determination, from these two views, of the following basic measurements (Fig. 3–16A and B): (1) the long diameter (L) and the broad diameter (B) from the posteroanterior roentgenogram, and (2) the greatest anteroposterior diameter (D) from the lateral view. From these three measurements the relative heart volume (RHV) is determined in accordance with the formula given in Figure 3–16C, which employs additionally the surface area (SA) of the patient obtained from chart values, knowing the height and weight of the patient. Figure 3–16C (Tables 3–2A and

Text continued on page 76

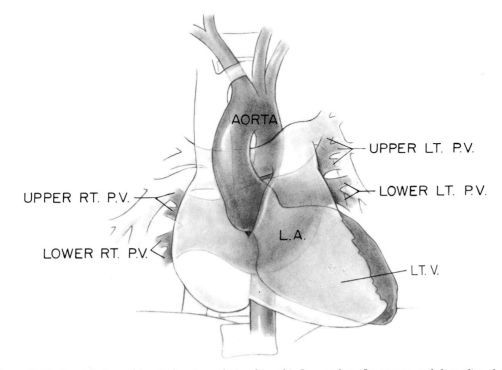

Figure 3–14. Frontal view of heart showing relationship of inflow and outflow tracts to left cardiac chambers. RT. P.V. = right pulmonary vein; L.A. = left atrium; LT. V. = left ventricle (shaded); LT. P.V. = left pulmonary veins. (After Schad, N., et al.: Differential Diagnosis of Congenital Heart Disease. New York, Grune & Stratton, 1966. Used with permission of Grune & Stratton.)

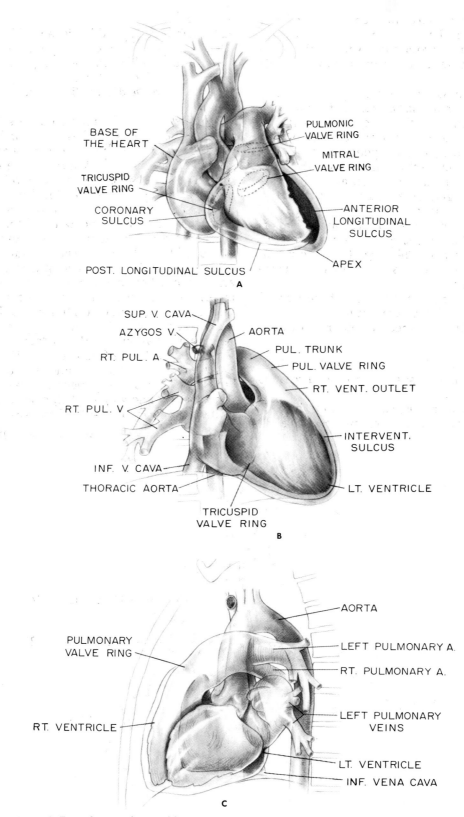

Figure 3–15. *A,* Frontal view of normal heart (transparent) showing relationship of inflow and outflow tracts to chambers. *B,* Normal heart in right posteroanterior oblique projection, rotation 60 degrees, showing the relationship of inflow and outflow tracts to the chambers of the heart by translucency of the chambers. (Note that in both projections there is some superimposition of the right and left ventricles.)

Illustration continued on opposite page

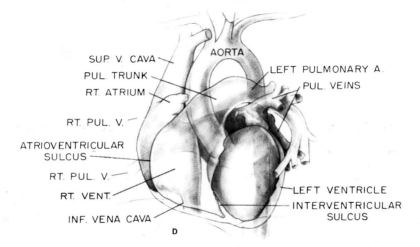

SUP. V. CAVA
PUL. TRUNK
RT. ATRIUM
RT. PUL. V.
ATRIOVENTRICULAR
SULCUS
RT. PUL. V.
RT. VENT.
INF. VENA CAVA

AORTA
LEFT PULMONARY A.
PUL. VEINS

LEFT VENTRICLE
INTERVENTRICULAR
SULCUS

D

Figure 3–15 *Continued. C,* Lateral view of normal heart showing inflow and outflow tracts to the ventricles and atria. *D,* Heart in left posteroanterior oblique projection, rotation 30 degrees, showing the relative positions of the major vessels and the inflow and outflow tracts by translucency of overlying chambers. (*A-D* modified from Schad, N., et al.: Differential Diagnosis of Congenital Heart Disease. New York, Grune & Stratton, 1966. Used with permission of Grune & Stratton.)

Figure 3–16. *A,* Usual measurements employed in calculating relative cardiac volume. *B,* Lateral view of normal heart showing the method of obtaining D, the greatest anteroposterior measurement of the heart in calculation of relative heart volume. *C,* Normal heart volumes in children and adults, and formula for determining heart volume in adults.

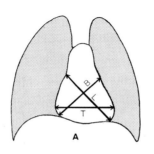

A

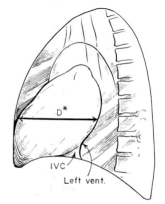

IVC
Left vent.

LATERAL VIEW OF NORMAL HEART

B

Normal Heart Volumes in Children and Adults		
Age	Volume/sq m Body Surface (RHV)	Standard Error of the Mean
0–30 days	196	22.6
30–90 days	217.8	33.9
90–360 days	282	35.8
1 to 2 years	295	30.4
2 to 4 years	304	41.5
4 to 7 years	310	36.2
7 to 9 years	324	28.6
9 to 12 years	348	33.6
12 to 14 years	369	53.8
14 to 16 years	398	61.9

Adapted from Mannheimer. In: Keats TE and Enge IP (eds.) Radiology 85:850, 1965.

In Adults	
Female (maximum normal)	450 − 490 ml/m²
Male (maximum normal)	500 − 540
Significant difference between sequential examinations	90 or more

$$\text{Relative Heart Volume (RHV)} = \frac{0.4 \ \text{X} \ \text{L} \ \text{X} \ \text{B} \ \text{X} \ \text{D}}{\text{Body surface area in meters}}$$

(Measurements from films obtained at film-to-target distance of 2 meters, or the lateral view at 1.5 meters)

Table 3–2A NOMOGRAM FOR THE DETERMINATION OF BODY SURFACE AREA OF ADULTS

Height	Body Surface	Weight
Feet and inches Centimetres	in square metres	Pounds Kilograms

Table continued on opposite page

Table 3–2B NOMOGRAM FOR THE DETERMINATION OF BODY SURFACE AREA OF CHILDREN

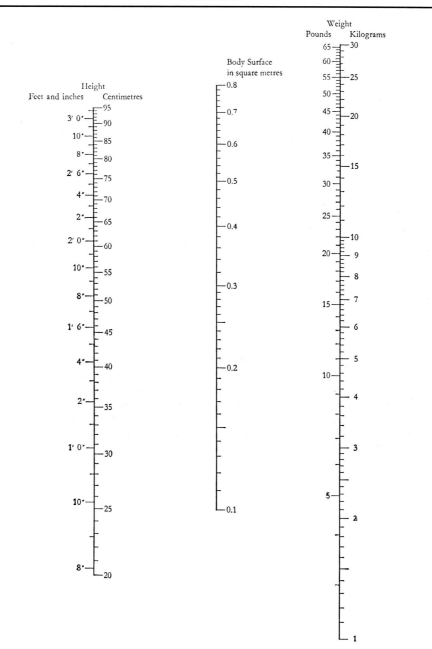

Key: The body surface area is given by the point of intersection with the middle scale of a straight line joining height and weight.

Table 3–3 ETIOLOGY OF HEART DISEASE AS DETERMINED BY CONFIGURATION CHANGES

Chambers Enlarged	Associated Intracardiac Pathology	Etiology
Left atrium	Mitral valvular disease (mitral stenosis particularly)	Rheumatic (occasionally other collagen diseases)
Left ventricle and left atrium	Mitral insufficiency +/− aortic insufficiency	Rheumatic (minimal left atrial enlargement whenever left ventricle is enlarged)
Left ventricle alone (virtually)	Aortic valvular disease	Rheumatic, hypertensive, aortic or subaortic stenosis
	Thick left ventricular wall	
	Aortic insufficiency only	Syphilis
Rounding of left ventricle suggesting hypertrophy	Coronary artery stenotic lesions	Atherosclerosis
Right ventricular hypertrophy	Marked thickening of right ventricular wall	Chronic obstructive pulmonary disease
		Pulmonary hypertension from any cause
		Congenital heart disease
		Thyrotoxic heart disease

B) gives the normal range of values. (It is estimated that RHV so obtained is 95% accurate in predicting the presence or absence of heart disease. Only the atherosclerotic heart and some types of congenital heart disease are exceptions.)

The *presence or absence of cardiac failure* can be deduced from the erect posteroanterior view of the chest by the flow pattern of the veins (especially in the upper lobes, where cephalization flow may be recognized). The interstitial and alveolar pattern, linear and acinar homogeneous shadows of increased density, and presence or absence of pleural effusion are also manifestations, usually somewhat later, of cardiac failure, especially when this information is coupled with cardiac size and shape.

The *etiology* of heart disease can usually be deduced from the configuration (Table 3–3). Special angiograms for coronary disease and angiocardiography for more detailed study of congenital heart disease are usually required. Pericardial, myocardial, coronary, and valvular *calcification* are readily detected with image amplifier fluoroscopy and occasionally on plain films. *Treatment planning* is the ultimate derivative of the foregoing evaluation. Whether it be medical or surgical, it can readily be outlined by the physician on the basis of findings.

Ultrasonography of the heart (echocardiography) and radionuclide studies of this area will be discussed under their respective sections.

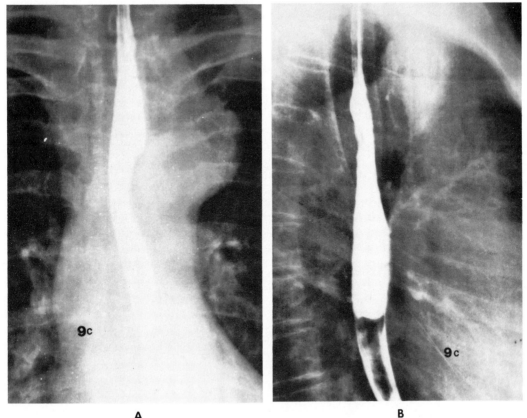

A   B

Figure E–31.

CLINICAL FINDINGS

This 60-year-old male was asymptomatic but came to his physician because he became aware of a swelling in his neck. Posteroanterior (Fig. E–31A) and lateral (Fig. E–31B) films of his lower neck and upper mediastinum were obtained.

Question

10–1. The MOST likely diagnosis is
A. Neurofibroma
B. Ganglioneuroma
C. Thyroid enlargement
D. Pseudocoarctation of the aorta
E. Mediastinitis

Radiologic Findings. The posteroanterior film (Fig. E–31*A*) and lateral films (Fig. E–31*B*) with barium in the esophagus show the lower neck region and upper two thirds of the cardiopericardial silhouette including the hili. The esophagus would appear to be deflected by the aortic knob in usual fashion; but *in the region of the aortic knob there is a double-contoured appearance* that extends up to the base of the neck, overlapping the medial edge of the clavicle in the frontal view. It is sharply circumscribed and imparts an inverted "3" appearance to the elongated aorta and its aortic knob. In lateral view, it would appear that there is a hemispherical knoblike shadow superimposed over the proximal portion of the aorta, with a slight tendency to intensification of the adjoining portion of the aortic arch. This lesion has no effect on the esophagus or trachea. It does, however, extend slightly above the clavicle, especially on its medial aspect and anteriorly.

The pulmonary arteries and remaining portions of the visualized superior mediastinum do not appear remarkable.

Discussion. The most likely diagnosis of the five indicated possibilities is **pseudocoarctation of the aorta.** To prove this diagnosis, an aortogram was done following injection of contrast agent through a catheter inserted into the ascending portion of the aorta, as shown in Figure E–32.

Prior to the injection of the contrast agent, it should be noted that the mass lesion is anteriorly situated. *Neurogenous lesions* involving the thoracic cage either superiorly or inferiorly *are almost invariably posterior.*

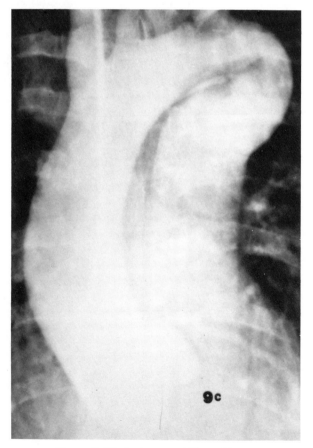

Figure E–32. Aortogram of Figure E–23.

Figure E–33 *A* and *B* show the classic appearance of *large thyroid enlargement of the neck.* This is an anteriorly situated lesion that displaces and compresses the trachea significantly and in the lateral view (Fig. E–33*B*). It is apparent that the mass lesion is anterior to the trachea, displacing both the trachea and esophagus posteriorly. Occasionally the thyroid gland will encircle the trachea and impose itself between the trachea and esophagus, but that is not exemplified in this case. There is minimal substernal extension on the right side to the level of the inferior margin of the right fourth rib posteriorly or right first rib anteriorly.

The radiographs shown in Figure E–34*A* and *B* are posteroanterior and lateral radiographs of a patient who had a *gunshot wound of his neck* that had penetrated the esophagus and produced a *mediastinitis.* The metallic foreign body of the bullet is visualized in Figure E–34*A* (b), overlying the first thoracic vertebra, and barium in the esophagus is shown to be fistulating into the superior mediastinum at the level of the aortic knob. The usual radiographic appearances of a mediastinitis are as follows: 1) a shaggy mediastinum suggesting an inflammation of the paramediastinal structures; 2) free air in the mediastinum extending up into the neck, resulting either from fistulation or gas production by the offending organism; and 3) an accumulation of purulent material or blood, which most frequently caps the left lung apex (as in this case). The history, of course, would be entirely different in this instance; but even if the film were shown without history and without the metallic foreign body, a somewhat irregular appearance above the aortic knob as well as the capping of the left lung apex would suggest a leakage of either blood or exudate from the mediastinal structures. *A patient with such a lesion would not be asymptomatic.*

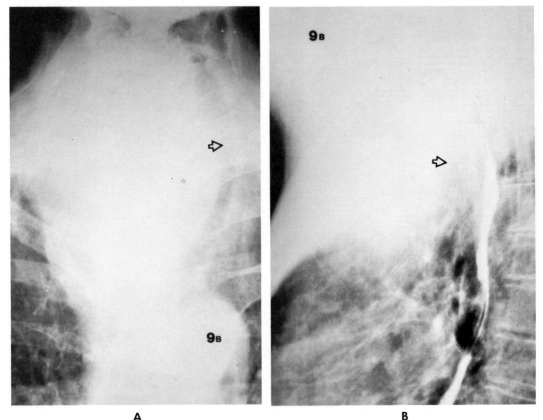

A   B

Figure E–33. Substernal thyroid.

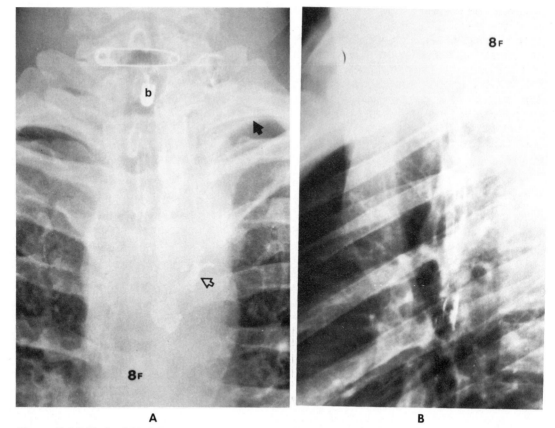

A   **B**

Figure E–34. Mediastinitis following a bullet wound. (Open arrow = esophageal fistula; closed arrow = leakage of blood around left apex.)

===== Exercise 11: Adult Male with a Crushing Blow to the Mediastinum =====

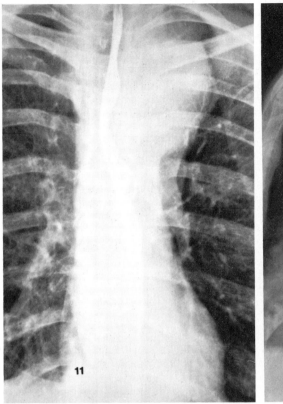

A

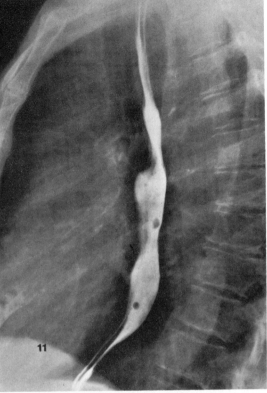

B

Figure E–35.

CLINICAL FINDINGS

This 50-year-old male was brought to the emergency room after an auto accident in which he appeared to have sustained considerable soft tissue lacerations and bruising of his face and chest. He was perfectly conscious, and complained of numerous aches and pains which were not localizing. His face had a somewhat ashen hue, but his pulse and blood pressure were normal.

A posteroanterior film of the chest (Fig. E–35 A), with barium in the esophagus and a lateral film of the chest, likewise with barium in the esophagus (Fig. E–35 B) were obtained, and a plastic surgeon was called to repair his facial lacerations.

Questions

11–1. Indicate which of the following radiographic findings in the films of the chest shown are MOST significant.
A. Widening of the aortic knob
B. Fracture of a rib
C. Irregularities and impressions on the esophagus
D. Irregularities in the contour of the descending thoracic aorta
E. Compression of a midthoracic vertebra

11–2. In order to interpret the most significant radiologic findings further, which of the following procedures would you perform in next sequence?
A. Repeat the chest radiographs in about 15 minutes to one-half hour

B. Perform a pleural tap of this patient's chest
C. Follow the patient, with careful attention to his vital signs, but do no more than repair his facial lacerations
D. Request that an aortogram be performed
E. Nothing special beyond repair of the facial lacerations

11–3. On further examination of this patient's radiographs, which of the following roentgen signs can you detect?
A. Fracture of the sternum
B. Calcium sclerosis in the arch of the aorta
C. Left apical pleural capping
D. Enlargement of the right atrium
E. Evidence of a lower thoracic paraspinous mass

11–4. On the basis of all the above findings and others not alluded to above which you believe are positive, which ONE of the following diagnoses would you consider as *most likely and important clinically?*
A. Atherosclerosis, with elongation and tortuosity of the aorta
B. Aortic stenosis with poststenotic dilatation of the aorta
C. Paraspinous abscess
D. Traumatic tear and dissection of the aorta
E. Atherosclerotic heart disease with calcium sclerosis of the coronaries

81

Radiologic Findings. On the posteroanterior view of the mediastinum, with barium in the esophagus (Fig. E–35 *A*) what appears to be the aortic knob is very markedly enlarged, extending upward to the extreme left apex. On closer inspection it is possible that there is a slightly double-contoured appearance of this aortic knob in that there is a shadow of greater opacity contained within it which more closely simulates the usual appearance of the aortic knob. There is an area of irregular laminated calcium near the periphery of the larger shadow. There is a double-contoured appearance of the descending thoracic aorta and a shadow just outside and lateral to that of the left pulmonary artery extending down toward the region of the left auricular appendage. There is a pleural opacification of the extreme left apex.

In the lateral view (Fig. E–35 *B*), the descending aortic shadow has an undulating appearance posteriorly and even anteriorly as it impresses itself on the barium-filled esophagus. There is apparently a change in caliber of the descending thoracic aorta about two vertebral segments above the left hemidiaphragm, where it appears easily one half the diameter of the descending thoracic aorta in the extreme left apex. There is a slight anterior bowing of the esophagus and trachea in the superior aspect of the thoracic cage.

Also in the lateral view (Fig. E–35 *B*), careful inspection of the sternum immediately below the manubriosternal junction shows an oblique fracture of the body of the sternum with a slight thickening of the pleura immediately underlying this apparent fracture. The anterior mediastinal space, however, is clear with no significant abnormalities beyond this undulatory appearance of the substernal pleura.

There is no other indication of fracture in those portions of the bony thoracic cage that are visualized. One might, however, raise question about the slight asymmetry of the manubrioclavicular joints on the posteroanterior view (Fig. E–35 *A*) in that the right clavicle appears slightly cephalad to the left.

Discussion. This patient illustrates an extremely important problem in relation to the emergency handling of traumatized patients. Not infrequently when they appear in the emergency room after an auto accident, the most important aspect of the injury is not immediately apparent. They are perfectly conscious, and there is complete maintenance of normal vital signs. They may have lacerations, widespread throughout the body, but none that appear life-threatening.

This was the case in the patient being discussed at this time. On the chest films at hand, in answer to **Question 11–1, the widening of the aortic knob** with a slight separation of the calcium sclerosis in the aortic knob from the adventitial outline is an extremely important finding. There is also a slight suggestion of "double contouring" of the aortic knob. A specific fracture of a rib is not detected but there are undulations and indentations on the barium-containing esophagus that are difficult to explain, except that at autopsy this patient was found to have blood in his pericardium, and hence this is a significant finding. The marked irregularity in the diameter of the descending thoracic aorta from its cephalad to caudad portions is most significant. It will be noted that in the immediate vicinity of the aortic knob it is markedly widened and irregular and scalloped. This elongation and tortuosity, however, tend to diminish to normal caliber just above the diaphragm. Such narrowness of midthoracic vertebrae as might be seen here is of no pathologic significance at this time and merely represents degenerative change in the thoracic vertebrae characteristic of a person of this age group.

Question 11–2: In the handling of this patient, the *appearance of the aortic knob,* the *separation of the calcification in the aortic wall at the knob level* from the outermost adventitia, and the pleural capping suggesting that there may be fluid and/or blood extending around the left pleural apex are most important. Also, the undulation and widening of portions of the descending thoracic aorta strongly suggest that this patient has sustained a **traumatic tear and/or dissection of the thoracic aorta.** It would therefore be most important, if one did not proceed immediately with an aortogram, to **follow the patient carefully so that**

his vital signs were recorded. Such patients can take a turn for the worse very quickly, and, having observed the radiologic findings described above, it would be appropriate to request that an aortogram be performed as soon as possible. A pleural tap would not be in order, since there is no indication on the lateral view of significant accumulation of fluid and/or blood above the diaphragm, although it is true that the costophrenic sinuses are not shown clearly in either film. If one were to choose not to do an aortogram immediately, one would certainly repeat the chest radiographs in about 15 to 30 minutes to be certain whether the findings were progressive or stationary with respect to a potential tear and dissection of the thoracic aorta.

Question 11–3: On further examination of the radiographs, one notes a fracture of the sternum about one inch below the manubriosternal junction and an indentation of the pleura immediately beneath this fracture, to suggest some blood just outside the visceral pleura at this level in conjunction with the sternal fracture. The calcium sclerosis in the arch of the aorta being slightly irregular and at a slightly greater distance from the adventitia than would normally be anticipated is most significant and further suggests dissection in the aortic arch. The left apical pleural capping has already been noted, and this is one of the important signs of a torn or traumatized thoracic aorta with bleeding surrounding the left lung apex. There is no indication of the enlargement of the right atrium in this instance, and the shadow behind the left ventricle extending toward the left, as seen on the lateral view, is most likely to be related to elongation and tortuosity of the aorta. There is certainly no evidence of a lower thoracic paraspinous mass.

Question 11–4: On the basis of all the above findings, the most likely diagnosis is traumatic tear and dissection of the aorta, and this is illustrated by the aortogram obtained in Figure E–36 A and B. In this aortogram there is an escape of the contrast agent into the left pleura overlying the left lung apex, and in Figure E–36 B, one notes the typical findings of injection of the contrast agent into the channel in the thoracic aorta created by the tear at the level in the arch where it most frequently occurs—the origin of the left subclavian artery. Here the contrast agent descends in the thoracic aorta in a second lumen created by the tear, beginning where one would expect the left subclavian to originate.

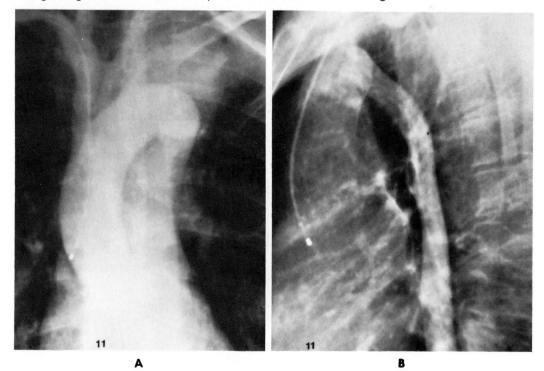

A									B

Figure E–36. Aortograms of patient in Figure E–35, demonstrating the aortic tear and dissection.

Exercise 12: Congenital Heart Disease in Adults, with and without Cyanosis

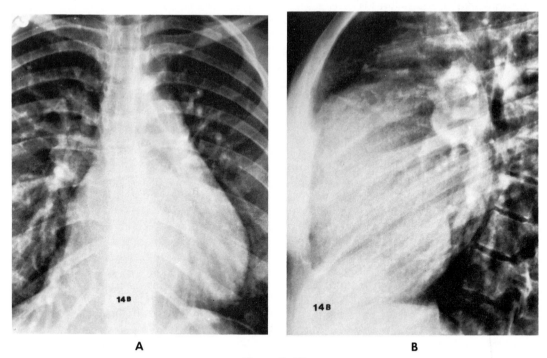

A   B

Figure E–37.

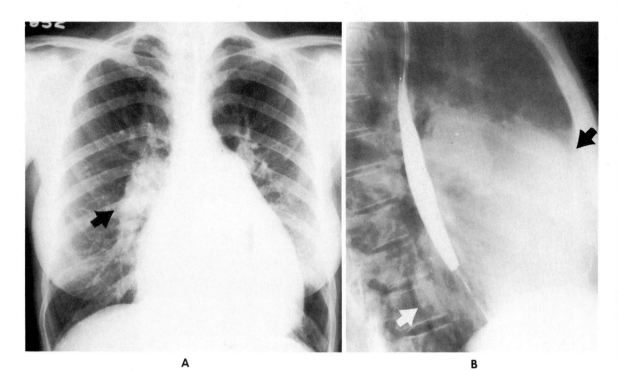

A   B

Figure E–38.

CLINICAL FINDINGS

The patient in Figure E–37A and B was a 42-year-old female who was beginning to note shortness of breath and increasing fatigability. She had had a relatively normal childhood. She had been pregnant twice with completely normal pregnancies and delivery of healthy babies. She recollected that the obstetrician had heard a "soft midsystolic murmur over the pulmonic area," but her symptoms were only noted recently. She had also noted increasing "palpitations" over her heart area, which concerned her.

The second patient (Fig. E–38A and B) was also a female but somewhat younger when she sought medical help. She was 28 years of age at that time, and in addition to increasing shortness of breath and fatigability began to notice a somewhat purplish hue to her lips and skin. Physical examination revealed that she had a more prominent midsystolic murmur over the pulmonic area and was cyanotic. There was no history of prior pregnancy.

Questions

12–1. Which of the following roentgen signs are applicable to Figure E–37A and B?
A. Prominent pulmonary vascularity
B. Normal pulmonary vascularity
C. Diminished pulmonary vascularity
D. Normal aortic knob
E. Small aortic knob

12–2. Although an esophagogram is not shown with Figure E–37A and B, which of the following statements are most expressive of what you see?
A. The left ventricle is significantly enlarged, more so than any of the other cardiac chambers.
B. The right ventricle is the most significantly enlarged cardiac chamber.
C. The pulmonary arteries "taper" rapidly, such as occurs with pulmonary hypertension.
D. The "goose-neck" appearance of the pulmonary artery is appropriately descriptive in this case.
E. If an esophagogram were obtained in these films, you would expect the esophagus to be displaced to the left and posteriorly.

12–3. With regard to Figure E–38A and B, which of the following statements are applicable?
A. The black arrow in A points to enlarged bronchopulmonary lymph nodes, indicating intercurrent lymphogenous disease.
B. From the appearance of the more peripheral pulmonary arteries you would expect this patient to have an Eisenmenger physiology.
C. The white arrow in B points to an enlarged left atrium.
D. You would expect this patient to have both enlarged left and right ventricles.
E. Patients with the clinical disorder depicted here are likely to have frequent bouts of pneumonia.

12–4. Since both patients have the same congenital basic cardiac lesion, the MOST likely diagnosis is:
A. Patent ductus arteriosus
B. Patent interventricular septum
C. Patent interatrial septum
D. Idiopathic dilatation of the pulmonary artery
E. Endocardial fibroelastosis

Radiologic Findings. In Figure E–37A and B, there is prominent pulmonary vascularity with a small aortic knob. In the lateral view, the right ventricle is markedly enlarged, encroaching cephalad on the sternum and diminishing the inferior extent of the anterior mediastinal clear space. There is a peculiar "goose-neck" appearance of the pulmonary arteries in the lateral projection. The pulmonary infundibulum is definitely identified extending from the superior aspect of the right ventricle to the aortic knob. Although barium in the esophagus is not available, there is no indication of encroachment on the retrocardiac space of an enlarged left atrium or a prominent interatrial groove. The aortic knob is on the left, and the gas bubble is beneath the left hemidiaphragm.

In Figure E–38A and B, there is an enlarged right pulmonary artery which tapers rather quickly to Zone B of the lung, suggesting an Eisenmenger physiology. Although the right ventricle appears somewhat enlarged (less than in Fig. E–37A and B), it is the left ventricle that is particularly prominent in Figure E–38B.

It is important to note that both patients are female. Both patients exhibit enlargement of the *right ventricle,* while *in the second patient* a significantly enlarged *left ventricle also* can be seen. The aortic knob is small, with preservation of the pulmonary infundibulum. *In neither instance does the left atrium appear enlarged.*

Discussion. Figures E–37A and B present a 42-year-old female with a **patent interatrial septal defect** who was physically quite well even through two pregnancies with this intracardiac congenital defect.

On the other hand, the second, younger patient (Fig. E–38A and B), who also had a **patent interatrial septal defect,** did not fare so well. At the age of 28, she was sustaining an **Eisenmenger's physiology with pulmonary hypertension.**

Thus, the answer to **Question 12–4** is **Patent Interatrial Septal Defect.**

To answer the questions in turn: **Question 12–1:** In Figure E–37A and B there is a **prominent pulmonary vascularity** with a **small aortic knob.** These are frequent findings with *intracardiac* shunting.

In answer to **Question 12–2,** the **right ventricle is definitely the most significantly enlarged cardiac chamber.** Unlike the second patient, the pulmonary arteries do not "taper" rapidly, and hence, one would not expect pulmonary hypertension—at least of clinical significance. **The "goose-neck" appearance** as seen on the lateral view is typical of patients with a patent interatrial septal defect and, when not seen on plain films, is often identified with angiocardiography. If an esophagogram were to be obtained, there would be *no significant displacement of the esophagus* in the region of the left atrium, which is one of the characteristics of patent interatrial septal defect, in contrast with a patent interventricular septal defect, in which slight enlargement of the left atrium is frequent.

With regard to **Question 12–3,** the black arrow in A points to an **enlarged right pulmonary artery** and there is rapid tapering of the more peripheral blood vessels in this case, indicating that an **Eisenmenger physiology with pulmonary hypertension** has supervened. The **white arrow** in B points to **an enlarged left ventricle** and not a left atrium. In a patient with patent interatrial septal defect and an Eisenmenger's physiology one may expect **enlargement of both the left and right ventricles.** Also, patients with this clinical disorder have **frequent bouts of bronchopneumonia.**

The interatrial septal defects are described in accordance with their sites in the atrial septum. These sites may be categorized into five types: 1) at the level of the fossa ovalis, often referred to as "the ostium secundum," the most common variety; 2) a defect inferior to the fossa ovalis between the fossa and the inferior vena cava; 3) in the uppermost part of the atrial septum near the sinus venosus; 4) in the lowermost part of the interatrial septum, which is referred to as the "ostium primum"; 5) in a position normally occupied by the coronary sinus.

The third type is sometimes referred to as a "sinus venosus" defect.

Ostium primum defects are located in the lower part of the septum near the area of formation of the endocardial cushion. This is where the atrial and ventricular septa join the two atrioventricular valves. Very often abnormalities of the contiguous parts are associated, such as a cleft mitral valve. Although the first patient represented an ostium primum defect, no other associated valvular abnormality was demonstrated. Generally, when ostium primum atrial septal defects occur as isolated entities, the physiological consequences resemble those of an isolated ostium secundum atrial septal defect. Down's syndrome in a child with congenital heart disease should immediately arouse suspicion of an endocardial cushion defect—an incidence estimated as high as 50%.

Since the isolated ostium primum defect was indeed the only component of this patient's endocardial cushion defect, and since generally the x-ray is indistinguishable from that of ostium secundum atrial septal defect unless Eisenmenger's physiology supervenes, the remainder of our discussion will relate to the ostium secundum defect with superimposed Eisenmenger's physiology.

Ostium secundum atrial septal defects occur more often in females, with a sex ratio ranging from 1.5 to 3.5 to 1. The mode of inheritance of this defect is thought to be either autosomal dominant or recessive. The defect often goes unrecognized for years unless a soft pulmonic midsystolic murmur of the atrial septal defect type becomes evident, and even this may be absent in early infancy. These patients are subject to recurrent lower respiratory infections, and the cardiac murmur may be discovered at the time of an examination for pneumonia. Although life expectancy is shortened in these patients, there are some who live to advanced ages.

Survival is significantly more limited in young adults who develop the complications displayed by the second patient with progressive pulmonary hypertension—but even in these patients longevity averages more than 40 years. Thus, the majority of children and young adults with atrial septal defects, particularly of the secundum type or the pure primum type, are relatively well and pass through the third and fourth decades with little or no detectable handicap. Even pregnancy is endured with relatively little difficulty unless pulmonary hypertension supervenes. All patients who survive to the sixth decade are usually symptomatic.

Even the pulmonary hypertension may occur with very few symptoms, although generally dyspnea and fatigue are present. Cyanosis appears or increases with effort and the patient may develop chest pain resembling angina. Hemoptysis occurs in about 25% of pulmonary hypertension patients.

Symmetrical cyanosis and digital clubbing occur when the pulmonary hypertension supervenes and reverses the interatrial shunt.

In the congenital syndrome spoken of as the "Holt-Oram syndrome," the ostium secundum atrial septal defect is the commonest cardiac anomaly, although other cardiac anomalies may occur. In the Holt-Oram syndrome, the thumb is either hypoplastic or there is an accessory phalanx, and apposition of the thumb with the fifth finger is very difficult. The thumb may indeed be rudimentary or even absent. Osseous anomalies range from those that are just barely perceptible to complete absence of an arm (abrachia) or absent arms with persistent underdeveloped hands (phocomelia).

Exercise 13: Congenital Cyanotic Heart Disease in the Adolescent and in the Infant

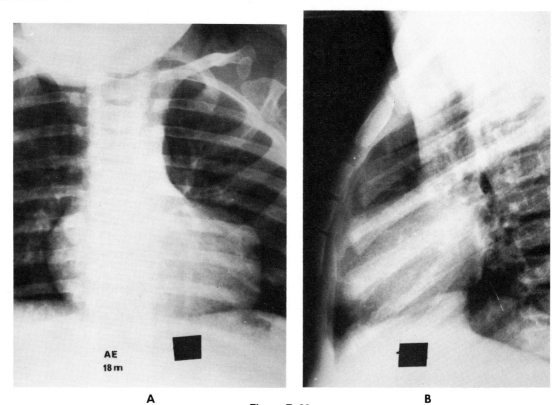

A

B

Figure E–39.

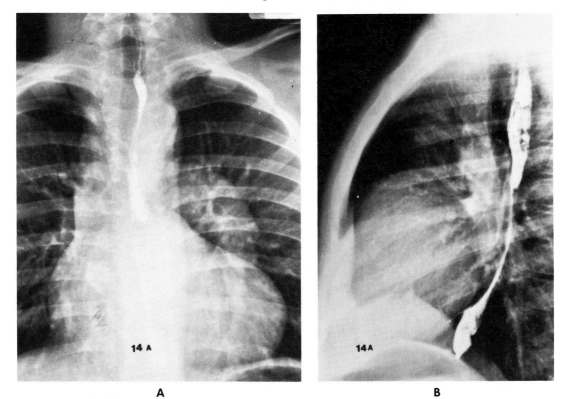

A

B

Figure E–40.

CLINICAL FINDINGS. The first two radiographs are posteroanterior and lateral (Fig. E–39 *A* and *B*) projections of an 18-month male patient who had been cyanotic from about 3 weeks of age, who was stunted in growth, and whose general tolerance for activity was diminishing.

The second set of posteroanterior projections (Fig. E–40 *A* and *B*) are those of an 18-year-old who also had been cyanotic since about 3 weeks of age and whose clinical appearance and history were very similar.

Questions

13–1. Given a teenager who has been cyanotic from birth, which of the following clinical diagnoses in relation to congenital heart disease would be MOST likely?
A. Patent ductus arteriosus
B. Tetralogy of Fallot
C. Tricuspid atresia
D. Patent interventricular septum
E. Patent interatrial septum of the secundum type

13–2. Given a teenager with congenital heart disease, which of the following clinical diagnoses in relation to congenital heart disease would be MOST likely, whether the patient is cyanotic or not?
A. Patent ductus arteriosus
B. Tetralogy of Fallot
C. Tricuspid atresia
D. Patent interventricular septum
E. Patent interatrial septum of the secundum type

13–3. In both of the above patients, which of the cardiac chambers or other intracardiac structures named is MOST likely maximally involved?
A. Right atrium
B. Right ventricle
C. Left atrium
D. Left ventricle
E. Interatrial septum

13–4. Indicate which of the following roentgen signs are most helpful in arriving at an accurate diagnosis in both cases.
A. Boot-shaped lower left cardiac contour
B. Narrow cardiac waist
C. Position of the "gas-bubble of the stomach"
D. Appearance of the pulmonary vasculature
E. The appearance of the bony structures of the thoracic cage

Radiologic Findings. In the posteroanterior view of the mediastinum of Figure E–39A, the heart is boot-shaped in contour with an elevation of the apex, and a "squared-off" appearance. The waist of the heart is very narrow, and the pulmonary arteries are small and barely in evidence. The aortic knob is visualized to the left, as is the gas bubble of the stomach. The bones of the thoracic cage are not remarkable.

In the lateral view (Fig. E–39B), a primary encroachment of the cardiac silhouette is anteriorly upward on the sternum toward the anterior mediastinal clear space, suggesting that the right ventricle is enlarged. The straightened appearance on the anterior aspect of the heart above the right ventricle and below the aortic knob is completely lacking and the anterior mediastinal clear space as a result is considerably enlarged in its anteroposterior dimension. There is no indication of encroachment of the cardiopericardial silhouette on the posterior mediastinum.

The sternum is segmented in relatively normal fashion for a child of 18 months of age, and the thoracic spine also appears normal.

In Figure E–40A, a posteroanterior view of the mediastinum, again there is a somewhat "boot-shaped" appearance of the heart, with elevation of the rounded contour of the outermost left portion of the cardiopericardial silhouette. Enlargement of what appears to be a left pulmonary artery by virtue of the branching contained from it is significant. The aortic knob is in normal position and the gas bubble of the stomach is likewise normally beneath the left hemidiaphragm. The right pulmonary artery is quite small, and there is a paucity of vasculature in the peripheral lung fields despite the prominence of the left pulmonary artery. In the lateral view (Fig. E–40C), there is an encroachment of the right ventricle on the anterior mediastinal clear space, indicating enlargement of this chamber, and once again there is a lack of the straightened appearance of what ordinarily would be considered the pulmonary infundibulum between the right ventricle and the shadow of the aorta itself. Thus, in anteroposterior dimension, the anterior mediastinal clear space is increased and rather triangular in configuration, with the base of the triangle at the sternum. The prominent left pulmonary artery can be clearly identified. Although there is a slight undulatory appearance of the esophagus containing barium, it is not notched above the aorta as might be expected with an anomalous right subclavian artery. There is a very slight indentation of the esophagus in the region of the left atrium, with a prominent angulation at the level of the interatrial groove on the posterior margin of the heart, suggesting minimal enlargement of the left atrium itself.

Discussion. Tetralogy of Fallot is the most common cause of cyanotic congenital heart disease after the immediate neonatal period. The anomaly consists mainly of the following four elements: 1) a high interventricular septal defect; 2) some form of pulmonary stenosis, usually infundibular; 3) over-riding of the aorta; 4) right ventricular hypertrophy. It is true that occasionally the pulmonary stenotic element is associated with valvular stenosis as well, but pure pulmonic valvular stenosis is rarely seen.

Other abnormalities of the pulmonary artery or its branches are also frequently seen (as in Fig. E–40 A and B), such as 1) poststenotic dilatation of one of the pulmonary arteries; 2) peripheral pulmonary artery coarctations; 3) hypoplasia of a pulmonary artery, usually the left; 4) complete absence of the pulmonary artery; and 5) a bicuspid pulmonary valve. Even tricuspid valvular abnormalities are occasionally seen.

Physiologically, with the severe infundibular pulmonic stenosis and over-riding aorta, almost all the blood from both ventricles is delivered to the aorta. It is considered now, however, that the right-to-left shunting is probably the most important factor, with direct emptying of the right ventricle into the aorta being of minor hemodynamic significance.

In addition to the symptoms indicated, these patients very often present with a history of "squatting."

As the result of these hemodynamic factors, the **right ventricle** is the most prominent radiologic feature in both cases presented herein.

There is, of course, a wide variation both clinically and radiologically. Because of the infundibular stenosis, the **cardiac waist is narrowed,** even extremely shallow or concave, as in both patients presented. The cardiac apex is displaced laterally and upwardly, largely because the right ventricle imposes itself over this aspect of the heart in frontal perspective, giving the classic **coeur en sabot** configuration. In the lateral view, the enlargement of the right ventricle is readily perceived in both instances by the cephalad encroachment of the right ventricular silhouette, squaring off its appearance in conjunction with the sternum anteriorly.

In approximately 25% of cases, the aorta is right-sided with a deflection of the esophagus to the left, instead of to the right at the level of the aortic knob. In both of our cases the aorta was left-sided. **The gas bubble is on the left side** also in both instances, a point of paramount importance in analysis of all congenital heart diseases to exclude some form of the rotatory abnormality of the heart or an outright *situs inversus.*

Even though the aorta drains both ventricles, it varies considerably in size.

The *pulmonary blood flow is diminished* as is true with other congenital heart lesions, such as hypoplastic right heart syndrome and transposition of the great vessels with pulmonary stenosis. A right-sided aortic arch is extremely infrequent in these two entities.

Unfortunately for roentgen analysis, the pulmonary vascularity is difficult to evaluate in all cases, and it may be unequal on the two sides. Thus, the pulmonary vascularity is definitely diminished in the first of the two cases presented here. From the illustrations given, the pulmonary vascularity would be difficult to evaluate in the second case.

Were it not for the ages of the two patients, differential diagnosis from other, unrelated conditions would be difficult by virtue of the associated abnormal anatomy and hemodynamics. These include 1) Type 4 persistent truncus arteriosus, occurring in infants; 2) the various transpositions with pulmonary stenosis, also occurring in infants; 3) single ventricle with pulmonary stenosis, another infantile congenital heart lesion; and 4) some cases of tricuspid or pulmonary atresia or hypoplastic right heart syndrome. In the infant, angiocardiography is usually necessary to differentiate these various lesions.

To answer **Question 13–2,** the **most frequent congenital heart lesion encountered in adolescents and adults is patent interventricular septum.** This, of course, is a very common congenital heart abnormality and may be either isolated or associated with other abnormalities. When isolated, it is consistent with good longevity. Three types have been identified: 1) that which occupies the muscular septum; 2) that which is situated in the membranous portion of the septum; and 3) that which is very high in the membranous portion of the interventricular septum and which is seen most frequently with a persistent truncus arteriosus and tetralogy of Fallot.

Only when an interventricular septal defect gives rise to a right-to-left shunt, excessive pulmonary blood flow, and active pulmonary vascular engorgement with resultant diastolic overloading and enlargement of the left atrium and left ventricle does the lesion become clinically significant. In small defects, such shunting does not occur and no right ventricular enlargement is seen.

When pulmonary hypertension with pulmonary vascular disease is superimposed upon the above, the right-sided pressure becomes very high and biventricular or even predominantly left ventricular enlargement yields to right ventricular hypertrophy, and overall cardiac size decreases.

It is important to note that in all types of interventricular septal defect, the right atrium does not become enlarged and *only the left atrium may be seen to impress itself upon the esophagus in the right anterior oblique or lateral projections when barium is present in the esophagus.* When the lesion is large, symptoms usually arise within the first year or two of life, and thus become readily apparent, such as dyspnea, fatigue, growth failure, recurrent pneumonia, and even congestive heart failure.

Another important difference is the diminutive appearance of the aortic knob in view of the intracardiac shunt. This is also true of the interatrial septal defect.

In older patients, when pulmonary hypertension supervenes and becomes severely fixed, an Eisenmenger's physiology with pulmonary hypertension is derived. Cyanosis becomes apparent, and a pattern of almost pure right ventricular hypertrophy supervenes.

Rarely, there is a communication between the left ventricle and right atrium, resulting from a high interventricular septal defect, which involves either a tricuspid valve annulus or the right atrium just above it. In these instances, the septal leaflet of the tricuspid valve is usually cleft and the valve is frequently insufficient.

In answer to **Question 13–3, the right ventricle is most prominent in both cases.** This is readily apparent on the lateral views, where considerable encroachment on the anterior mediastinal clear space and "climbing of the sternum" are apparent.

In answer to **Question 13–4,** it will be noted that 1) the heart is boot-shaped in its lower left cardiac contour owing to the **enlargement of the right ventricle** and the coeur en sabot appearance previously described. 2) **The cardiac waist is narrow because of the infundibular pulmonic stenosis.** This is modified in the second case by a poststenotic dilatation of the left pulmonary artery, which is readily apparent on the frontal perspective. 3) The **gas bubble** is in evidence **under the left hemidiaphragm** in both cases, indicating that a situs inversus is not present in either instance, although we know that statistically anywhere from 20 to 30% of patients with tetralogy of Fallot will have a right-sided aorta. 4) Comment has already been made of the usual appearance of **diminution of pulmonary vasculature,** but occasionally this may be apparent unilaterally or may be very difficult to detect, as in the second case. 5) The bony structures of the thoracic cage are completely normal in this instance, except that there is a persistence of segmentation of the sternum in the first case, as detected in the lateral view. In general, patients with congenital heart disease often have delayed ossification.

This is highly variable and is not very helpful in this particular instance, since the four segments below the manubrium form a single bone between 12 and 25 years of age in most individuals. The manubrium and sternum become fused in about 10% of adults.

ADDENDUM

It is probably also noteworthy that in addition to poststenotic dilatation of the left pulmonary artery, the second patient *had a hypoplastic right pulmonary artery unilaterally,* verified by angiocardiography.

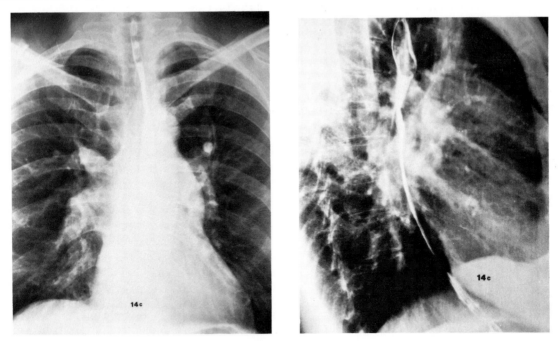

Figure E–41.

CLINICAL FINDINGS (Fig. E–41 A and B)

This 47-year-old male was normal at birth, but when he was one month old, his mother noted a palpable thrill over the precordium and a loud systolic murmur was heard at the age of one month. His chest radiograph at that time was considered normal.

He had chest fluoroscopic and radiographic examinations in adolescence that were said to show a "left atrial enlargement," but he was otherwise asymptomatic until the recent past.

Recently, he began to note increasing shortness of breath and increasing fatigue, was told that his heart seemed to be undergoing configuration changes (although persistently abnormal), and became cyanotic.

You are shown posteroanterior and lateral (Fig. E–41 A and B) radiographs of his chest obtained very recently, when he sought help.

Questions

14–1. Which of the following roentgen signs do you observe?
 A. Enlargement of both pulmonary arteries equally
 B. Enlargement of the right pulmonary artery predominantly
 C. Enlargement of the right atrium
 D. Enlargement of the left atrium
 E. A normal or diminutive aortic knob peripherally

14–2. With regard to the pulmonary vasculature peripherally, would you regard this as
 A. Increased
 B. Decreased
 C. "Tapered," as with pulmonary hypertension
 D. Complicated in its appearance by the associated presence of pneumonia or lymphadenopathy
 E. Complicated by the presence of passive hyperemia of the lungs

14–3. Which of the following diagnoses would you consider very likely, all factors considered, including his history?
 A. Patent ductus arteriosus
 B. Patent interventricular septum
 C. Patent interatrial septum
 D. Corrected transposition
 E. Coarctation of the aorta

14–4. This patient has a history of a palpable thrill and loud systolic murmur shortly after birth but had a normal-appearing heart radiographically and remains relatively asymptomatic, but he is told that in adolescence he had an enlarged left atrium radiographically. Assuming that his left atrium appears to be of relatively normal size but his physical condition is deteriorating, which of the following diagnoses is MOST likely?
 A. Patent ductus arteriosus
 B. Patent interventricular septum
 C. Patent interatrial septum
 D. Corrected transposition
 E. Coarctation of the aorta

93

Radiologic Findings. In the posteroanterior view (Fig. E–41*A*) there is very marked enlargement of the right pulmonary artery, especially that leading to the lower half of the right lung field, including the right middle lobe. There is rapid tapering of the blood vessels as they approach Zone B of the lungs. In the more peripheral portions of the lungs the blood vessels assume a normal configuration.

The left pulmonary artery is not nearly as markedly enlarged as is the right, but the "rapid tapering" at Zone B of the arterial vessels is again noted.

The aortic knob is either diminutive or normal in size but certainly is not enlarged. There is, however, a marked enlargement in the pulmonary sector of the heart in frontal view but no significant enlargement of the cardiopericardial silhouette below this level. In the lateral view (Fig. E–41*B*), the barium in the esophagus shows no significant displacement in the region of the left or right atrium, and the ventricular silhouette, both anteriorly and posteriorly, is well within normal limits. The prominence of the pulmonary arteries and infundibular portion of the right ventricle is still noteworthy, with some encroachment upon the anterior mediastinal clear space.

The radiologic findings in Figure E–42*A* and *B* are somewhat similar except that 1) the pulmonary vasculature is prominent throughout the lungs and not nearly so prominent centrally; 2) there is enlargement in the region of the left atrium by displacement of the esophagus posteriorly, with a small notch visible in the region of the inter-atrial groove; and 3) it is probable that there is a greater prominence of the right ventricle.

The main differences noted in Figure E–43 are that 1) the aortic knob is definitely either normal or slightly enlarged; 2) the pulmonary sector in the left cardiac contour is prominent. There is an increase in pulmonary vascularity.

In Figure E–44 *A* and *B*, the main differential findings are 1) the aortic knob and that portion of the aorta immediately below the aortic knob impress themselves upon the esophagus, producing an inverted "Figure 3" appearance; 2) the left ventricle appears quite prominent; and 3) there is a definite notching of the

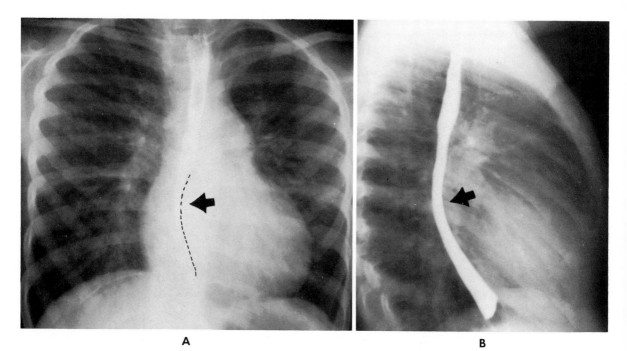

A   **B**

Figure E–42. Ventricular septal defect. Posteroanterior (*A*) and lateral (*B*) views of the chest in a patient with a patent interventricular septum. Note the enlargement of the left atrium as indicated on both the frontal and lateral esophagram views. This is an important differential feature between the interventricular and interatrial septal defects.

inferior margins of the ribs (Fig. E–44*B*). The pulmonary arterial pattern is not unusual.

Discussion. In answer to the various questions:

In **Question 14–1** there would appear to be **enlargement of the right pulmonary artery predominantly.** The **aortic knob** is probably on the **diminutive** side or, at the most, **low normal.**

Despite the fact that he was told some years earlier that he had an enlarged left atrium, there is no indication on the present film studies of an enlarged left or right atrium.

With regard to **Question 14–2,** the more peripheral blood vessels are not increased, nor are they decreased. **They are tapered** as one extends from the markedly enlarged right pulmonary artery to the mid-zone of the lung, but more peripherally beyond this tapering of the pulmonary artery, especially to the right upper lobe, the pulmonary vasculature does not appear to be abnormal.

In consideration that this patient had a history of a palpable thrill and loud systolic murmur shortly after birth but was normal otherwise, even during the adolescent period, with only an enlarged left atrium noted radio-

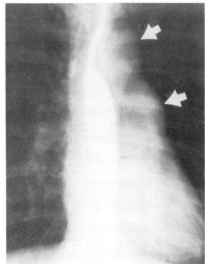

Figure E–43. Patent ductus arteriosus. Posteroanterior view of the chest in a patient with a patent ductus arteriosus. Note the enlargement of both the aortic knob and the pulmonary artery. With patency of interatrial or interventricular septum, the aortic knob is ordinarily small or diminished in size. The left atrium may be slightly enlarged with a patent ductus arteriosus.

graphically by a physician, the diagnosis that should come to mind immediately upon noting the roentgen findings above is **patent interventricular septum.** The factor to be explained is the apparent resumption of a normal-appearing left atrium on these films, obtained at the time his physical condition was deteriorating.

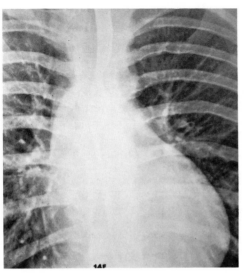

A

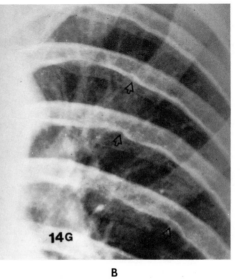

B

Figure E–44. Coarctation of the aorta. *A,* PA film of the heart; *B,* coned-down view of the upper ribs.

All of these findings are quite typical of a patent interventricular septum, except for the fact that his deterioration began as late in life as it did. Although individuals with a patent interventricular septum frequently survive and have a relatively normal life expectancy, the normal life expectancy is usually the result of a spontaneous closure of the patent interventricular septum; in patients with a large ventricular septal defect, mortality is highest in early childhood, especially the first year.

A relatively characteristic sequence of events such as occurred here suggests that *this patient was beginning to sustain an Eisenmenger physiology with increased pulmonary hypertension*, and, when the shunt was reversed from right-to-left, symmetrical cyanosis began to occur. Actually, little or no cardiac enlargement may be present when a larger interventricular defect is associated with Eisenmenger physiology. It is not unusual for an occasional patient to demonstrate increased vascularity of the right lung and relatively normal vascularity of the left. As the intrapulmonary hypertension proceeds, the "pruning" or "tapering" of the pulmonary arteries becomes more prevalent. Indeed, when the shunt has been reversed since early childhood, the peripheral pulmonary bed may appear relatively normal.

In a ventricular septal defect, the aortic knob is either normal or small, since the shunt is intracardiac.

The left atrial enlargement occurs when there is a sizable right-to-left shunt causing a volume overload of the left heart. Even under these circumstances, however, the left atrial dilatation is usually moderate but it can, in older patients, resemble organic mitral valvular disease. When the pulmonary hypertension becomes very high and the predominantly left ventricular enlargement yields to right ventricular hypertrophy, the heart may actually decrease in size. Thus, when the shunts become larger, there is a less dominant pattern of left-sided cardiac enlargement, left atrial enlargement may virtually disappear with only minimal indentation on the esophagus in the lateral view persisting.

Because of the marked prominence of this patient's right pulmonary artery, and because of the lack of indentation of the esophagus in the region of the left atrium at the time he was examined, clear differentiation from an atrial septal defect would not be possible and angiocardiography would be necessary.

Figures E–42A and B **(patent interventricular septum)** show the enlarged left atrium clearly, the diminutive aortic knob, and only a minimal plethora of the lung.

Figure E–43 shows a typical **patent ductus arteriosus** in which the aortic knob is indenting the esophagus significantly and is thus different from the intracardiac shunts of the interatrial and interventricular types.

With regard to **coarctation of the aorta** (Fig. E–44A and B), the radiographic distinction from the patient in Figure E–41 is marked. Figure E–44 illustrates a coarctation of the aorta of the adult type, in which the area of coarctation is located just distal to the level of the ductus arteriosus (a rarer type in the infant is observed proximal to the ductus arteriosus). It will be noted from the films that there is a double indentation of the esophagus at the site of coarctation, with the aortic knob above it and the poststenotic dilatation below. This type of poststenotic dilatation is, of course, not present in all cases. It is known as the "inverted Figure 3 sign."

Figure E–44 also demonstrates *rib notching* involving the posterior fourth to eighth ribs, best shown in the magnified view (*B*). Such rib notching is rarely seen in patients under the age of 7 or 8. Although it is often stated that such rib notching is pathognomonic of coarctation of the aorta, there are a number of other entities that may be associated with similar rib notching, and confusion may result.

Exercise 15: Swollen, Painful Joints at Age 10 Years; Heart Disease at 23

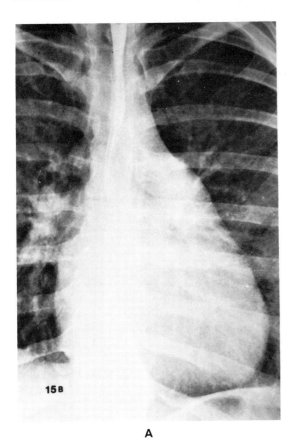

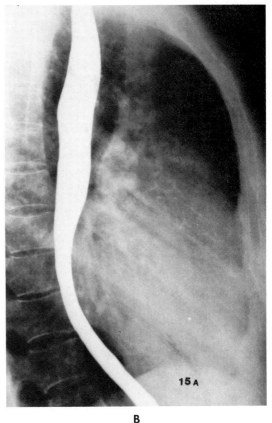

A   **B**

Figure E–45.

CLINICAL FINDINGS (Fig. E–45 *A* and *B*)

This 23-year-old male at the age of 10 noted that his joints were somewhat swollen and painful; he was taken to a physician by his mother, who was told that a diastolic murmur over the heart could be heard. He was given appropriate medication and told to remain in bed for approximately 3 months, during which time his joint swelling receded and no further recurrence of joint involvement was noted. The diastolic murmur, however, persisted to the present.

Questions

15–1. What is the MOST likely etiology of the heart disease sustained in this patient?
A. Heart disease associated with rheumatoid arthritis
B. Rheumatic heart disease
C. Thyrotoxic heart disease
D. Congenital heart disease
E. Cor pulmonale in relation to tuberculous pericarditis

15–2. What is the MOST likely lesion within the heart as depicted?
A. Aortic valvular disease
B. Tricuspid valvular disease
C. Pulmonic valvular disease
D. Mitral valvular disease
E. None of the above

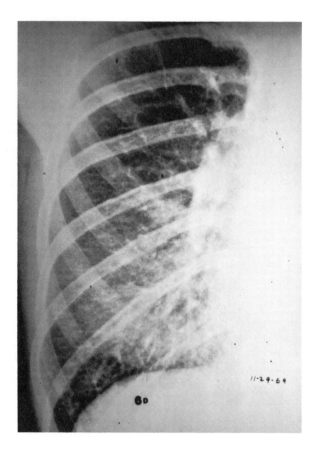

Figure E–46. Rheumatoid lung showing Kerley "B" lines at right lung base.

Radiographic Findings. In Figure E–45A and B, the heart is diffusely enlarged with a tendency to increased convexity in the pulmonary sector. There is enlargement of the heart to the right as well. There is an impression upon the barium-filled esophagus from its left aspect toward the right, with posterior displacement.

The right half of the heart has a double-contoured appearance.

Pulmonary vasculature is within normal limits.

(The costophrenic sinuses revealed very faint interstitial horizontal lines extending into the costophrenic sinuses bilaterally (Fig. E–46).)

Discussion. The patient in Figure E–45A and B had **mitral valvular disease due to rheumatic heart disease.** The convexity of the left cardiac margin indicates that stenosis is predominant. In most cases there is both mitral stenosis and mitral insufficiency, with one or another of the elements of this physiology predominating. The left ventricle is also greatly enlarged when mitral insufficiency is significantly associated.

There is an enlarged left atrium. The presence or absence of insufficiency cannot be judged by the size of the left atrium alone.

The lines in the costophrenic sinus (Fig. E–46), which are very often associated with mitral stenosis, are "Kerley B lines"—thought by Dr. Kerley to be rather specific for mitral stenosis. We have since learned that these lines merely represent accentuations of the interstitium, and they have been called "septate" or "interstitial" lines because of this.

In about one half of the patients there is coexistent involvement of the aortic valve, which might give rise to an aortic insufficiency or stenosis or both, and allow a rather complex cardiac contour on the basis of this additional valvular involvement (Fig. E–47). In some patients there is even tricuspid valvular

CARDIAC PATHOLOGY: VALVULAR DISORDERS
(Rheumatic, syphilitic,arterio-
sclerotic) (aortic valve insufficiency and
stenosis)

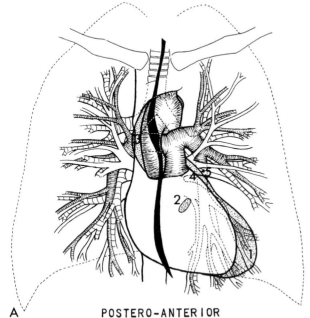

1. Enlargement left ventricle
   Apex directed to left,
   Apex rounded,
   Pulsations markedly increased.
2. Aortic valve and/or ring may be
   calcified.
3. Aorta is diffusely enlarged with
   increased amplitude of pulsations,
   especially in syphilis; slight
   enlargement with rheumatic aortic
   heart disease.
4. Cardiac waist deeper.
5. "Mitralization" occurs secondarily
   with damming back of blood and
   approaching failure.

A   POSTERO-ANTERIOR

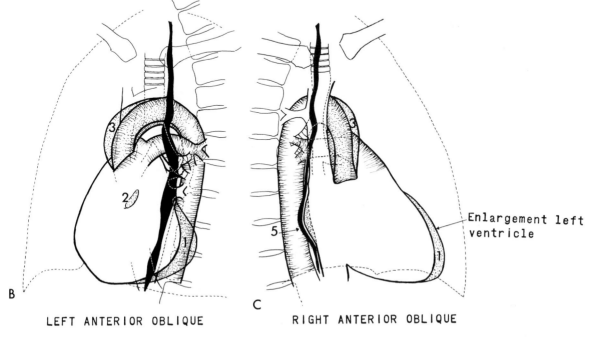

Enlargement left
ventricle

B

LEFT ANTERIOR OBLIQUE   C   RIGHT ANTERIOR OBLIQUE

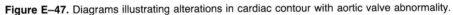

Figure E–47. Diagrams illustrating alterations in cardiac contour with aortic valve abnormality.

involvement, which produces enlargement of the right heart as well as the left and does not fully resemble the above described findings.

In tuberculous pericarditis, a tentlike appearance of the heart is produced so that it loses its curvatures on both the left and right aspects, and usually an adhesive pericarditis results. Under these circumstances, the heart sounds become distant, and very often there is a **Pick's triad** with *partial obstruction of the superior vena cava, elevation of the right hemidiaphragm* due to enlargement of the liver, and *ascites,* none of which are present in this patient.

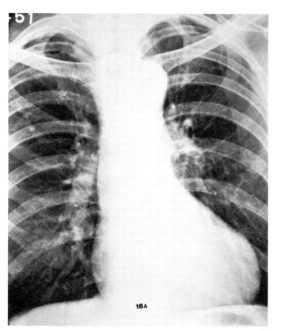 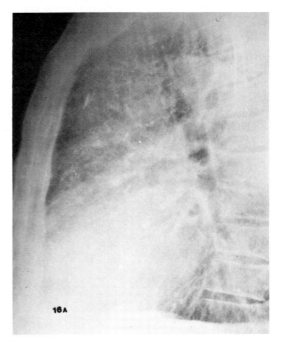

Figure E–48.

CLINICAL HISTORY (Fig. E–48 *A* and *B*)

This patient is a 62-year-old male who is asymptomatic, but who, on routine physical examination, was found to have a blood pressure of 170/105.

You are shown two chest radiographs, a posteroanterior (Fig. E–48*A*) and a lateral view (Fig. E–48*B*).

Questions

16–1. What is the MOST important radiographic finding in this patient?
A. Elongation and tortuosity of the aorta
B. Enlargement of the left ventricle
C. Calcium sclerosis of the aorta
D. Passive hyperemia of the lungs
E. Active hyperemia of the lungs

16–2. The MOST likely diagnosis in this patient is
A. Hypertensive heart disease
B. Arteriosclerotic heart disease
C. Aortic valvular disease
D. Mitral valvular insufficiency
E. Left ventricular aneurysm

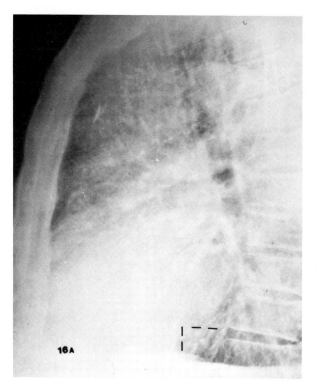

Figure E–49. Lateral view of the chest demonstrating the measurements utilized for left ventricular enlargement.

Radiologic Findings. The most important radiologic finding is **enlargement of the left ventricle.** This is indicated by identifying the inferior vena cava on the lateral projection as it penetrates the right hemidiaphragm, measuring 2 cm. cephalad, and horizontally to the outer margin of the left ventricle as depicted in the lateral view (Fig. E–49). This is also indicated in Figure E–50A, by the enlarged, boot-shaped configuration of the heart.

In the lateral view, the measurement should not exceed 18 mm.

In the posteroanterior view, apart from being "boot-shaped," the shadow of the left ventricular apex should not extend beyond the midpoint of the left hemidiaphragm (assuming a perfectly positioned film, and that the patient does not have a pectus excavatum).

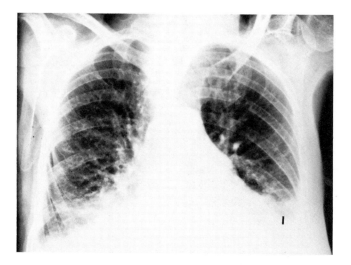

Figure E–50. PA film of the chest demonstrating redistribution of flow (cephalization). The other indicators of cardiac failure here are pleural effusion (especially left), interstitial pulmonary edema, and cardiac enlargement.

Discussion. This patient also has elongation and tortuosity of the aorta due to arteriosclerosis. These findings, however, would not be as important with respect to this patient's longevity as the finding of an **enlarged left ventricle.** There is no indication of passive or active hyperemia of the lungs. With passive hyperemia of the lungs there is a redistribution of flow in the lungs, often called "cephalization of flow," due to dilatation of the veins in the upper lobes *when the patient is in the erect position,* and a constriction of lower lobe veins. These occur in the first stage of cardiac failure (Fig. E–50). In a later stage of passive hyperemia of the lungs, there is not only diffuse dilatation of venous pattern with redistribution of flow but also an accentuation of the interstitial and alveolar pattern of the lungs, suggesting distention of these structures by fluid. Ultimately a pleural effusion may result.

The etiology of this patient's heart disease is **hypertensive heart disease** with marked enlargement of the left ventricle due to dilatation and hypertrophy. There is no indication of a left ventricular aneurysm either on frontal or lateral perspectives. There could be an associated arteriosclerotic heart disease in which the coronary arteries are involved, but if this were the paramount disorder, very likely the heart would not be quite as enlarged. Among the various disease entities that produce cardiac failure, arteriosclerotic heart disease, when paramount, does not allow as much dilatation and hypertrophy because of a relative lack of blood supply.

If this patient had aortic stenosis, he might also have a markedly enlarged left ventricle (Fig. E–51A and B), but often in these cases fluoroscopy will identify calcification of the aortic valve, and there will be a poststenotic dilatation of the ascending aorta, as is shown in Figure E–51A. One may not be able to see the calcification in the aortic valve on routine radiography, but image amplification will very accurately show the presence of such calcification, since these "dancing" aortic valve leaflets can be readily identified under image intensifier fluoroscopic

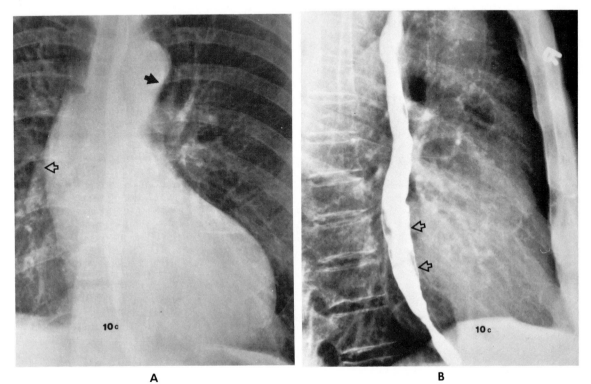

A   B

Figure E–51. Aortic valvular stenosis, poststenotic dilation, and left ventricular enlargement.
Illustration continued on following page

vision. Likewise, the pulsation of the aortic valve ring itself, if calcified, is synchronous with cardiac pulsations and thus can be readily seen.

In the barium-filled esophagus of the patient with calcific aortic stenosis, there is often a slight diffuse displacement of the esophagus posteriorly but *not selectively* in the region of the left atrium. This is not unusual when there is diffuse enlargement of the left heart, since the esophagus itself is displaced posteriorly by the markedly enlarged heart. With calcific aortic stenosis, there is poststenotic dilatation of the ascending aorta but the remainder of the aorta is not involved, even though there is calcium sclerosis in the aortic knob itself (black arrow, Fig. E–51*B*).

Figure E–51*C* shows the different locations for calcification as seen radiographically in the valves of the heart.

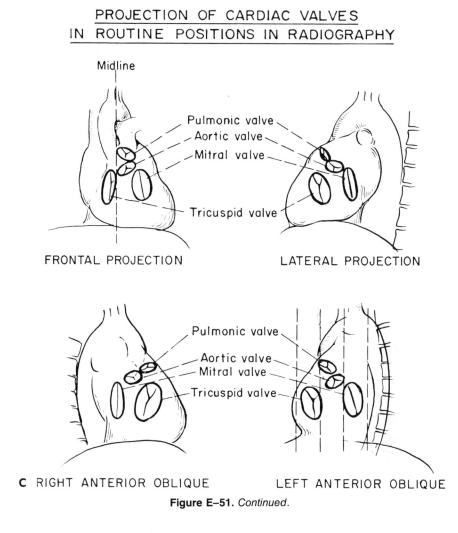

PROJECTION OF CARDIAC VALVES
IN ROUTINE POSITIONS IN RADIOGRAPHY

Midline

Pulmonic valve
Aortic valve
Mitral valve

Tricuspid valve

FRONTAL PROJECTION   LATERAL PROJECTION

Pulmonic valve

Aortic valve
Mitral valve
Tricuspid valve

C   RIGHT ANTERIOR OBLIQUE   LEFT ANTERIOR OBLIQUE

Figure E–51. *Continued.*

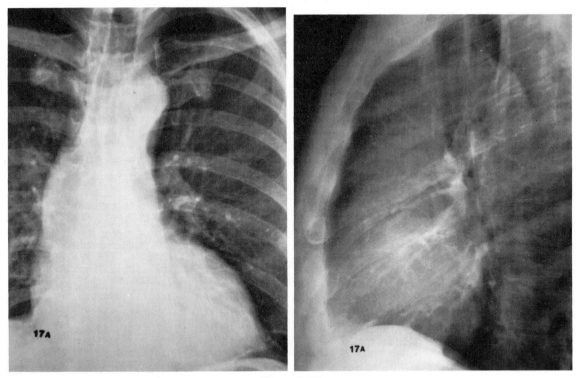

Figure E–52.

CLINICAL HISTORY (Fig. E–52 *A* and *B*)

This 60-year-old male was experiencing increasing pain in his left chest radiating down his left arm, especially after exertion of any type. At times his pain would occur quite spontaneously after a heavy meal. He had mild exertional dyspnea.

You are shown two films, posteroanterior and lateral radiographs of the heart (Fig. E–52*A* and *B*).

Questions

17–1. The MOST important radiologic finding is
A. The elongation and tortuosity of the aorta.
B. A double-contoured appearance of the aortic knob.
C. Increased convexity and moderate enlargement of the left ventricle.
D. Enlargement of the right ventricle.
E. Poststenotic dilatation of the aorta.

17–2. The MOST likely cardiac diagnosis in this case is
A. Hypertensive heart disease.
B. Arteriosclerotic heart disease.
C. A dissecting aneurysm of the aorta.
D. Cor pulmonale.
E. Aortic insufficiency.

Radiologic Findings. There is a **rounding and convexity of the left ventricle,** which is only slightly enlarged, as indicated by the method of measurement illustrated in Fig. E–49.

There is possibly an enlargement of the right ventricle, as indicated by the slight cephalad encroachment upon the anterior mediastinal clear space and moderate elongation and tortuosity of the aorta. There is no indication of passive hyperemia of the lungs. The shadow of the manubrium can be identified at the level of the aortic knob and accounts for a slightly double-contoured appearance of the aortic knob, which, however, is not further exemplified by other findings in relation to the aorta.

There is no evidence of passive hyperemia of the lungs.

Discussion. The most important radiologic finding in this patient with angina-like pains is that his heart has an **increased convexity and slight enlargement suggesting moderate cardiac hypertrophy and dilatation of the left ventricle,** such as one might see with **arteriosclerotic heart disease.** Ordinarily with coronary atherosclerosis there is a deficiency of nutrition to the heart, so that it does not undergo the marked concentric hypertrophy and dilatation of other disease entities that give rise to heart failure, such as hypertensive heart disease. Although this patient's right ventricle is moderately enlarged, this, too, may occur with arteriosclerotic heart disease and does not suggest the presence of a cor pulmonale, wherein one would expect increased pulmonary resistance and chronic obstructive pulmonary disease. There is no indication of this on these films.

With aortic insufficiency one would expect a much more marked boot-shaped contour to the left ventricle, greater enlargement, and probably more indication of dilatation of the ascending aorta.

The appearance of the manubrium at the level of the aortic knob must not be confused with double-contouring, such as occurs with dissection of the aorta, and there is no indication of pleural capping over the left lung apex to suggest the escape of blood into the left pleural space by such a dissection.

These findings are typical of **arteriosclerotic heart disease** in a patient with evidence of *concentric hypertrophy of the left ventricle* with a moderate degree of enlargement.

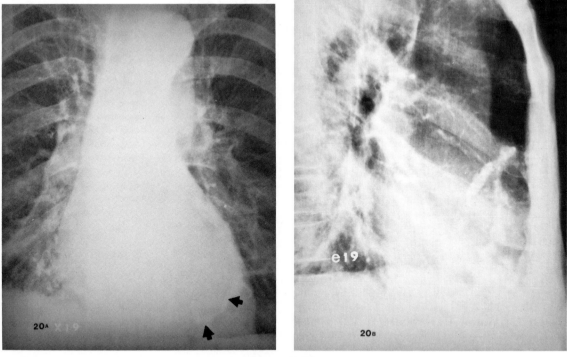

Figure E–53.

CLINICAL HISTORY

You are shown PA and lateral radiographs of the cardiopericardial silhouette (Fig. E–53A and B). This patient was asymptomatic at the time these films were obtained. His heart sounds were distant.

Questions

18–1. The MOST likely diagnosis is
A. Calcification in a myocardial aneurysm
B. Calcification of the endocardium
C. Calcification of the mediastinal pleura
D. Calcification of the pericardium
E. Calcification of the myocardium without an aneurysm being present

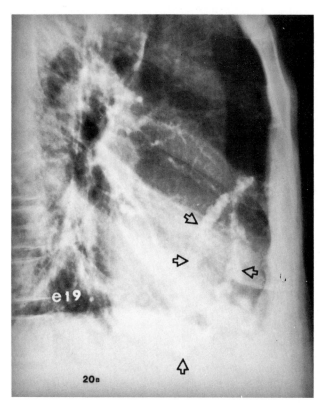

Figure E–54. The arrows point to calcification of the pericardium in lateral perspective.

Figure E–55. The arrows point to calcification of the left ventricle in lateral view.

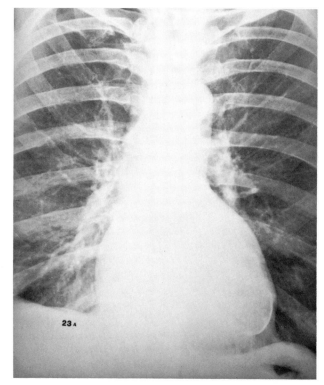

Radiologic Findings. In Figure E–53A and B, an area of calcification is identified that is ovoid in configuration in the lateral view (Fig. E–54); its superior aspect extends to the superior cephalad margin of the cardiopericardial silhouette and the inferior margin of this ellipsoid calcific shadow extends down below the visualized portion of the diaphragm for a distance of approximately 2 cm.

The calcification, as projected in the posteroanterior projection, is indicated by the arrows in Figure E–53A and may be confused with calcification of the myocardium (Fig. E–55). With myocardial calcification, the ring of calcification lies well cephalad to the left hemidiaphragm, whereas with pericardial calcification, it would appear to rest upon the diaphragm.

Discussion. The patient in Figure E–53 demonstrates **calcification in the pericardium.** The symptoms sometimes associated with calcification of the pericardium are the so-called "Pick's triad," which consists of 1) *a small quiet heart with distant heart sounds,* 2) *increased superior vena caval pressure and edema of the upper extremities* with elevation of the diaphragm, and 3) *marked ascites.* The symptoms related to a calcified pericardium will depend upon whether or not the contiguous structures are impressed upon or constricted sufficiently to affect blood flow. If the superior vena cava is impressed upon and constricted, there will be edema of the upper half of the body; if the calcification extends down to involve the inferior vena cava, there will be ascites with an elevation of the hemidiaphragm. Removal of these calcific plaques is imperative to restore normal function and normal venous pressure relationships.

Many areas of calcification can occur in and about the heart, as indicated in Figure E–56A, B, and C, in which calcification is demonstrated to occur in the sinus of Valsalva whether or not there is an aneurysm present; in the aortic or mitral valves and/or ring; in the coronary arteries (especially the anterior descending branch of the left coronary artery), readily recognized by image amplification fluoroscopy; in a patent ductus arteriosus; in a myocardial infarct; in a left ventricular aneurysm; and in the left atrium, especially if the calcium deposit is within an atrial thrombus.

In general, areas of calcification in and around the heart are best recognized by image amplification, where the fluoroscopic image intensifies the differential absorption of radiation by the calcification as against the adjoining epicardial or pericardial fat and myocardium. The movement of pulsatile valves and/or ring as well as calcifications contained within pulsating structures elsewhere in the heart are readily identified as pulsating areas. A single radiograph may not depict these, since the time of the radiographic exposure may be too long to obtain more than a "blurred" appearance of the area, which would blend with the surrounding tissues, and hence, not be visualized clearly on the radiograph. It is imperative that for most accurate detection of calcification of the heart and its adjoining structures, *image amplification fluoroscopy coupled with computed tomography* compose the most effective and accurate imaging modalities available for this purpose.

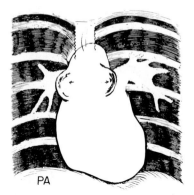

CALCIFIED SINUS OF VALSALVA
ANEURYSM

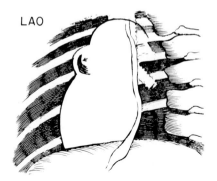

LAO

CALCIFIED SINUS OF VALSALVA

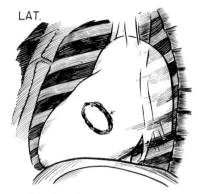

LAT.

CALCIFIED MITRAL RING

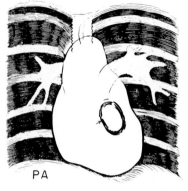

PA

CALCIFIED MITRAL RING

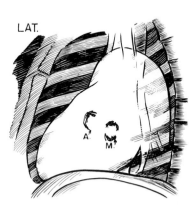

LAT.

CALCIFIED MITRAL VALVE

A   CALCIFIED AORTIC VALVE

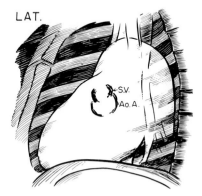

LAT.

CALCIFIED SINUS OF VALSALVA
CALCIFIED AORTIC ANNULUS

Figure E–56. *A* to *C*, Cardiopericardial structures that may contain calcium as depicted radiographically.

Illustration continued on opposite page

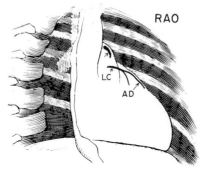
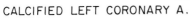

RAO

LC

AD

CALCIFIED LEFT CORONARY A.

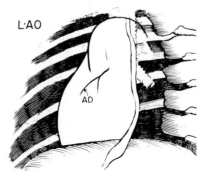

L·AO

AD

CALCIFIED LEFT CORONARY A.

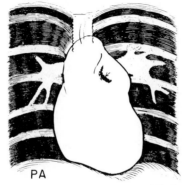

PA

CALCIFIED PATENT DUCTUS

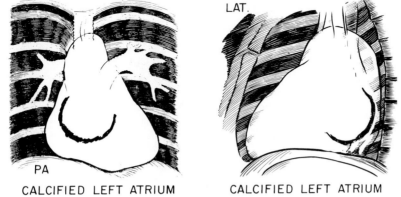

PA

B CALCIFIED LEFT ATRIUM

LAT.

CALCIFIED LEFT ATRIUM

Figure E–56 *Continued*

Illustration continued on following page

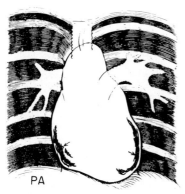

PA
CALCIFIED PERICARDIUM

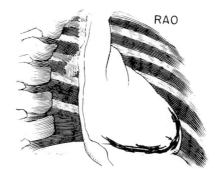

RAO

CALCIFIED PERICARDIUM
WITH CONSTRICTIVE PERICARDITIS

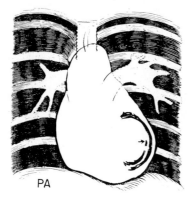

PA
CALCIFIED
MYOCARDIAL INFARCT

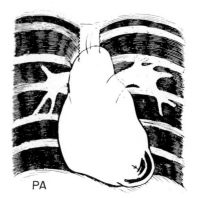

PA
CALCIFIED
LEFT VENTRICULAR ANEURYSM

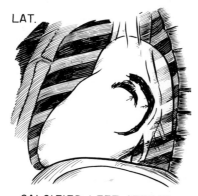

LAT.

CALCIFIED LEFT ATRIUM
WITH CALCIFIED THROMBUS

C

Figure E–56 *Continued*.

4

Abdomen

The most frequently obtained single view of the abdomen is an anteroposterior view with the patient supine. When acute abdominal disease is suspected clinically, an erect film of the abdomen and posteroanterior view of the chest are also obtained. If the patient cannot stand for a posteroanterior view of the chest, then horizontal beam studies of the abdomen are obtained with the patient either supine or on one side—preferably his left. If there is free air in the abdomen, it will rise to the uppermost portion of the abdomen, permitting the visualization of the free air in the peritoneal space to the extent that even 1 or 2 ml of free air may be identified if the films are appropriately obtained. The posteroanterior view of the chest is necessary because acute abdominal pain often is the referred type, related to an abnormality in the chest rather than the abdomen (Fig. 4–1).

Historically, the supine anteroposterior view of the abdomen has been called the KUB film, probably because the study was originally designed to emphasize the kidney, ureter, and urinary bladder for visualization of urinary calculi.

The routine for study of a supine KUB film is indicated in Figure (Fig. 4–2 A and B). After defining the kidney by the contrast of the fatty envelope around the kidney (Gerota's fascia) and attempting to delineate the position of the ureters on either side as they are normally distributed over the psoas musculature, the urinary bladder is delineated by virtue of the perivesical fat surrounding it. Thereafter the soft tissue structures of the flank are carefully evaluated. It will be noted that the flank shadows contain several layers of fat. A particularly important layer is the one immediately juxtaposed to the peritoneum. This is the so-called "properitoneal fat layer." Further defining this fatty layer and extending the eye cephalad, an angle delineating the lower margin of the posterior liver is seen. This is the "hepatic angle." The liver substance is very homogeneous, and the liver is probably the densest soft tissue structure contained within the abdomen. As the eye extends across the liver to the left side, a somewhat similar angular structure is identified beneath the spleen and spoken of as the "splenic angle." Ordinarily the flank shadows are concave medially, but in obese people various creases and folds are obtained or minimal convexity. Absolute symmetry is necessary. In most people there is a space between the flank shadow and the gas in the ascending colon on the right side and descending colon on the left. These are spoken of as the "right-sided and left-sided gutters."

After delineation of these structures, the retroperitoneal structures, which thus far have not been visualized, are studied, particularly the fatty envelope of the psoas muscles, which should be symmetrical; the quadratus lumborum muscles, which are likewise symmetrical; and the fatty envelope of the obturator internus muscle on the inner aspect of the pelvic inlet.

Emphasis is then placed on the bony structures contained on the films of the abdomen. These comprise the ribs superiorly, the lumbar spine, and the pelvis, with the hips ordinarily included. The basic roentgen signs are sought in all these structures.

Attention is directed thereafter to the gas pattern of the abdomen. Normally gas is contained within the stomach and the large intestine, except in the very young and very old. Except in these two extreme age groups, gas contained within the small intestine is usually an indication of some abnormality, either of a reflex or mechanical obstructive

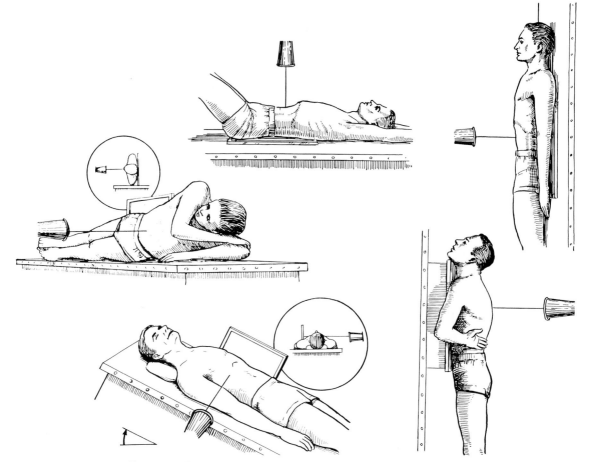

Figure 4–1. Routine projections obtained in acute abdominal disease.

origin. Minimal gas in the small intestine may at times be normal. The identification of these gas shadows is extremely important (Fig. 4–3). The stomach, large intestine, ileum, and jejunum can be recognized readily with practice. If gas shadows are inordinately dilated, mechanical obstruction should be suspected. If gas shadows are displaced, a soft tissue mass may be suspected. A mass causing such displacement may be either inflammatory or neoplastic. The presence of fluid levels in distended loops of small intestine, with the patient in the erect position, suggests mechanical obstruction. Fluid levels within the stomach or colon are ordinarily of no pathologic significance, since fluid in these areas may be readily introduced just prior to the examination either by the oral administration of fluid or by enemas, which are so frequently given prior to the examination of the patient with acute abdominal disease.

Space does not permit an elucidation of all the various gas patterns that take on pathologic significance. Suffice it to say, however, that extraluminal gas occurs not only beneath the diaphragm but also within the retroperitoneal structures; within various fossae in the retroperitoneal space, such as the gutters and adjoining the ascending and descending colon; in the lesser omental bursa; in a subhepatic site; in the paraduodenal fossae; in the pericecal or periappendiceal areas; and in the pelvis minor proper (Fig. 4–4).

The shadow of the aorta often can be identified because of the calcification contained therein. Even its branches may be calcified at times, supporting a diagnosis of abdominal angina, if clinical symptoms are correlated.

After this routine, the abdominal area is carefully surveyed for major areas of calcification or opacification. The most significant

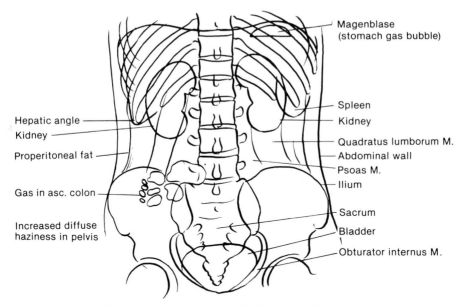

Magenblase (stomach gas bubble)

Hepatic angle
Kidney
Properitoneal fat

Gas in asc. colon

Increased diffuse
haziness in pelvis

Spleen
Kidney
Quadratus lumborum M.
Abdominal wall
Psoas M.
Ilium

Sacrum
Bladder
Obturator internus M.

1. Kidney; 2. Ureter for calculi; 3. Bladder; 4. Flanks;
5. Liver, diaphragm and spleen; 6. Retroperitoneal Shadow;
7. Bony structures; 8. Gas shadows; 9. Mass shadows;
10. Calcific shadows.

A

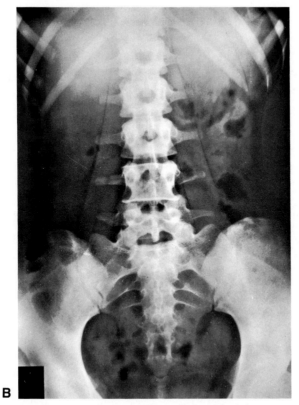

B

Figure 4–2. *A,* Routine for examination of the recumbent film of the abdomen. *B,* Anteroposterior projection of the abdomen (KUB film).

of these consist of calcified arteries, calculi in the urinary tract, biliary calculi, prostatic calculi, calcifications within the pancreas (which are practically always indicative of pancreatitis, with or without carcinoma), and calcifications within the appendix, where calcified fecaliths are practically always indicative of obstructive appendicitis (Fig. 4–5).

Calcification within the gallbladder occurs in only about 15% of gallstones, since about 85% of gallstones are radiolucent, and the introduction of contrast media within the gallbladder is necessary for their demonstration by conventional radiography. Stone defects in the gallbladder are also readily demonstrable by ultrasonography. On the other hand, 85 or 90% of calculi of the urinary tract are opaque, and only 10% are radiolucent.

Unfortunately in the examination of the infant abdomen, the properitoneal and fatty planes are not identifiable until the age of 5 in most instances, and sometimes not until the age of 10 years. Moreover, at times the infant's abdomen is best examined in the prone rather than the supine position for optimal delineation of gas shadows.

Additional views of the abdomen are obtained as follows:

1. *Inspiration and expiration films* for testing the mobility of the kidney. The kidney, if it is not surrounded by inflammatory tissue, moves approximately 5 cm. in the change from inspiration to expiration, or in the change from the erect to the supine view. Fixation of the kidney occurs if it is surrounded by a neoplastic or inflammatory process.

2. *Decubitus views* of the abdomen are obtained with the patient lying on one side or the other if he is too ill to stand for an erect film (Fig. 4–1). They are particularly useful in the assessment of flank shadows and to determine the presence of free air, which represents a ruptured hollow viscus. These films may also be used for detecting fluid levels and mechanical obstruction.

3. *Oblique views* of the abdomen are obtained especially in examination of the urinary tract where full delineation of the ureters and isometric depiction of the kidney collecting system is desirable. Likewise oblique studies of the urinary bladder are helpful in delineating abnormalities contained therein.

4. An *inverted view* of the abdomen has been utilized for demonstration of such structures as an imperforate anus in the newborn or neonate. These, however, are not necessary if one employs water-soluble contrast agents for visualization of fistulas when fistulas to the region of the perineum exist.

SCHEMATIC ILLUSTRATION OF DISTENDED BOWEL

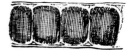

JEJUNUM
(NO INDENTED SEROSA;
COILED SPRING APPEARANCE)

ILEUM
(NO INDENTED SEROSA)

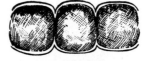

COLON
(NOTE INDENTED SEROSA BY
HAUSTRAE)

Figure 4–3. Schematic illustration of distended bowel, showing differences among jejunum, ileum, and colon.

POTENTIAL SPACES

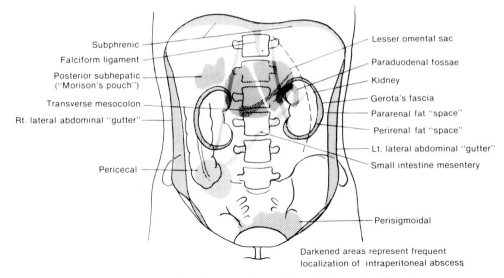

Subphrenic
Falciform ligament
Posterior subhepatic ("Morison's pouch")
Transverse mesocolon
Rt. lateral abdominal "gutter"
Pericecal

Lesser omental sac
Paraduodenal fossae
Kidney
Gerota's fascia
Pararenal fat "space"
Perirenal fat "space"
Lt. lateral abdominal "gutter"
Small intestine mesentery

Perisigmoidal

Darkened areas represent frequent
localization of intraperitoneal abscess

Figure 4–4. The usual localization of intra-abdominal free air and/or abscesses.

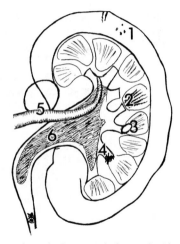

1. Calcification in renal cortex
    a. Granuloma infection
    b. Infarction
    c. Xanthogranuloma
    d. Neoplasm
        Calcification may be punctate, powdery, amorphous, mulberry, or circumlinear
2. Calcification in renal pyramids
    a. Medullary sponge kidney
    b. Nephrocalcinosis
    c. Renal tubular acidosis
3. Renal papillary necrosis
4. Calcification in calyces, pelvis, or ureter common in hypercalcemic states
    a. Hyperparathyroidism
    b. Sarcoidosis
    c. Cushing's disease
5. Renal artery calcification (aneurysm)
6. Staghorn calculus—not common with hypercalcemic states
7. Calcification in tuberculosis often occurs throughout kidney or ureter

Figure 4–5A. Line diagram showing how determination of the location of a calculus may help to elucidate the basic disease process.

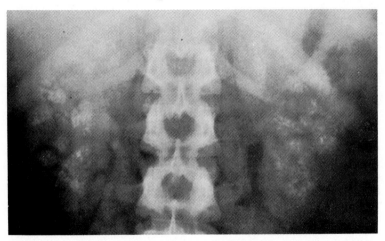

Figure 4–5B. Medullary sponge kidney and calcifications in collecting tubules.

117

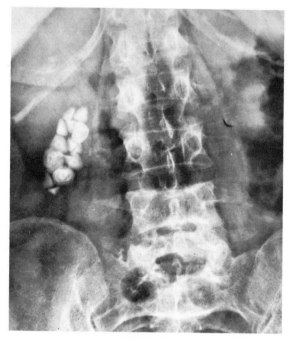

Figure E–57.

CLINICAL HISTORY

Case 19–1: 45-year-old woman with right upper quadrant pain (Fig. E–57)

Case 19–2: 52-year-old-alcoholic man with epigastric pain (Fig. E–58)

Case 19–3: 30-year-old woman with flank pain and pyuria (Fig. E–59)

Case 19–4: 65-year-old woman with intermittent claudication (Fig. E–60)

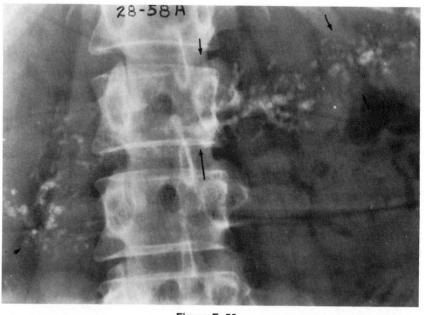

Figure E–58.

Questions

19–1. The MOST likely diagnoses in Cases 19–1 and 19–2, respectively, are:

A. Calcified gallstones—chronic pancreatitis.
B. Calcified gallstones—acute pancreatitis.
C. Kidney stones—chronic pancreatitis.
D. Kidney stones—acute pancreatitis.
E. Calcified gallstones—kidney stones.

19–2. Which of the following statements are true?

A. About 15–20% of gallstones are radiographically calcified.
B. Most gallstones are composed of pure cholesterol.
C. Alcoholism is the most common cause of pancreatic calcification.

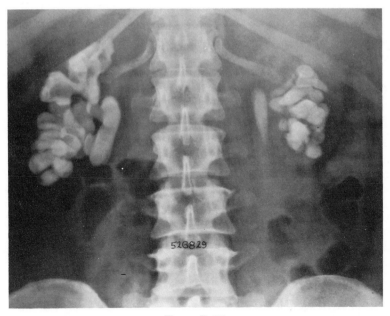

Figure E–59.

D. Cholelithiasis is a cause of acute pancreatitis.
E. Cholelithiasis frequently causes pancreatic calcification.

19–3. The MOST likely diagnoses in Cases 19–3 and 19–4, respectively, are:
A. Abdominal aortic aneurysm—pancreatic calcification.
B. Staghorn calculi—abdominal aortic aneurysm.
C. Staghorn calculi—pancreatic calcification.
D. Abdominal aortic aneurysm—staghorn calculi.
E. Pancreatic calcification—abdominal aortic aneurysm.

19–4. Which of the following statements are true?
A. About 85% of all renal calculi are radiographically calcified.
B. Staghorn calculi are uncommonly related to urinary tract infection.
C. A lateral abdominal film is a poor view for identifying an aortic aneurysm.
D. Plain films accurately detect abdominal aortic aneurysms.
E. Abdominal ultrasound is more accurate than plain films for diagnosing aortic aneurysm.

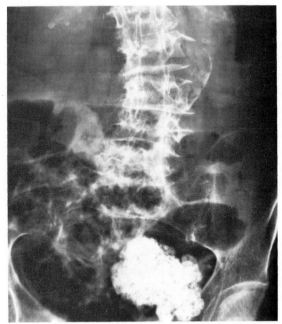

Figure E–60A.

Radiologic Findings. Case 19–1 demonstrates multiple laminated calcifications in the right upper quadrant, projecting in part over the lower pole of the right kidney,. The faceted appearance of these densities is characteristic of gallstones. Case 19–2 shows multiple calcifications in the expected location of the pancreas. In an alcoholic patient, pancreatic lithiasis from chronic pancreatitis would be the most likely diagnosis **(A is the correct answer to Question 19–1).**

Case 19–3 demonstrates antler-shaped densities outlining both renal collecting systems, consistent with staghorn calculi. In Case 19–4, curvilinear calcification is seen just to the left margin of the midlumbar spine. This appearance suggests the presence of an aortic aneurysm, which was confirmed by abdominal ultrasound **(B is correct for Question 19–3).** Incidentally, the large mottled density in the left pelvis of Case 19–4 is a calcified uterine fibroid.

Discussion. Up to 20% of gallstones are sufficiently calcified to be radiographically visible **(Question 19–2 A is true).** Gallstones are composed of many substances including cholesterol, bile salts, and biliary pigments. However, pure cholesterol and pure pigment stones are uncommon **(Question 19–2 B is false).** Most gallstones contain a mixture of components, including calcium salts which make them radiographically opaque.

In the United States, 85–90% of patients with pancreatic lithiasis are alcoholics **(Question 19–2 C is true).** Conversely, less than half of patients with chronic alcoholic pancreatitis will develop radiographically visible pancreatic calcification. Although gallstones passing through the biliary tract can cause acute pancreatitis **(Question 19–2 D is true),** chronic calcific pancreatitis is rarely due to cholelithiasis **(Question 19–2 E is false).**

Most renal calculi are radiographically opaque because calcium salts are common components of kidney stones **(Question 19–4 A is true).** Renal calculi are usually small in size and lie within the pelvocalyceal system. They may be multiple in number and bilateral in location. When calcifications are seen projecting over the renal shadows on routine films of the abdomen, oblique views are frequently needed to localize the densities to the kidneys. A staghorn calculus partially or completely fills the renal collecting system, thereby resembling the "antlers of a deer." Most are composed predominantly of magnesium ammonium phosphate ("struvite") and form in an infected urine rendered alkaline by urea-splitting organisms **(Question 19–4 B is false).**

Calcification in an aortic aneurysm may be difficult to appreciate on the supine abdominal film because of obscuration from the overlying bony structures of the lumbar spine. A lateral abdominal film may be necessary and will often show calcification in the anterior and posterior walls of the aneurysm **(Question 19–4 C is false).** Unfortunately, not all aortic aneurysms are sufficiently calcified to be demonstrated on plain abdominal films **(Question 19–4 D is false).** In recent years, ultrasound has emerged as an alternate means to image abdominal aortic aneurysms, and has been shown to be superior to plain films of the abdomen for making this diagnosis **(Question 19–4 E is true).**

Calcium shadows in the abdomen have been well summarized by McAfee and Donner (as shown); and some abdominal extra-urinary shadows are shown in Figure E–60B.

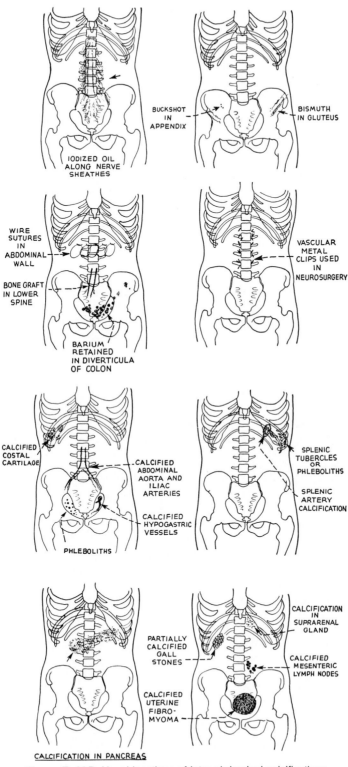

BUCKSHOT
IN
APPENDIX

BISMUTH
IN GLUTEUS

IODIZED OIL
ALONG NERVE
SHEATHES

WIRE
SUTURES
IN
ABDOMINAL
WALL

BONE GRAFT
IN LOWER
SPINE

BARIUM
RETAINED
IN DIVERTICULA
OF COLON

VASCULAR
METAL
CLIPS USED
IN
NEUROSURGERY

CALCIFIED
COSTAL
CARTILAGE

CALCIFIED
ABDOMINAL
AORTA AND
ILIAC
ARTERIES

CALCIFIED
HYPOGASTRIC
VESSELS

PHLEBOLITHS

SPLENIC
TUBERCLES
OR
PHLEBOLITHS

SPLENIC
ARTERY
CALCIFICATION

CALCIFICATION
IN
SUPRARENAL
GLAND

PARTIALLY
CALCIFIED
GALL
STONES

CALCIFIED
MESENTERIC
LYMPH NODES

CALCIFIED
UTERINE
FIBRO-
MYOMA

CALCIFICATION IN PANCREAS

Figure E–60B. Usual locations of intra-abdominal calcifications.

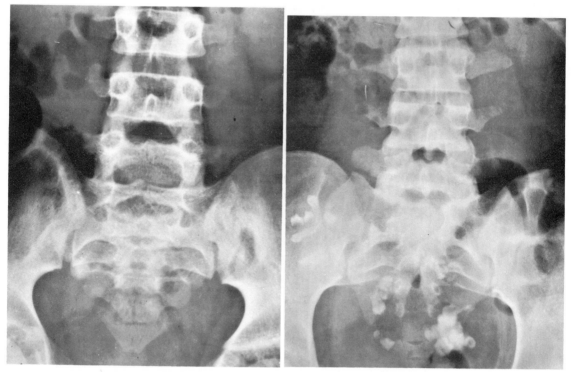

Figure E–61.

Figure E–62.

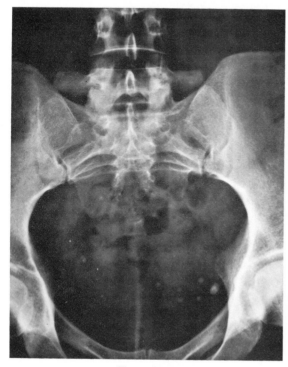

Figure E–63.

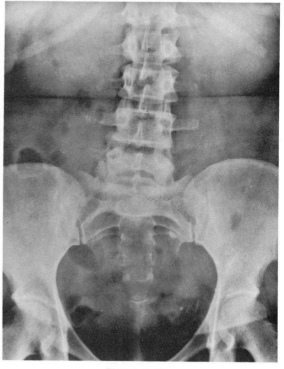

Figure E–64.

CLINICAL HISTORIES
Case 20–1: 9-year-old boy with right lower quadrant pain (Fig. E–61)
Case 20–2: 25-year-old woman with lower abdominal fullness (Fig. E–62).
Case 20–3: 40-year-old woman with epigastric pain (Fig. E–63).
Case 20–4: 35-year-old woman with hematuria (Fig. E–64).

Questions
20–1. In Case 20–1, what would be the MOST likely diagnosis?
A. Tuberculous spondylitis.
B. Sacral neoplasm.
C. Ureteral colic.
D. Pelvic phlebolith.
E. Acute appendicitis.

20–2. In Case 20–2, what would be the MOST likely diagnosis?
A. Dermoid cyst of the ovary.
B. Chondrosarcoma of the sacrum.
C. Swallowed dentures.
D. Cystadenoma of the ovary.
E. Uterine fibroids.

20–3. What is the MOST likely origin of the multiple pelvic calcifications in Case 20–3?
A. Multiple ureteral calculi.
B. Multiple phleboliths.
C. Multiple bladder calculi.
D. Bilateral ovarian dermoid cysts.
E. Multiple uterine fibroids.

20–4. In Case 20–4, what is the MOST likely diagnosis?
A. Renal tuberculosis.
B. Right ureteral calculi.
C. Left ureteral calculi.
D. Bladder calculus.
E. Appendicolith.

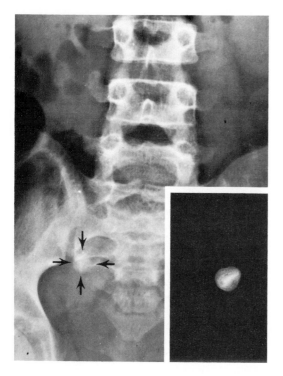

Figure E–65. An oval calcification (arrows) projects over the right sacroiliac joint. Calcified appendiceal stones are usually single and vary in size from 0.5 to 2.0 cm. The inset is a radiograph of the surgically removed appendicolith showing the typical lamination often seen.

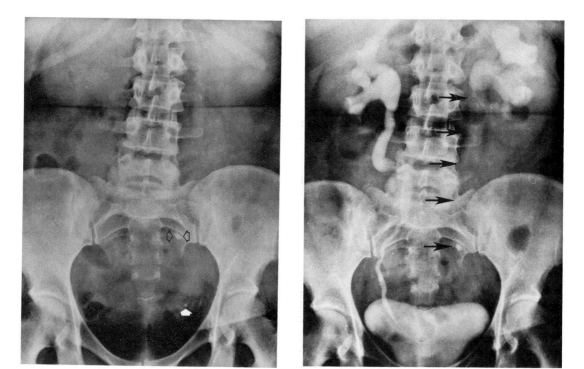

A   B

Figure E–66. *A,* Two densities are present along the expected course of the lower left ureter. The largest projects just medial to the left sacroiliac joint (open arrows), while the smaller is present in the left pelvis (closed arrow). *B,* Subsequent intravenous urogram shows urinary obstruction on the left. The dilated ureter (arrows) can be followed to the level of the larger ureteral stone.

Radiologic Findings. Case 20–1 is a boy with acute appendicitis **(E is the correct answer to Question 20–1).** An oval calcification measuring 1 cm in diameter projects over the inferior margin of the right sacroiliac joint (Fig. E–65). At surgery, appendicitis with perforation and an obstructing appendicolith were found.

In Case 20–2, multiple calcified densities are seen projecting over the midpelvis and right ilium. Many of these densities have the appearance of teeth, and in a young woman dermoid cyst of the ovary is the most likely diagnosis **(A is the correct answer to Question 20–2).** Actually, dermoid cysts of both ovaries were found at surgery.

Case 20–3 demonstrates multiple pelvic calcifications, many projecting below the level of the ischial spines. They are round and oval in shape and some have radiolucent centers. In the absence of specific urinary tract symptomatology, multiple phleboliths would be the best consideration **(B is the correct answer to Question 20–3).**

In Case 20–4, two calcific densities are present projecting respectively over the left mid-sacrum and within the left pelvis (Fig. E–66 A). With a history of hematuria, the most likely choice would be left ureteral calculi **(C is the correct answer to Question 20–4).** A subsequent intravenous urogram showed marked left ureteropelvocaliectasis with ureteral dilatation identified to the level of the larger and more superiorly situated calculus (Fig. E–66 B).

Discussion. Calcified appendiceal stones are present in only about 10% of cases; however, when seen they indicate at least a 90% chance of acute appendicitis in the symptomatic patient. In children being evaluated for suspected appendicitis, the finding of an appendicolith is virtually diagnostic of the disease. Indeed, because of the higher incidence of complicated appendicitis, especially gangrene and perforation, associated with appendiceal stones, prophylactic appendectomy has been recommended in the child having an incidentally discovered appendicolith.

Phleboliths are thrombi within the pelvic veins, explaining their usual circular shape. Calcification within these thrombi starts peripherally, and, if incomplete, accounts for the typical radiolucent center seen radiographically. Phleboliths have little clinical significance except for their confusion with other pelvic densities, particularly ureteral calculi. In general, ureteral stones lie above and medial to the ischial spines, lack a radiolucent center, and often have an irregular shape. Differentiation, however, is occasionally impossible. Close clinical correlation is necessary, and intravenous urography may be needed.

Dermoid cysts are cystic teratomas of the ovary and occur most frequently between the ages of 20 and 40 years. Some form of calcification or ossification is seen radiographically in about one half of patients with dermoid cysts, while the appearance of teeth or bone is present in nearly one third of cases.

Urolithiasis is always a consideration in the patient with hematuria. Since 80–90% of urinary calculi are radiographically opaque, the plain abdominal film is important in the initial evaluation. Close scrutiny of the abdominal film is crucial because ureteral calculi may be elusive, especially when they project over the lumbar transverse processes and the sacroiliac region. As well shown in this case (Fig. E–64), two natural sites for calculus impaction in the lower ureter are at its crossing over the iliac vessels and its junction with the bladder. However, not every calcification along the expected course of the ureter will prove to be a ureteral calculus. Intravenous urography is often needed to localize a density to the ureter. At times, this can be an exasperating problem in the pelvis in trying to determine, for example, whether a specific density is a stone or a phlebolith.

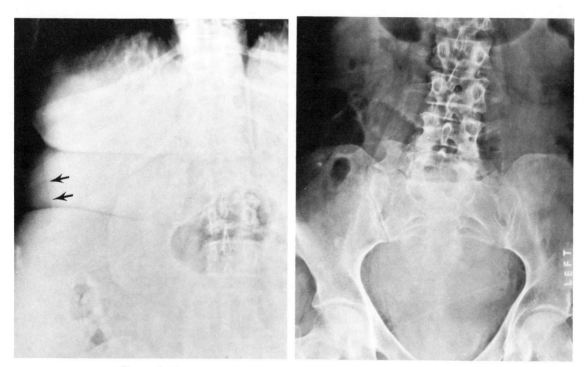

Figure E–67.

Figure E–68.

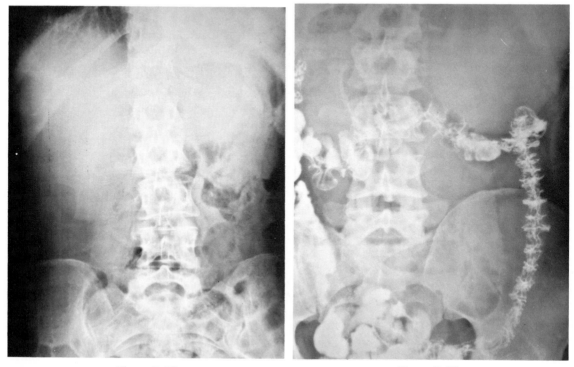

Figure E–69.

Figure E–70.

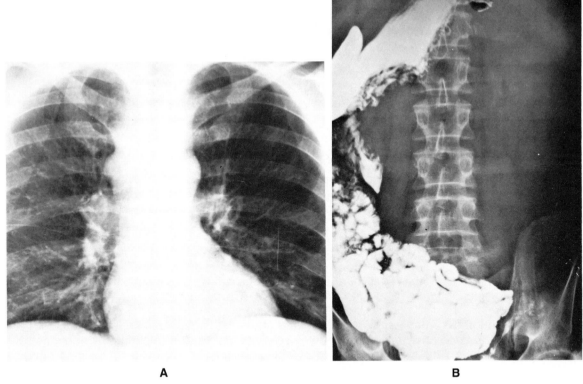

A   B

Figure E–71.

CLINICAL HISTORIES
Case 21–1: 55-year-old alcoholic woman with abdominal distention (Fig. E–67A).
Case 21–2: 45-year-old woman with lower abdominal fullness (Fig. E–68).
Case 21–3: 60-year-old woman with carcinoma of the lung (Fig. E–69).
Case 21–4: 35-year-old woman with fever and anemia. (Fig. E–70).
Case 21–5: 60-year-old man with lymphadenopathy. Frontal (Fig. E–71A and B) chest film (A) and small bowel film (B) are shown.

Questions
21–1. In Case 21–1, the medial displacement of the liver edge (arrows) is MOST likely due to
A. Excess flank fat from obesity.
B. Cirrhosis of the liver.
C. Ascites in the paracolic gutter.
D. Fatty infiltration of the liver.
E. Hemochromatosis of the liver.

21–2. In Case 21–2, what would be the MOST likely consideration?
A. Pelvic abscess.
B. Ovarian cyst.
C. Pelvic lymphoma.
D. Pelvic hematoma.
E. Ectopic pregnancy.

21–3. In Case 21–3, what would be the MOST likely consideration?
A. Hepatomegaly.
B. Splenomegaly.
C. Cirrhosis.
D. Nephromegaly.
E. Ascites.

21–4. In Case 21–4, the inferior displacement of the colon is MOST likely due to?
A. Gastric outlet obstruction.
B. Adrenal carcinoma.
C. Renal cell carcinoma.
D. Hepatomegaly.
E. Splenomegaly.

21–5. In Case 21–5, the findings in the abdomen and chest are MOST consistent with?
A. Splenomegaly and thoracic adenopathy from sarcoidosis.
B. Retroperitoneal sarcoma with thoracic metastases.
C. Renal cell carcinoma with thoracic metastases.
D. Splenomegaly and thoracic/retroperitoneal adenopathy from lymphoma.
E. Thoracic/retroperitoneal adenopathy from metastatic testicular carcinoma.

Radiologic Findings. In Case 21–1, the liver edge is visualized and displaced inward because of ascites in the right paracolic gutter **(C is the correct answer to Question 21–1).** In the absence of ascites, cirrhosis, fatty infiltration, and hemochromatosis of the liver would not be associated with hepatic displacement.

Case 21–2 shows increased density in the pelvis and a paucity of gas-containing structures. In a middle aged woman, an ovarian or uterine mass would be the most likely consideration. Ultrasound of the pelvis showed a large, fluid-filled mass, confirmed at surgery as an ovarian cyst **(B is the correct answer to Question 21–2).**

In Case 21–3, the right side of the abdomen shows increased density and is relatively gasless. Also, the gastroduodenal air shadows are displaced to the left (Fig. E–72A), confirmed by an upper gastrointestinal series (Fig. E–72B). These findings indicate hepatomegaly **(A is the correct answer to Question 21–3).** A radionuclide liver scan showed metastases from carcinoma of the lung.

Case 21–4 shows an oval soft tissue density in the left upper quadrant, displacing the transverse colon inferiorly on this postevacuation film following a barium enema. Adrenal and renal cell carcinoma rarely present as large masses in the upper abdomen. In gastric outlet obstruction, a distended stomach would project to the right of the midline. Therefore, the most likely diagnosis is splenomegaly **(E is the correct answer to Question 21–4).**

The findings in Case 21–5 are widening of the superior mediastinum from thoracic adenopathy and a huge abdominal mass markedly displacing the stomach and small bowel due to splenomegaly and retroperitoneal adenopathy. In a patient with peripheral lymphadenopathy, this combination of findings is most likely caused by lymphoma **(D is the correct answer to Question 21–5).**

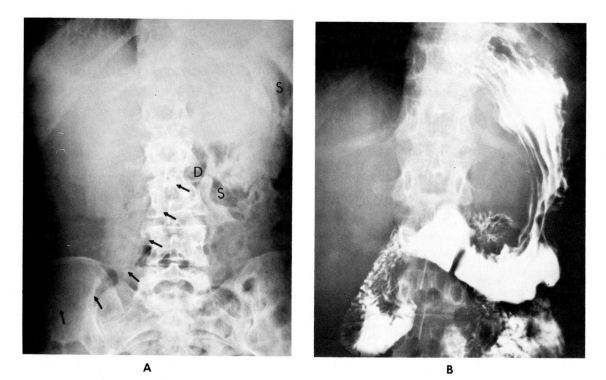

A   **B**

Figure E–72. *A,* Marked enlargement of the liver (arrows) with displacement of the duodenum (D) and stomach (S) to the left. *B,* Upper gastrointestinal series confirms the gastroduodenal displacement suspected on the plain film.

Discussion. The earliest radiographic findings in ascites include medial displacement of the liver edge (Fig. E–67), loss of definition of the hepatic angle, and inward displacement of the colon in the paracolic gutters. Later findings are abdominal haziness and central flotation of the small bowel loops (Fig. E–72C). The plain abdominal film, however, poorly detects small to moderate amounts of ascitic fluids, and abdominal ultrasound or computed tomography has been proven to be more sensitive (Fig. E–72D).

When the plain film suggests the presence of a pelvic mass, a specific diagnosis is often difficult to make. Intravenous urography and barium enema are useful in excluding a mass arising from the lower urinary tract or colon, or in showing extrinsic involvement of these structures. On the other hand, pelvic ultrasound or computed tomography best demonstrate the cross-sectional anatomy of the pelvis and show the interrelationships of the various pelvic organs.

Although abdominal plain films are helpful in detecting enlargement of the spleen, they are of little use in diagnosing hepatic disease, particularly if significant hepatomegaly is not present. Fortunately, other imaging modalities are available to evaluate for hepatic metastases, and include abdominal ultrasound and computed tomography, radionuclide liver scan, and hepatic angiography. From the standpoint of cost, however, ultrasound and the radionuclide scan are the best choices for initial screening.

In most cases, barium studies of the gastrointestinal tract are insensitive in evaluating for retroperitoneal disease. The intravenous urogram may be helpful only if renal, ureteral, or bladder displacement is evident. On the other hand, ultrasound and computed tomography of the abdomen have proven to be sensitive methods for assessing the retroperitoneum. Along with pedal lymphangiography, these methods most accurately evaluate the retroperitoneum for lymphoma.

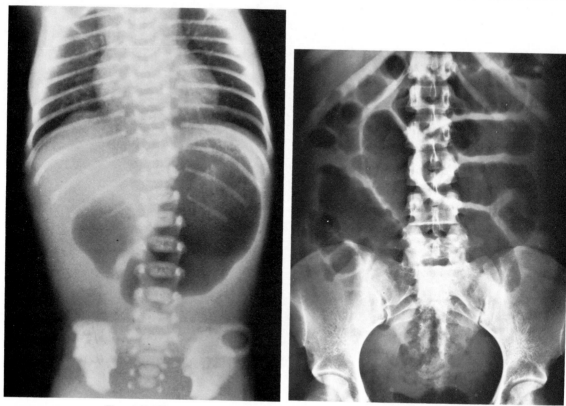

Figure E–73.

Figure E–74.

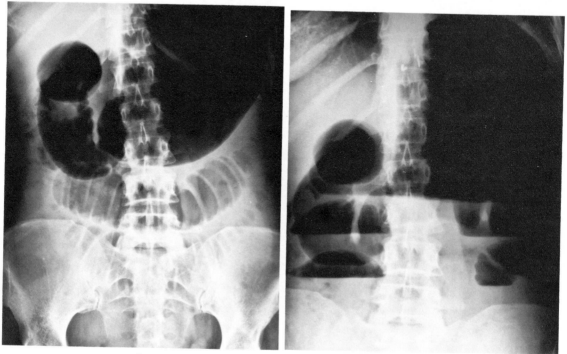

A

B

Figure E–75.

130

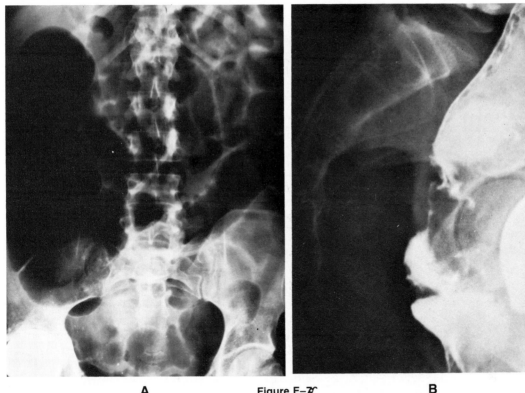

A   Figure E–7   B

CLINICAL HISTORIES

Case 22–1: An infant with abdominal disten-tion (Fig. E–73).

Case 22–2. 18-year-old girl with left lower lobe pneumonia (Fig. E–74).

Case 22–3. 35-year-old woman with previous abdominal surgery presents with distention. Supine (Fig. E–75A) and upright (Fig. E–75B) films of the abdomen.

Case 22–4. 65-year-old woman with increas-ing constipation. Supine abdominal film (Fig. E–76A) and lateral rectal view from a barium enema (Fig. E–76B).

Questions

22–1. In Case 22–1, which would be the MOST likely diagnosis?
A. Annular pancreas.
B. Duodenal atresia.
C. Hypertrophic pyloric stenosis.
D. Duodenal stenosis.
E. Jejunal stenosis.

22–2. In Case 22–2, the MOST likely diagno-sis would be?
A. Functional ileus of the bowel.
B. Mechanical small bowel obstruction.
C. Functional megacolon.
D. Right colon volvulus.
E. Sigmoid volvulus.

22–3. In Case 22–3, the MOST likely diag-nosis is?
A. Gastric outlet obstruction.
B. Functional ileus of the bowel.
C. Mechanical obstruction of the duodenum.
D. Mechanical obstruction of the jejunum.
E. Mechanical obstruction of the ileum.

22–4. Which of the following statements are true?
A. In adults, gastric outlet obstruction usually is due to neoplasm.
B. Air-fluid levels in the bowel are specific for mechanical obstruction.
C. Adhesions are the most common cause of small bowel obstruction.

D. Inguinal hernias are rarely associated with small bowel obstruction.
E. Small bowel intussusception is a common cause of obstruction.

22–5. In Case 22–5, the MOST likely conclu-sion would be?
A. Functional colon distention—normal barium enema.
B. Functional bowel distention—normal bar-ium enema.
C. Mechanical colon obstruction—sigmoid volvulus.
D. Mechanical colon obstruction—sigmoid di-verticulitis.
E. Mechanical colon obstruction—rectal car-cinoma.

22–6. Which of the following statements are true?
A. Carcinoma of the colon is a common cause of obstruction.
B. Sigmoid diverticulitis rarely causes colonic obstruction.
C. Cecal volvulus is more common than sig-moid volvulus.
D. Barium enema is useful in suspected colon obstruction.
E. Barium enema is contraindicated in toxic megacolon.

Radiologic Findings. Case 22–1 is duodenal atresia **(B is the correct answer to Question 22–1).** The film shows gaseous distention of the stomach and proximal duodenum, an appearance called the "double-bubble" sign. Duodenal stenosis and annular pancreas could give a similar appearance, except that bowel gas would be seen distally. Jejunal stenosis would also show distal bowel gas. Although gastric distention may be seen in hypertrophic pyloric stenosis, dilatation of the adjacent duodenum is not a feature.

Case 22–2 demonstrates a diffuse abnormal abdominal gas pattern with greatest distention of the centrally located small bowel loops. Although partial mechanical small bowel obstruction would be a consideration, the generalized distribution of gas is more indicative of a functional ileus **(A is the correct answer to Question 22–2).** Her abdominal distention was due to a reflex ileus secondary to left lower lobe pneumonia, and quickly disappeared following appropriate antibiotic therapy.

Case 22–3 shows marked gaseous distention of the stomach, duodenum, and proximal jejunum on the supine film, associated with multiple air-fluid levels on the upright projection. The localization of findings to the upper gastrointestinal tract suggests a mechanical obstruction. Gastric outlet or duodenal obstruction are unlikely, since the mesenteric small bowel is also dilated, making mechanical obstruction of the jejunum or ileum more likely. Since only several dilated loops of small bowel are seen, the jejunum would be the suspected site for obstruction **(D is the correct answer to Question 22–3).** At surgery, jejunal adhesions were found.

Case 22–4 demonstrates gaseous distention throughout the abdomen, with more significant dilatation of the right side of the colon. The barium enema shows an irregular, constricting lesion of the rectum, posterior to the right hip arthrodesis. This appearance is characteristic for rectal carcinoma. The near complete occlusion of the rectal lumen has led to colonic obstruction **(E is the correct answer to Question 22–5).** Distention of the small bowel has occurred secondarily to the colonic obstruction.

Discussion. Gastric outlet obstruction in adults is usually due to peptic ulcer disease **(Question 22–4 A is false).** The presence of air-fluid levels in the bowel simply indicates interference with the normal aboral progression of intestinal contents, and can be seen in either functional ileus or mechanical bowel obstruction **(Question 22–4 B is false).** The distribution of air-fluid levels is a more important observation with focal involvement favoring a mechanical obstruction. The two most common causes of small bowel obstruction are adhesions **(Question 22–4 C is true)** and external abdominal hernias, particularly inguinal hernia **(Question 22–4 D is false).** Small bowel intussusception is not a common cause of obstruction **(Question 22–4 E is false).** Ileocolic intussusception is more typical in children, while obstructing intussusception is uncommon in adults.

The two most common causes of colonic obstruction in adults are carcinoma of the colon **(Question 22–6 A is true)** and sigmoid diverticulitis **(Question 22–6 B is false).** Volvulus accounts for only about 10% of cases of colonic obstruction with the sigmoid colon being the most common site **(Question 22–6 C is false).** If plain films of the abdomen suggest colonic obstruction, the barium enema is an effective means of evaluation **(Question 22–6 D is true).** However, if peritoneal perforation is likely, such as in toxic megacolon, the barium enema is contraindicated **(Question 22–6 E is true).**

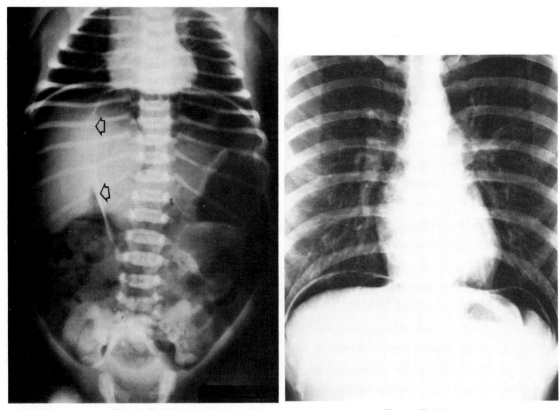

Figure E–77.   Figure E–78.

CLINICAL HISTORIES
   Case 23–1: Newborn with marked abdominal distention (Fig. E–77)
   Case 23–2: 25 year old woman with shoulder pain (Fig. E–78)

Questions
   23–1. In Case 23–1, the MOST likely diagnosis is?
   A. Necrotizing enterocolitis.
   B. Meconium ileus.
   C. Ruptured abdominal viscus.
   D. Duodenal stenosis.
   E. Duodenal atresia.

   23–2. In Case 23–2, the MOST likely diagnosis is?
   A. Tension pneumothorax.
   B. Pneumoperitoneum.
   C. Colon interposition.
   D. Bullous emphysema.
   E. Basilar pneumonitis.

Radiologic Findings. Case 23–1 shows bulging of the flanks and elevation of the hemidiaphragm associated with hyperlucency throughout the abdomen. The intestinal gas pattern, however, is unremarkable. The arrows outline the falciform ligament, which is radiographically visible only when surrounded by air. The most likely diagnosis, therefore, is ruptured abdominal viscus with resulting pneumoperitoneum **(C is the correct answer to Question 23–1).** All of the other listed possibilities would present with specific changes in the intestinal gas pattern.

Case 23–2 demonstrates crescent-shaped lucencies beneath both hemidiaphragms, outlining the liver on the right and the spleen and stomach on the left. Three days previously, the patient underwent abdominal surgery and had a postoperative pneumoperitoneum **(B is the correct answer to Question 23–2).** Lack of mediastinal shift and focal hyperlucency in the lung fields excludes tension pneumothorax and bullous emphysema, respectively. Colon interposition occurs on the right, with bowel interposed between the liver and hemidiaphragm. Haustrations are usually recognized without difficulty.

Discussion. The combination of oval distention of the abdomen with a visible falciform ligament has been labeled the "football sign" and is a reliable indicator of massive pneumoperitoneum in the newborn. Pneumoperitoneum in the neonate is often the result of spontaneous rupture of the stomach. However, colonic or small bowel perforations from many different causes are other considerations. Less commonly, pneumoperitoneum results from a complicating pneumomediastinum in infants being treated for respiratory distress.

In adults, the most common cause of pneumoperitoneum are the postoperative state, ruptured abdominal viscus, and peritoneal dialysis. Residual pneumoperitoneum may persist for 1 to 2 weeks. Serial abdominal films, however, should show a gradual reduction in the amount of free peritoneal air. Persistent or increasing postoperative pneumoperitoneum suggests a perforated viscus or ruptured surgical anastomosis. Spontaneous pneumoperitoneum is most often due to perforation of a duodenal ulcer. Less common causes include pneumomediastinum, pulmonary emphysema, pneumatosis intestinalis, and air entrance per vagina.

Pneumoperitoneum is most readily detected on the upright film of chest, especially if only small amounts of air are present. Decubitus films of the abdomen are also useful. The left lateral decubitus view is preferred because small air collections may be seen accumulating between the right lateral liver margin and the peritoneal surface. With proper radiographic technique, as little as 1–2 cc of free air may be seen within the peritoneum.

5

The Skeleton

Since trauma to the skeleton and body as a whole forms such a great and integral part of the practice of the physician, this will be dealt with separately from other skeletal diseases. Apart from trauma, study of the bony skeleton relates primarily to (1) determination of bone age, (2) a survey of the skeleton for metastases from a primary tumor, (3) a survey of the skeleton for study of congenital, infectious, or other neoplastic disease, (4) metabolic disease alterations such as hyperparathyroidism or nutritional deficiency states, and (5) the radiographic study of joints.

BONE AGE

Skeletal growth assessment is a valuable method for determining the normalcy of children, for detecting endocrinopathies (such as hypothyroidism) and chromosomal aberrations, and for distinguishing between small size on a genetic basis and retardation of stature from other causes (such as malnutrition, central nervous system disorders, chronic infections, congenital heart disease, renal disorders, hepatic disorders, pulmonary disorders, blood diseases, and intestinal disorders). Disorders that may cause large stature are largely related to hormonal influences such as pituitary hyperfunction, testicular hypofunction, adrenal cortex adenoma or carcinoma, genital hyperfunction, possibly pineal tumors, or tumors of the hypothalamus.

The major features that are studied in the assessment of skeletal maturation are (1) the ossification of the long and short bones, which is usually complete in utero with the exception of the secondary epiphyseal centers; (2) the onset of ossification of the epiphyses, which occurs in a rather regular fashion and has been tabulated; (3) completion of ossification with fusion of the epiphyses and metaphyses; and (4) maturation indicators in the wrist, hand, tarsus, foot, and knee.

Generally, epiphyses begin to appear at birth or shortly thereafter and are ordinarily completed by puberty. Ossification is usually complete by the twentieth year in the female and the twenty-third year in the male. Hence, in children under 5 years of age, skeletal age is measured by the time of appearance of the centers of ossification. For children 5 to 14 years of age, a study is made of maturation factors and the penetration of cartilaginous areas by reference to standards. For children 14 to 25 years of age, the skeletal age is registered by epiphyseal-diaphyseal union and reference to "completion of ossification" tables. In general, views of the hand and wrist are most valuable up to the age of 18; of the elbow up to the age of 14; of the shoulder to about 30 months of age in the infant and thereafter between the ages of 12 and 16. Views of the pelvis and hip are most valuable up to the age of 4½ years and thereafter between the ages of 12 and 17. Views of the knee in the lateral projection are most valuable up to the age of 6 and thereafter between the ages of 10 and 13½ years; of the foot, in the anteroposterior projection up to the age of 6 and in the lateral between the ages of 5 and 9½ years.

In the female the ossification onset and fusion occur somewhat earlier, by approximately one year to 18 months in each instance.

The "age-at-appearance" percentiles for the major postnatal ossification centers can be determined. Maturation indicators are studied by reference to standards for the various regions studied such as the hand,

135

wrist, tarsus, foot, and knee as indicated by the age of the child, and these are tabulated in relation to the mean age given plus the standard deviation.

All these data are interrelated to give the most probable **bone age.** *It is important to recognize that irrespective of the bone age assessment, one area may not suffice as a guide to the development of other bones or joints.* Also, the genetic pattern of the individual must be taken into consideration. Moreover, if the assessment is based on developmental data compiled from a population that is not comparable to the individual being evaluated, allowances must be made for moderate deviations. Premature fusion of one or more epiphyses may result as a complication of infection, trauma, or nutritional disturbances such as scurvy or pathologic fracture; in such metabolic disturbances as Cooley's anemia; and in the congenital adrenogenital syndrome with virilism.

METASTATIC BONE SURVEY
(Figure 5–1A and B)

Most metastases to the skeleton involve the spinal column and skull rather than the more distal portions of the extremities. There are exceptions, however. Hence, the routine metastatic survey usually includes *two films of the skull,* a posteroanterior film of the *chest* (for rib study particularly), films of the suspected portions of the *spine,* and an anteroposterior view of the *pelvis.* Films of the upper half of the upper and lower extremities may also be included if there is an element of pain in any of these areas.

A **radionuclide bone scan**, to be described subsequently, is probably a much more accurate way of demonstrating tumor metastases. Only about 5% of metastases are not demonstrated by means of radionuclide studies, even though they are not necessarily osteoblastic. Of course, those that are demonstrated with radionuclide studies may be subsequently studied radiographically to elucidate better definition and detail than can otherwise be obtained with the nuclear medicine study, and disease processes such as infections and Paget's disease may also be excluded.

CONGENITAL INFECTIOUS AND
NEOPLASTIC DISEASES

The subject of congenital and hereditary abnormalities of the skeletal system has be-

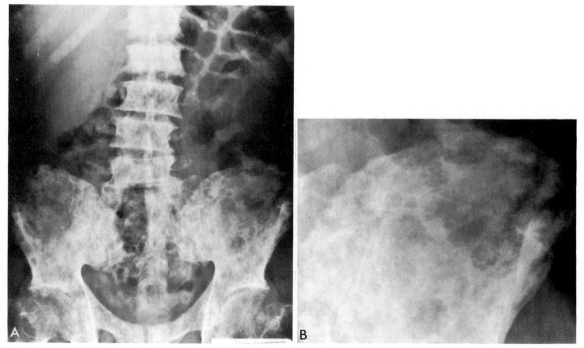

Figure 5–1. *A* and *B,* Anteroposterior views of the abdomen showing the lumbar spine and pelvis in a patient with widespread metastases from carcinoma of the prostate. In *A,* the entire lumbar spine and pelvis are shown. In *B,* a close-up view of the ilium is shown in better detail. Note the spotted lucency and marked dense sclerosis of the variety of tumor metastases.

come exceedingly complex and extends far beyond the scope of this text. Inborn errors of metabolism are more and more being identified as specific metabolic disorders, which in turn may be related to genetic mutations or chromosomal aberrations. Very often, these may be identified by the physician from a carefully obtained history and physical findings and usually are considered as either underdevelopments, overdevelopments, or maldevelopments of a single or multiple skeletal part or as diseases of bone related to a defect extrinsic to the bone but involving the bone secondarily. The individual consideration and diagnosis at hand is evolved by careful consultation with the radiologist and a pediatrician especially well versed in these phenomena.

INFECTIONS OF BONE

The widespread use of antibiotics has radically altered the radiologic diagnosis and medical treatment of pyogenic osteomyelitis. Actually, the spread of infections to adjoining joints is no longer as serious a problem, since antibiotic therapy significantly aborts or modifies the course of the disease.

The earliest radiologic manifestations of pyogenic osteomyelitis may not appear for 10 to 14 days following the onset of the disease, although the abnormality may be detected with radionuclide diagnostic imaging techniques signif-

icantly earlier, and this will be addressed in the section under nuclear medicine. The earliest radiologic manifestation as the infected bone undergoes pathologic change may be soft tissue swelling at the site, with or without periosteal elevation and thickening. It is during this phase that the bone is undergoing vascular and osteoclastic resorption, and as the process proceeds radiologically, localized bone resorption is manifest. As the periosteum is irritated it lays down new cortical bone. If this occurs, and if the process does not respond to antibiotics, one soon finds dead bone with sequestration, which radiologically may appear denser than the surrounding bone, with a zone of radiolucency due to adherent pus or infected granulation tissue (Fig. 5–2A and B). Unfortunately if this should occur, the time-honored surgical procedure of saucerization, removal of sequestra, and excision of sinus tracts must still be employed to supplement the limited beneficial effect of antibiotic therapy.

At this phase the appearance is that of chronic osteomyelitis, with or without chronic bone abscess formation. There are forms of chronic osteomyelitis unaccompanied by outright visible sequestration (Brodie's abscess), and sclerosing osteomyelitis and occasionally necrosis and abscess formation are very limited, with an abundant reparative fibrous tissue and bone regeneration.

The important points to remember are: (1) *the onset of the osteomyelitis antedates the*

Figure 5–2. Acute osteomyelitis affecting the distal metaphysis of the left femur.

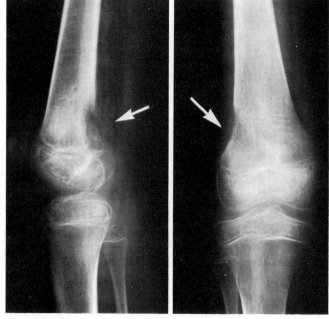

A   B

roentgenographic appearance by 10 days to two weeks, (2) nuclear medicine techniques to be described later precede these appearances, (3) amyloidosis at times develops in patients with neglected or unsuccessfully treated bone infections, (4) malignant tumors at times form in old sinus tracts, which may indeed necessitate amputation. These are usually squamous cell carcinomas but on rare occasions may be fibrosarcomas.

The osteomyelitis may be primary, in which case it is hematogenous in origin, or secondary to soft tissue infection adjoining the bone, as often occurs in diabetics.

Tuberculosis of bone and joints is always secondary to an established focus of tuberculosis elsewhere in the body—most commonly in the lungs. There are three forms of skeletal tuberculosis: arthritis, spondylitis, and osteomyelitis of the shafts of the long bones. With the advent of effective chemotherapy, the incidence and course of bone and joint tuberculosis have been distinctly modified, and although examples of this disease are not infrequently found in other countries, they have become rare indeed in the United States.

It is considered that other infectious skeletal involvement, such as may occur with fungal infestation, leprosy, syphilis, parasitic disease, and viral infections, are outside of the scope of this text, except to mention that they do occur and must be considered in the clinical assessment of the patient.

BENIGN AND MALIGNANT BONE NEOPLASMS

Tumors of bones are infrequently encountered in clinical practice, but because of their malignant potential, they should be seriously considered whenever the potential exists. Primary bone tumors may arise from any of the tissue elements that are indigenous to bone, including the bone marrow and neural tissues. These include benign and malignant neoplasms originating in bone proper, cartilage, the marrow elements, vascular blood vessels, and lymph vessels; neurogenic tumors; and even the notochord. In the marrow, the most important malignant diseases of hematopoietic cells are the plasma cell myeloma (Fig. 5–3*A,B,C,D*), Ewing's sar-

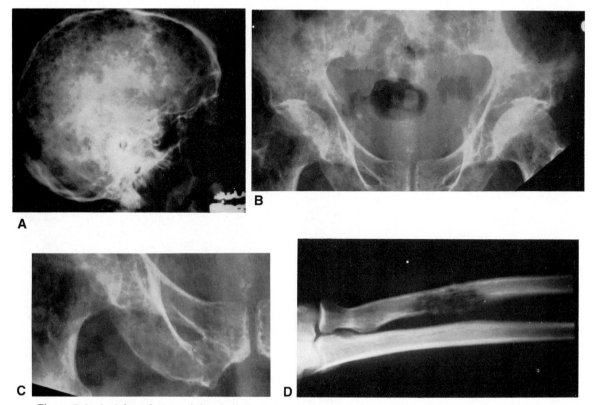

Figure 5–3. *A,* A lateral view of the skull. *B,* An anteroposterior view of the pelvis. *C,* A coned-down view of the right pubis and ischium. *D,* A more localized form of the disease in involvement of the radius of the forearm.

coma, and reticulum cell sarcoma. In the marrow, however, one must also consider fat cells, fibrous connective tissue, and smooth muscle. The giant cell tumor is of uncertain origin and may at times be classified as either benign or malignant, with about 10 to 30% following a malignant course. Because of the relative rarity of bone neoplasms, no further comment is justified in this text.

SKELETAL CHANGES IN ENDOCRINE DISORDERS

Hypo- and hyperfunction of the endocrine glands are known to produce skeletal changes. There is a vast literature on this subject, and this will be touched upon very briefly. For example, *pituitary basophilism* or basophil cell adenoma of the anterior lobe of the pituitary gland was at one time thought to be responsible for Cushing's syndrome, with its pronounced osteoporosis, backache, round shoulders, and multiple fractures, especially of the ribs. *Hyperfunction of the eosinophil cells* of the anterior lobe of the pituitary gland produces an excess of growth hormone, which stimulates chondrogenesis and osteogenesis in skeletal tissues, producing human gigantism or acromegaly. Before puberty, particularly, there is marked excessive growth of this type, and after puberty acromegaly results. *Hypopituitarism,* most often caused by tumors of Rathke's pouch, results during childhood in a dwarfism and an arrest or retardation of ossification. The bone age of children affected by this disorder lags behind the chronologic age.

With regard to the adrenal glands, *hypercorticism* results in a marked thinning of bones, osteoporosis, and, in the female, a masculinizing effect. In a male child, sexual precocity and inordinate muscular development are produced, with considerable acceleration of growth in the skeleton at first, but in the end there is premature fusion of epiphyses and small stature. In the adolescent or adult male, virility and striking hirsutism may result.

Actually 40% of primary adrenocortical tumors are malignant. It is also important to note that Cushing's syndrome may develop occasionally in patients with bronchial carcinoma, ovarian tumors of various types, and thymic tumors.

Hyperthyroidism induces osteoporosis, especially of the calvaria, ribs, and spine. There is excessive excretion of calcium and phosphorus. If the process begins before the end of adolescence, there is an accelerated skeletal growth. Later, however, it leads to bone wasting. Untreated *hypothyroidism* leads to myxedema in the adult and to cretinism in young children, with dwarfism resulting. In this instance there is a delayed appearance and retardation of the centers of ossification.

Primary hypogonadism apparently has no skeletal effects after the growth period except that it may favor osteoporosis in women. In female children, ovarian agenesis produces a stunted growth or dwarfism often associated with other anomalies, such as a webbed neck or coarctation of the aorta. In the male child, hypogonadism results in eunuchism, and the skeleton is relatively tall, the extremities are long and slender with thin cortices and the epiphyseal cartilage plates persist beyond the normal age and remain active.

It is possible that *teratomas of the pineal gland* are responsible for precocious puberty, as manifested by an advanced ossification of these centers causing the long bones to be large and heavy in relation to the age of the subject.

With regard to the *pancreas,* diabetes mellitus may alter skeletal development in children. The centers of ossification may be advanced so that initial body height is above average for the age of the patient, but with longstanding disease, the centers of ossification eventually are retarded and the bones appear thin, narrow, and osteoporotic. In adults one sees advanced arteriosclerosis with partial occlusion of peripheral arteries and a tendency to gangrene and infection, especially in the feet and lower limbs.

The *parathyroid glands* are significantly involved in skeletal metabolism, the three major functions being (1) to mobilize calcium from the skeleton, (2) to induce phosphate diuresis, and (3) to increase absorption of calcium from the intestines. Thus, parathyroid adenomas sometimes induce a striking demineralization of the bones, whereas at other times they may be biologically inactive. The most obvious changes are in the cancellous bone of vertebrae, the small bones of the hands such as the phalanges, the ends of the long bones, and the tables of the calvaria (Fig. 5–4A,B,C,D,E).

In the kidneys one may observe renal stones composed of calcium phosphate or oxalate and nephrocalcinosis, especially in

HYPERPARATHYROIDISM

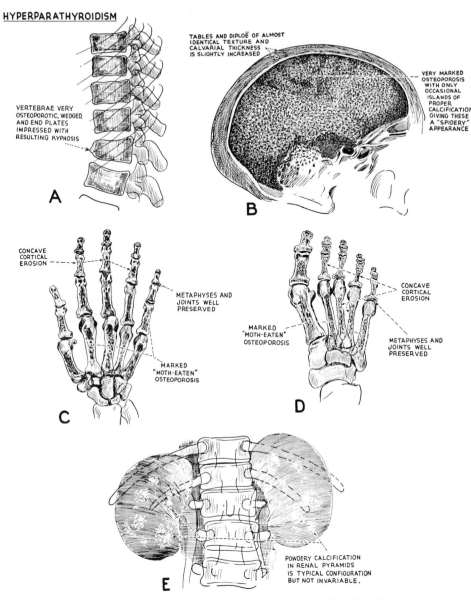

Figure 5–4. Hyperparathyroidism due to a parathyroid adenoma. *A* to *E*, Labeled tracings of the spine, skull, hand, foot, and kidney areas in a patient with a parathyroid adenoma. Note the powdery calcification in the renal pyramids rather typical of the type of nephrocalcinosis that occurs in this condition.

the pyramids and medulla. There is practically always an elevated serum alkaline phosphatase. In some instances the bone appears pseudocystic (osteitis fibrosa cystica). Actually, these are localized areas of marked skeletal resorption appearing radiographically as a rather circumscribed lucent defect of varying size and location—especially in the jawbones, calvaria, hands, and long bones.

Hyperparathyroidism may also be secondary to renal disease or osteomalacia, similar in its physiology to rickets in children.

Pseudohyperparathyroidism has the biochemical and clinical manifestations of hyperparathyroidism and is observed in a number of malignant tumors, such as carcinomas arising in the lung, kidney, pancreas, and esophagus, as well as malignant lymphoma and stromal cell sarcomas of the uterus among other sites. As many as 30 to 40% of patients with Zollinger-Ellison syndrome with nonbeta-pancreatic islet cell tumors are believed to have hyperparathyroidism due to a parathyroid adenoma, carcinoma, or hyperplasia.

A

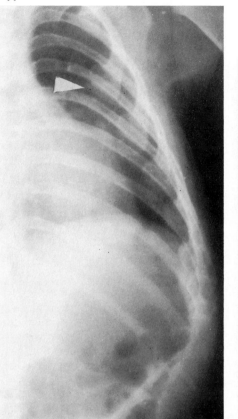

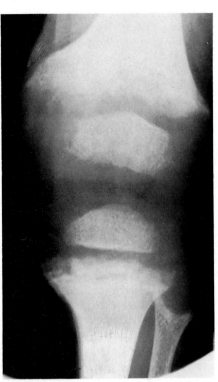

B

HYPOVITAMINOSIS D
(RICKETS - CHILDREN) (OSTEOMALACIA - ADULT)

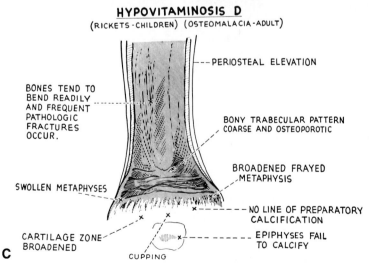

PERIOSTEAL ELEVATION

BONES TEND TO BEND READILY AND FREQUENT PATHOLOGIC FRACTURES OCCUR.

BONY TRABECULAR PATTERN COARSE AND OSTEOPOROTIC

BROADENED FRAYED METAPHYSIS

SWOLLEN METAPHYSES

NO LINE OF PREPARATORY CALCIFICATION

CARTILAGE ZONE BROADENED

EPIPHYSES FAIL TO CALCIFY

CUPPING

C

Figure 5–5. *A,* View of the ribs showing the flared appearance at the costochondral junctions corresponding with a rachitic rosary. *B,* Closeup view of the knee showing the frayed expanded appearance of the metaphyses of the femur and tibia and the poorly ossified epiphyses of the femur and tibia. *C,* Labeled tracing demonstrating the most significant radiographic findings

Hypoparathyroidism results in a low serum calcium level whereas the serum phosphorus level is elevated and the tubular reabsorption of phosphorus is correspondingly high. Clinically there is a relationship to tetany, cataract formation, calcification of basal ganglia, and mental retardation. There may be stunting of stature, and a variety of other skeletal changes have been noted.

In pseudohypoparathyroidism there are the manifestations of hypoparathyroidism, as previously described. However, there is no deficiency in the glands themselves, but rather a failure of the renal tubule to respond to the phosphouretic action of parathyroid hormone. It is genetic in origin, recessive, and unresponsive to parathormone. The skeletal abnormalities include short stature, round face, and short metacarpal and metatarsal bones. There may also be calcification in the basal ganglia and metastatic calcification in the skin. When the skeletal manifestations are lacking and the biochemical abnormalities are present, or when the serum calcium and phosphorus levels are normal and the skeletal alterations are present, the condition may be known as pseudo-pseudo-hypoparathyroidism. The more recent concept of pseudo-pseudohypoparathyroidism is that it is a cyclic phase of pseudohypoparathyroidism and not a separate clinical entity.

SKELETAL CHANGES IN METABOLIC DISORDERS GENERALLY

Many metabolic disorders result in skeletal changes. Primary disorders of lipid metabolism result in Gaucher's disease and xanthoma tuberosum multiplex; purine metabolism disorders result in gout particularly; amino acid metabolism abnormalities result in hereditary ochronosis, which produces marked bone and joint disease with excessive calcification in cartilage; abnormal mucopolysaccharide metabolism results in gargoylism and Hurler's disease, and disorders of pigment metabolism result in porphyria. Other metabolic disorders result in scurvy (deficiency of vitamin C), rickets (Figure 5–5A,B,C) (resulting from nutritional, absorptive deficiency, or renal deficiency), and osteomalacia, the counterpart of rickets in the adult. Renal insufficiency may occur with or without secondary hyperparathyroidism, aminoaciduria, and other manifestations of renal tubular transport disease. Sprue, stea-

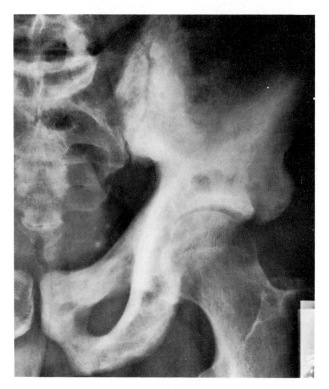

Figure 5–6. Radiograph illustrating the roentgen findings in Paget's disease of the hip. Note the coarsened and somewhat mosaic appearance of the ilium, ischium, and pubis, with a tendency toward thickening and a similar mosaic appearance of the trabecular pattern. This mosaic appearance corresponds with the pathologic appearance of the osseous matrix.

torrhea, and pancreatic insufficiency may also be listed in this category. There is little doubt that the physician should be familiar with such skeletal changes as these and be alert to these occurring in his patient population. Space does not permit a complete elucidation of the skeletal changes resulting from these.

Skeletal changes may occur in neurotrophic disorders associated with spinal cord disease and in neuroarthropathies such as tabes dorsalis, which in the knee produces the "bag of bone" appearance. Destructive neural changes may occur in the foot, especially from poorly controlled diabetes mellitus of long standing, and neuroarthropathy may occur as the result of injury to peripheral nerves.

Skeletal changes may occur in certain blood diseases such as hemophilia and other coagulation deficiency states, in chronic hemolytic anemias, in sickle cell anemia, in thalassemia major, and in spherocytic anemia.

Paget's disease of bone (Fig. 5–6) occurred in over 3% of a sizeable series of subjects past 40 years of age whose skeletons were thoroughly examined at autopsy. Radiologically, there is an initial phase of bone resorption, and this in turn is followed by alternating cycles of bone formation with renewed resorption over many years. This ultimately leads to gross alterations of architecture, imparting a "mosaic" appearance to the bone microscopically and a markedly coarsened and somewhat sclerotic appearance of bone radiologically. It is probably more important in this context to observe that the disease occurs mainly in middle-aged or older patients in the upper and lower extremities, pelvis, lumbar spine, and skull. The main aid to a laboratory diagnosis of this condition is the markedly elevated serum alkaline phosphatase. The disease may even be found in such sites as the sternum, clavicle, hand, and foot. Occasionally it is complicated by alteration to osteogenic sarcoma in the adult. Malignant transformation may not only be to that of osteogenic sarcoma but also to fibrosarcoma or an anaplastic tumor containing many multinuclear tumor cells, simulating a malignant giant cell tumor. When malignant disease results, survival is rarely beyond one year.

Text continued on page 149

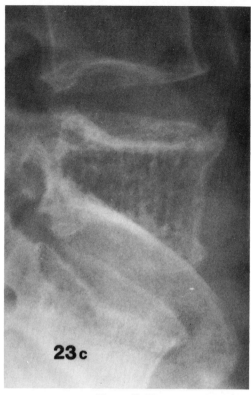

Figure E–79.

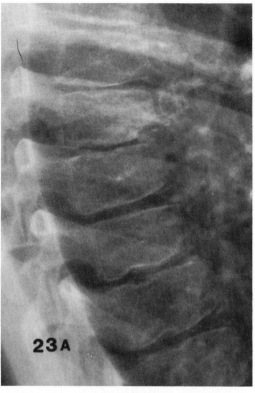

Figure E–80.

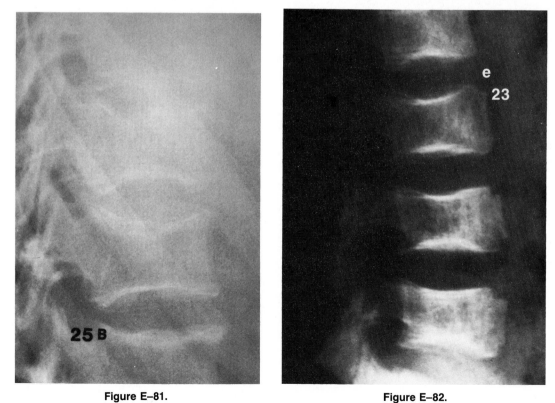

Figure E–81.

Figure E–82.

CLINICAL HISTORIES

Figure E–79 is a lateral view of the fourth lumbar vertebra of a 55-year-old female.

Figure E–80 is the lateral view of the lower thoracic spine of a 13-year-old female who complained of mild pain in the back for a period of several months.

Figure E–81 is the lateral view of the lumbar spine of a 54-year-old female who likewise complained of pain in her back.

Figure E–82 is the lateral view of the lumbar spine in a 30-year-old female who had no complaints referable to her back; the radiographic appearance was coincidental in respect to examination of her urinary tract. A lateral view of the lumbar spine was obtained.

Questions

24–1. The MOST likely diagnosis in Figure E–79 in this patient is
A. Paget's disease of the spine
B. Metastatic disease from a tumor elsewhere
C. Eosinophilic granuloma
D. Malignant lymphoma
E. Hemangioma

24–2. With regard to Figure E–80, the MOST likely diagnosis is
A. Tuberculosis spondylitis
B. Cretinism
C. Morquio's disease
D. Scheuermann's osteochondrosis of the thoracic spine
E. Heavy metal poisoning

24–3. With regard to Figure E–81, the *diagnostic possibilities* are
A. Osteoporosis from involutional change
B. Multiple myeloma
C. Deforming spondylosis
D. Osteomalacia
E. Renal insufficiency with secondary hypoparathyroidism

24–4. What are the *possible diagnoses* in Figure E–82?
A. Aseptic necrosis with infarction, as in sickle cell disease
B. Schmorl's nodes
C. Erythroblastic anemia
D. Hemolytic anemia
E. Hodgkin's disease

Radiologic Findings. The intrinsic architecture of L-4 vertebra in Figure E–79 is characterized by longitudinal striations arranged in a cephalocaudad direction. There are interspersed zones of lucency with remarkable regularity. The endplates are well preserved, although there are spurs along the anterior aspects both superiorly and inferiorly. There is no extension of the architectural change of this vertebral body into the pedicular region of the neural arch.

In Figure E–80, the secondary centers of ossification forming the end-plates of the lower thoracic vertebral appear to be fragmented in several instances. There are undulations of the end-plates of the vertebrae bodies. The vertebral bodies appear to be somewhat deficient in height and there is a tendency to kyphosis at the thoracolumbar junction.

In Figure E–81, there is an apparent diffuse radiolucency of all of the vertebrae, with a considerable concavity of a smooth type of the adjoining end plates of the several lower thoracic and lumbar vertebrae. The vertebral bodies are diminished in height. The ellipsoid nature of the intervertebral discs is increased in every instance. There is no actual significant narrowness of the anterior margins of the vertebrae with respect to the posterior; this shape for the vertebral bodies has been described "codfish" in type. There are no apparent foci of localized destruction or proliferation of bone. There is however, a *diffuse cloudy appearance of the trabeculae,* so that the individual trabeculae of these vertebrae are not clearly defined.

In Figure E–82A, the following roentgen signs are most apparent: 1) the end-plates appear increased in density in comparison with the texture of the vertebral bodies; 2) there is a steplike appearance in the superior and inferior end-plates of adjoining vertebrae, giving this the so-called "H" appearance (Fig. E–83), where the nuclei pulposi may be projecting into the vertebrae but the squared-off appearance is quite unusual. The texture of the vertebral bodies other than the sclerotic appearance of the end-plates shows a coarsening of the trabeculae as well as a tendency to lucency between the coarsened trabeculae.

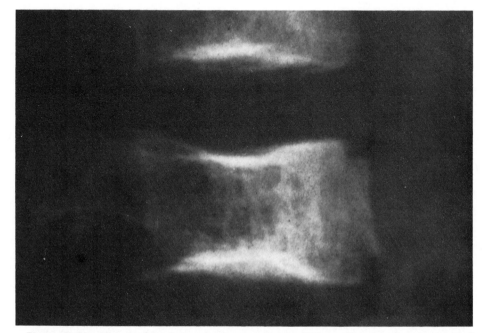

Figure E–83. Close-up lateral view to demonstrate the "H" configuration described and the coarsened trabeculation.

Discussion.* The diagnosis in Figure E–79 is classic **hemangioma of the vertebra.**

In *Paget's disease* the sclerosis of the vertebral body tends to form a "picture frame" around the periphery of the vertebral body in lateral and anteroposterior perspectives.

In *metastatic disease* there is evidence of outright destruction of the vertebra involved, with no preservation of its internal trabecular architecture and very frequently an associated pathological collapse.

If this were an *osteoblastic type metastasis,* such as occurs from carcinoma of the prostate, the vertebral body would be very densely sclerotic.

With *eosinophilic granuloma,* a lytic process of the vertebra is observed and very often associated collapse, giving rise to the appearance known as "vertebra plana."

With *malignant lymphoma* there is usually a cloudy, ill-defined sclerosis of the vertebral body with the trabecular pattern ill-defined.

Occasionally, patients with hemangioma of the vertebra will suffer some pain as the result of the lesion if the spine is subjected to trauma and minimal collapse, even though not detectable radiographically. In most instances, hemangioma of the vertebra is a coincidental finding when the spine is radiographed.

The correct answer for Figure E–80 is **Scheuermann's osteochondrosis** in an adolescent spine. This is characterized by aseptic necrosis and fragmentation of the secondary ossification centers. It is also characterized by a "juvenile kyphosis." The vertebrae most frequently involved are the lower and midthoracic and occasionally the uppermost lumbar.

With *cretinism* there is also a tendency to fragmentation of the secondary ossification centers, but this fragmentation extends across the entire end-plate and does not involve the anterior aspect of the secondary growth centers preferentially. Moreover, the appearance of the secondary ossification centers in an *adult with cretinism would simulate that of the adolescent* with a markedly delayed bone age.

With regard to Morquio's and Hurler's mucopolysaccharidoses, usually the most involved vertebrae are the uppermost lumbar, especially L-1, and there is a tendency to relative posterior displacement of L-1 with respect to T-12. There is a tongue-like protrusion of the vertebral body involved in its midsection, with some of the mucopolysaccharidoses or accentuated tongue-like protrusion of the inferior aspect of the vertebral body.

With *heavy metal poisoning* there may be diffuse increase in density at the metaphyseal ends of the long bones particularly, but the effect on vertebrae is seen beneath the cartilaginous portion of the growth plate rather than in the secondary ossification center itself. In some types of "heavy metal poisoning" such as in fluorosis, there is a diffuse sclerosis of the entire vertebral body due to a shell-like covering of the vertebral body with dense sclerotic bone.

With regard to Figure E–81, the following diagnoses would be considered tenable: (1) **osteomalacia;** (2) **osteoporosis:** (3) **multiple myeloma** of certain types; and (4) **certain types of secondary hyperparathyroidism,** but less frequently found with renal insufficiency. With renal insufficiency, there is a tendency to the "rugger jersey" appearance, with dense sclerosis of the uppermost and lowermost end plates of the vertebrae and a marked lucency in the midsection of the vertebrae in many cases.

The fact that the trabeculae appear clouded and ill-defined would favor a diagnosis of **osteomalacia** of some type, since with osteomalacia the trabeculae tend to be indistinct, in comparison with osteoporosis, in which the trabeculae retain distinct margination, although they are fewer in number, being replaced by unossified osteoid. In *multiple myeloma,* approximately one third of cases are characterized only by diffuse radiolucency of the vertebrae rather than by the punched-out appearance so often associated with this disorder. Approximately one third of the cases are recognized by diffuse hyperlucency, one third by punched-out lucent foci of defective ossification with replacement by plasmacy-tomas and in one third there is no specific radiologic appearance demonstrable. With *deforming spondylosis,* degenerative changes are found at the end-plates and usually spur formation with osteophyte bridging of interspaces is recognizable. These differ from the syndesmophytes so characteristic of ankylosing spondylitis, which is due to a calcification of the paraspinous ligaments overlying the vertebrae. Actually, the *single diagnosis that would definitely be unlikely would be a deforming spondylosis,* with the other diagnoses coming into consideration as described above, but **osteomalacia** being the most likely.

With regard to Figures E–82 and E–83, the most likely diagnoses are 1) an **aseptic necrosis with infarction** centrally in the region of the nuclei pulposi, as in **sickle cell disease;** or 2) **erythroblastic anemia.** In view of the greater frequency of **sickle cell disease,** the "H"-like appearance of the end-plates of the vertebrae (magnified in Figure E–83) is most often associated with sickle cell disease, and this was a patient with this disorder. However, it has been clearly demonstrated that patients with erythroblastic anemias of the Mediterranean type also may have this appearance and it is indistinguishable in the two abnormalities.

Schmorl's nodes, on the other hand, are central or eccentric defects of the end-plates, but have a rounded rather than a squared-off appearance. They usually imply degenerative change in the end-plate, or occasionally are found with the aseptic necrosis of osteochondrosis, but the appearance is not squared-off to form a figure "H," as in this instance. With hemolytic anemias, there is no tendency to such "H" configuration, although the vertebral bodies may be markedly lucent and the intervertebral discs may be ellipsoid with partial collapse of the vertebral bodies in their central sections.

With *Hodgkin's disease* there is a tendency to an intermixture of longitudinal sclerosis of an irregular type, and to osteopenia, with the overall appearance of moderate osteosclerosis of the vertebrae affected. There would be no appearance suggestive of sickle cell disease.

DISORDERS OF SYNOVIAL JOINTS

Radiologic diagnostic imaging is basic to abnormalities of synovial joints. The radiographic method of analyzing joint disease without the introduction of contrast media calls for a careful study of **(1) the alignment of the bones on either side of the joint, (2) the capsular and pericapsular soft tissue, (3) the character of the subchondral bone, (4) the width of the joint space, (5) the status of the bony structures on either side of the joint in both the epiphyses and diaphyses, and (6) further elucidation by arthrography with contrast media if necessary.** This procedure will be discussed separately.

In the pathogenesis of the disease process that affects joints, there is considerable overlap in the appearances of these several areas radiographically, and it is extremely important to correlate the history and physical findings with some laboratory studies if they are available, in order to arrive at a diagnosis. In fact, in the historical sequence, it is extremely important to reconstruct the pathogenesis of the disease process, referring back to the very first examination of the joint for the present complaint.

The linings of the synovial joints react to a wide variety of noxious influences, both locally and from elsewhere in the body. As a result of these noxious influences, some diseases are characterized by capsular distention without bony involvement. Some are characterized by subchondral and capsular proliferation with bony spur formation, calcification, and even ossification to variable degrees. Some diseases of joints are characterized by osteoporosis of neighboring bone and narrowness of the joint space with even subchondral bone resorption. Others demonstrate periarticular bone resorption without significant adjoining osteoporosis. In the course of the pathogenesis of many of these diseases, ankylosis results, but this is usually a nonspecific late change in a destructive joint disease process. Some diseases are characterized by loose bodies within the joint (joint mice) and articular irregularities, and still other diseases show evidence of synovial, cartilaginous, capsular, pericapsular, bursal, or peritendinous calcification.

In some instances different diseases result in identical radiologic appearances, and often the interpretation depends on the stage of the disease process, as determined radiographically. For example, traumatic arthropathy, degenerative arthritis, and hemophilic arthritis may at times appear the same. Likewise, when there is considerable osteoporosis of neighboring bone and narrowness of the joint space, tuberculous arthritis and rheumatoid arthritis may closely resemble each other. Even pyogenic arthritis, which produces less surrounding osteoporosis, may present a confusing radiographic appearance.

Tuberculosis is one of the common expressions of skeletal involvement in both children and adults—the knee joint in adults and the hip in children, although other joints such as the shoulder, elbow, or wrist may be affected. In correlation with the roentgen image one must determine the duration of symptoms, the presence or absence of a febrile illness, pulmonary disease, blood chemistry and reactivity to certain serologic agents, and the character of fluid in the joint if present.

Degenerative arthritis (osteoarthritis) (Fig. 5–7A,B,C,D) is probably the most common joint disease encountered in the adult. Damage to the articular cartilage eventually results, and osteophyte formation occurs at the bony ends surrounding the joint, with a slight tendency to pseudocystic absorption of the subchondral bone. In the hip this results in a narrowed joint space, pseudocystic subarticular bony resorption, and osteophyte formation at the joint margins. In the spine, spondylosis deformans occurs when the vertebral bodies tend to be almost fused by exostoses extending across the altered intervertebral discs. In the terminal phalanges, the marginal exostoses are often reflected by Heberden's nodes.

Rheumatoid arthritis (Fig. 5–8A,B,C) is another common disease entity that affects the young and the old alike. It is a disease process resembling closely other so-called "collagen" diseases, which include rheumatic fever, disseminated lupus erythematosus, periarteritis nodosa, dermatomyositis, systemic sclerosis, and possibly other conditions characterized by arteritis. In this form of arthritis the linings of the synovial joints are the principal target sites, although tendon sheaths, bursal sacs, and other organs such as the eye, lungs, pleura, and heart may be affected. Subcutaneous rheumatic nodules develop at one time or another in about 20% of all cases. In general, the roentgenographic appearances reflect the pathologic changes with soft tissue swelling, thickening of the affected joint capsule, significant osteoporosis, and perhaps inflammatory hyperemia. As the disease process progresses, there is

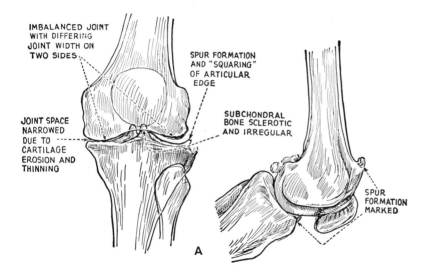
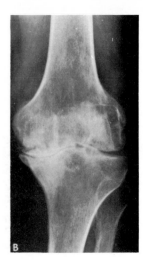
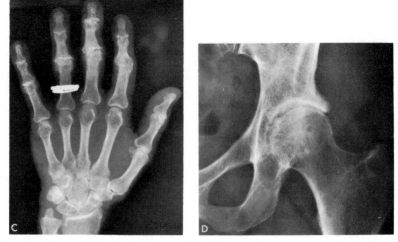

Figure 5–7. Hypertrophic arthritis. *A,* Pathogenesis in diagram. *B,* Anteroposterior view of the knee showing marked hypertrophic arthritis. *C,* Posteroanterior view of the hand showing marked hypertrophic arthritis affecting the small joints of the finger. The proximal interphalangeal joints of the index, third, and fourth fingers are maximally involved. Note the good texture, however, of the surrounding bones. *D,* Minimal to moderate radiographic evidence of hypertrophic arthritis of the left hip. Notice the eburnation and sclerosis of the shelving portions of the bone, the narrowness of the joint space, and the asymmetry of the joint space with zones of lucency interspersed among those of sclerosis in the adjoining margin of the acetabulum.

destruction of articular cartilage with narrowness of the joint and denudation of cartilage. Osteoporosis of the bone adjoining and distant from the joint may also ensue. Eventually subluxation, contractures, ankylosis, and other deformities may occur. Supervening degenerative changes may even at times mask the rheumatoid arthritis, and only a good clinical history with reconstruction of the pathogenesis can resolve the issue.

Rheumatoid arthritis may be associated with psoriasis in approximately 3% of cases, and psoriatic arthritis radiologically may have a somewhat similar appearance, although different joints frequently are involved. For example, it is the distal interphalangeal joints most frequently involved with psoriatic ar-

thritis, whereas the more proximal joints of the hand are involved in the rheumatoid.

SUMMARY REGARDING PLAIN FILM INTERPRETATION IN SKELETAL INVOLVEMENT

Thus it may be seen that plain film diagnostic imaging plays an extremely important part in skeletal diagnosis with important aspects reflected in bone age determination; congenital, infectious, and neoplastic demonstration, both primary and secondary; metabolic disturbances; and finally, the correlation of the history and physical findings with joint abnormalities.

150

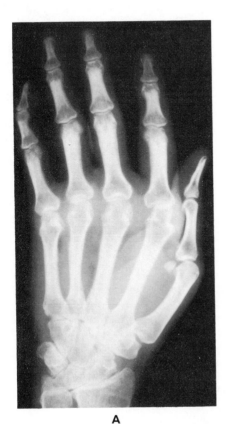
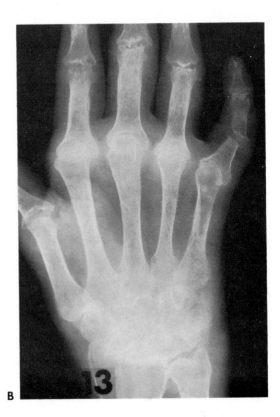

A

B

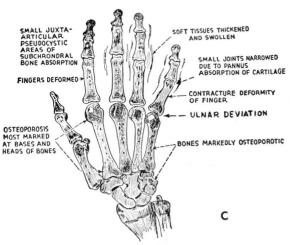

C

Figure 5–8. Rheumatoid arthritis of the hand. *A*, Radiograph of early phase. *B*, Very late phase, approaching arthritis mutilans. *C*, Line diagram illustrating the major roentgen manifestations.

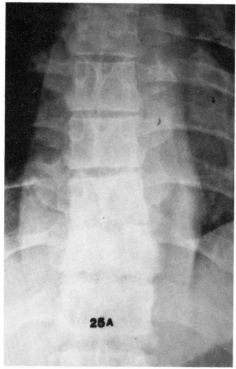
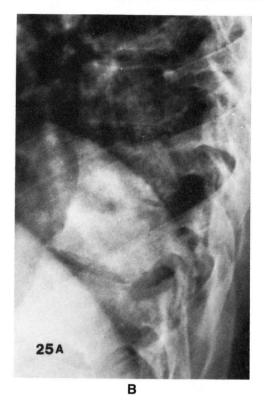

A

B

Figure E–84.

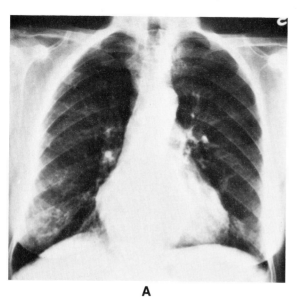
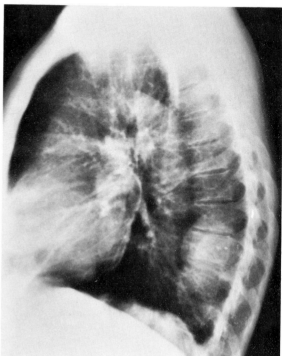

A

B

Figure E–85.

CLINICAL HISTORIES

Case 25–1. Anteroposterior (Fig. E–84A) and lateral (Fig. E–84B) views of the lower thoracic spine in a patient who was febrile and complained bitterly of lower thoracic pain and immobility.

Case 25–2. Posteroanterior (heavy exposure) (Fig. E–85A) and lateral (Fig. E–85B) views of the chest in a patient who had no pain or fever, but had an enlarged liver and spleen and was told by his physician that he was anemic.

Questions

25–1. Which of the following radiologic pathologic entities are similar in both cases?
A. They both have evidence of destruction in the lower thoracic vertebrae.
B. They both have a paraspinous mass.
C. They both have rib destruction.
D. They both have collapsed vertebrae.
E. They both have narrowness and almost complete disappearance of an interspace.

25–2. What is the MOST probable diagnosis in Case 25–1, Fig. E–84A and B?
A. Aortic aneurysm.
B. Metastatic neoplasm with destruction in vertebrae.
C. A chronic infectious spondylitis with a psoas abscess.
D. A neurogenic posterior mediastinal tumor.
E. A mesothelioma.

25–3. What is the MOST probable diagnosis in Case 25–2, Fig. E–85A and B?
A. A paraspinous mass related to a process such as extramedullary hematopoesis.
B. A neurogenic posterior mediastinal tumor.
C. A chronic infectious spondylitis.
D. An aortic aneurysm.
E. A bronchogenic cyst.

Radiologic Findings. In Figure E–84A and B there is a large paraspinous mass extending well below the lowermost thoracic vertebra and continuous with the retroperitoneal structures—most likely the psoas musculature. This paraspinous mass is smoothly contoured and yet somewhat double-contoured. It is separable from the aortic knob, which is at the uppermost part of the anteroposterior film (Fig. E–84A). Paraspinous ligamentous structures that should be visualized here are not in evidence. The descending thoracic aortic shadow is also obliterated from view. There is evidence of end-plate destruction of T-10 and T-11, particularly in their anterior two thirds, and extension of the destruction into the vertebral bodies, and these are surrounded by sclerotic bone within the vertebral bodies proper. The posterior margins of these vertebrae are preserved. There is a slight kyphus deformity at these levels.

In Figure E–85A and B there is a somewhat similar paraspinous mass visualized in the PA film of the chest (Fig. E–85A), but in this instance the shadow of the descending thoracic aorta is well preserved. There is extension of a mass to the right, producing a minimal "double contouring" in the shadow of the right atrium. In the lateral view (Fig. E–85B), the ellipsoid mass is identified in the posterior gutters of the thoracic cage but it is definitely separable from the shadow of the descending thoracic aorta and is not associated with a destructive process of vertebrae or diminution in size or involvement of the end-plates of the vertebral bodies in the immediate vicinity.

Discussion. The correct answer to Question 1 is that both cases have a **paraspinous mass.** Although there is vertebral body and intervertebral disc destruction in Figure E–84A and B, there is no involvement of the vertebrae in Figure E–85A and B. Only Figure E–84A and B have narrowness and almost complete disappearance of the interspaces involved. There is no such involvement of bone or the interspaces in Figure E–85A and B.

The most probable diagnosis in Case 1—Figure E–84A and B—is C, chronic infectious spondylitis with a psoas abscess. This proved to be a **tuberculous spondylitis**. The most important roentgen findings to indicate this diagnosis were the destruction of the end-plates and intervertebral space at T-10 and T-11 with the posterior gibbus and the adjoining involvement of the vertebral bodies. The surrounding abscess is evident on Figure E–84A, and it obviously extends below the lowermost margin of the film to involve the psoas musculature. Metastatic neoplasm in a vertebra does not ordinarily cause destruction of the intervening interspace, and in this respect this is most likely an infectious spondylitis and not metastases from any neoplastic process. A neurogenic tumor in a somewhat similar location is shown in Figures E–86 and E–87. A neurogenic tumor impresses itself upon the posterior margins of the vertebrae, as in Figure E–87, but does not destroy the interspaces, and the intervertebral cartilage is highly resistant and remains intact. A neurogenic tumor, of course, may be present without destruction of the bony contiguous structures such as the vertebral bodies or the laminae or intervertebral foramina. Occasionally there also is destruction of the pedicles. None of these findings are present.

A bronchogenic cyst is shown in Figure E–88A and B, which also appears posteriorly but has its origin ordinarily near the bifurcation of the trachea and extends posteriorly from this point of origin. It may extend directly posteriorly or hang as a droplet from its point of origin. There is no indication of obliteration of the descending thoracic aorta or paraspinous ligamentous structures. It may or may not contain air.

In answer to Question 3, the most probable diagnosis in Case 2 (Fig. E–85A and B) is a **paraspinous mass related to a process such as extramedullary hematopoiesis**. Although in frontal perspective a paraspinous mass is demonstrated, in the lateral view, Figure E–85B, there is no involvement of the vertebrae, their pedicles, the interspaces, or end-plates. The patient was known to have hepatomegaly, splenomegaly, and a chronic hemolytic anemia. The extramedullary hematopoiesis is usually compensatory under these circumstances because of an inadequate production or excessive destruction of red blood cells. Under

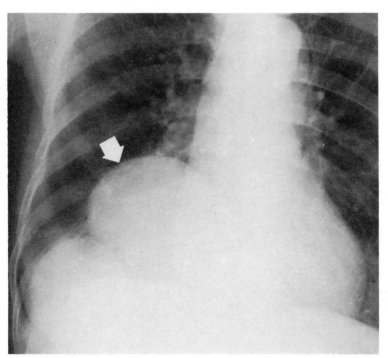

Figure E–86. PA film of the chest demonstrating a neurofibroma affecting the posterior inferior mediastinum.

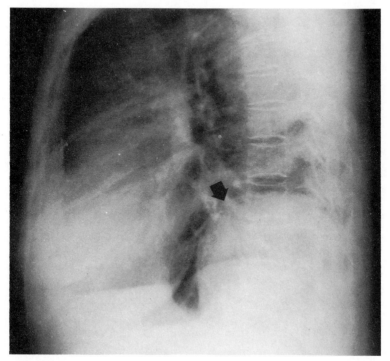

Figure E–87. Lateral films of the chest demonstrating a neurofibroma affecting the posterior inferior mediastinum. Although Figures E–86 and E–87 were not obtained for bone detail, the erosion of the intervertebral foramina in the lower thoracic region is quite readily demonstrated.

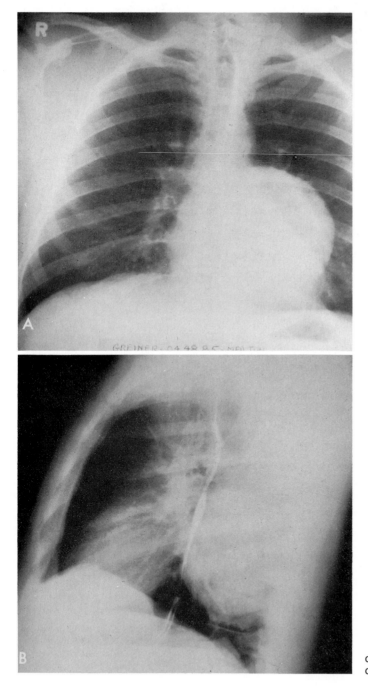

Figure E–88. *A* and *B*. Bronchogenic cyst of the mediastinum in characteristic location.

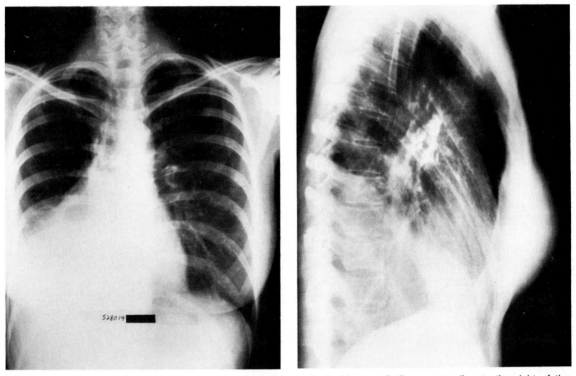

Figure E–89. PA and lateral views of the chest in a patient with mesothelioma extending to the right of the cardiopericardial silhouette, and in lateral view into the major fissure.

these circumstances, a tumorlike mass may be present in the thoracic paravertebral area, as was the case in this instance. Local symptoms are rarely present. The findings in this case are characteristic in that the mass is smooth (although it may be lobulated) and it is in the posterior thoracic gutter region bilaterally. The diagnosis may be corroborated by administering a radiopharmaceutical to this patient—^{99m}technetium sulfur colloid in a dose of approximately 2 to 5 microcuries and obtaining an image of the posterior lower thoracic region in about 15 minutes. This agent is phagocytized by the reticuloendothelial cells and would demonstrate a relative paucity of such cells in the liver and spleen and an abudance in the suspected tumor mass. A mesothelioma is illustrated in Figure E–89*A* and *B*. Although in the posteroanterior view, a tumor mass can be seen as projected through the heart, it extends toward the right predominantly, and in the lateral projection (Fig. E–89*B*) it is seen to be situated inferiorly and anteriorly. Mesotheliomata may be single or multiple and may occur anywhere in the pleural space, being derived either from the mesothelium itself or from the underlying stromal connective tissues. They ordinarily present as masses of this type but can, on occasion, be demonstrated primarily as a pleural hemorrhagic effusion with no masses grossly demonstrable. There is ordinarily no bony erosion contiguous to these masses. There is usually no associated metastatic involvement of the liver and spleen to produce hepatomegaly and splenomegaly as well as chronic anemia.

Trauma to the Skull, Thorax, and Abdomen

One of the most important indicators for radiographic imaging is a history of recent or remote trauma. Although the skeletal system is particularly subject to this mode of examination, often the most serious injury is that sustained by the brain within the calvaria; the globe of the eye within the orbit; the lungs, heart, and aorta within the chest (Fig. 6–1); both intraperitoneal and retroperitoneal abdominal viscera (Fig. 6–2); and muscles, ligaments, and tendons. There is probably no occasion in the practice of medicine in

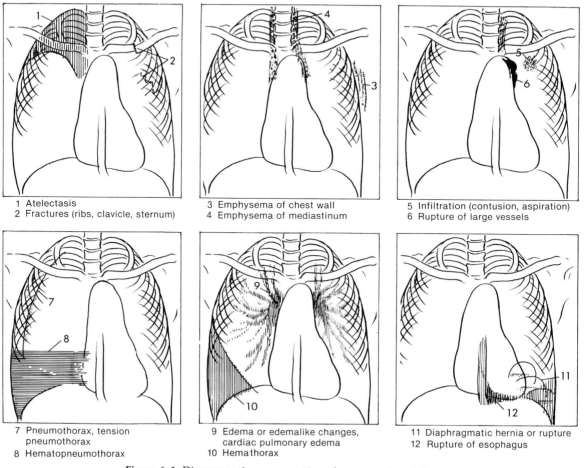

1 Atelectasis
2 Fractures (ribs, clavicle, sternum)

3 Emphysema of chest wall
4 Emphysema of mediastinum

5 Infiltration (contusion, aspiration)
6 Rupture of large vessels

7 Pneumothorax, tension pneumothorax
8 Hematopneumothorax

9 Edema or edemalike changes, cardiac pulmonary edema
10 Hemathorax

11 Diaphragmatic hernia or rupture
12 Rupture of esophagus

Figure 6–1. Diagrammatic representation of common chest injuries.

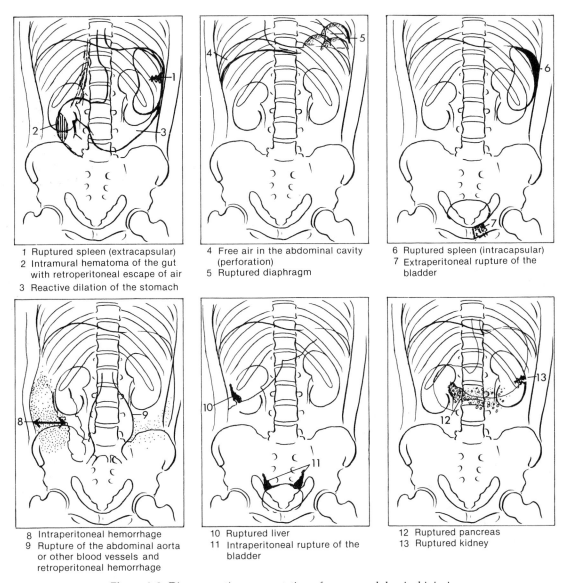

1 Ruptured spleen (extracapsular)
2 Intramural hematoma of the gut
  with retroperitoneal escape of air
3 Reactive dilation of the stomach

4 Free air in the abdominal cavity
  (perforation)
5 Ruptured diaphragm

6 Ruptured spleen (intracapsular)
7 Extraperitoneal rupture of the
  bladder

8 Intraperitoneal hemorrhage
9 Rupture of the abdominal aorta
  or other blood vessels and
  retroperitoneal hemorrhage

10 Ruptured liver
11 Intraperitoneal rupture of the
   bladder

12 Ruptured pancreas
13 Ruptured kidney

Figure 6–2. Diagrammatic representation of common abdominal injuries.

which a closer relationship must exist between the physician who orders a plain film x-ray examination and the radiologist who conducts the examination as that which exists following trauma. The patient must be spared pain, potential hazard, and unnecessary expense; yet the ultimate result from this modality of diagnostic imaging must ensure that the patient receives the optimal medical care.

The patient must not be moved any more than is absolutely essential until the extent of the injury has been ascertained and it is known that movement will not aggravate the injury. Although there may be a strong desire on the part of the radiologist to obtain the clearest and best diagnostic image, this can-

not be done until the hazard of movement of the patient is carefully evaluated. Moreover, the patient must always be treated for a life-threatening process such as shock or hemorrhage before diagnostic imaging is undertaken.

VARIOUS INDICATIONS FOR RADIOLOGIC EXAMINATIONS AFTER INJURIES

In summary, the indications for plain film radiologic diagnostic imaging are:

1. Any suspected bony injury •
2. Potential injuries to the central nervous system •

3. Blunt or open trauma to the thorax with potential injury to major vascular structures such as the aorta or even chambers of the heart •
4. Blunt or open trauma to the abdomen •
5. Contusions of solid organs such as the spleen or kidney, which may be bleeding into the retroperitoneal space •
6. Foreign body injury or massive injury of soft tissues, with associated involvement of internal organs •
7. Legal and insurance implications for injuries at work •

It is unacceptable to document injuries on the basis of fluoroscopic examinations alone if image intensifiers are available. All injuries must be documented by films and not fluoroscopy.

Even if the patient is dead on arrival in an emergency room, a postmortem radiograph must not be neglected to establish a correct diagnosis after injuries are acknowledged. Indeed, any death that occurs within 24 hours following injury is usually considered a "coroner's case" and is required by law to have a postmortem study. The results of x-ray imaging are of inestimable value in relation to explanations to the patient's family, and the medicolegal implications for the decision indeed may help solve a crime.

TRAUMA TO THE SKULL

Although the skull is involved in approximately 65% of all injured persons and in roughly 70% of all individuals killed in accidents, there is no indication of fracture of the skull found in about 25% of all victims of traffic accidents. There is no direct correlation between the severity of the brain damage and the degree of an existing skull fracture. When intracranial hemorrhage does occur, approximately 65% are subdural hematomas; 25% epidural hematomas; and 10% intracerebral hemorrhages within the brain proper. Clinically, it is difficult to differentiate between intracranial hemorrhage, edema of the brain without hemorrhage, and contusion of the brain stem. Hence, referral to neurosurgical expertise, involving neuroradiologic special procedures, is recommended. The advent of computed axial tomography has made early differentiation of these various injuries possible at a radiation exposure to the patient virtually identical to

that associated with skull films with most equipment, and at a cost only moderately greater.

The primary treatment should, of course, be directed toward brain edema, hemorrhage, shock, central respiratory depression, aspiration, and disturbances of temperature regulation. Thereafter, x-ray investigation should be carried forward as rapidly as possible. Computed tomographs yield far more information than the conventional five views of the skull. If conventional views of the skull are obtained, they must include a posteroanterior film, anteroposterior in Townes' projection, both laterals, posteroanterior Water's, and lateral films especially designed to show the facial structures in greatest detail. Special attention may be given to the zygomatic arch, the petrous bone, the base of the skull, the mandible, the temporomandibular joint, and the teeth, depending upon clinical indications.

Skull radiographs are difficult to interpret because of the normal anatomic variations in vascular channels, sutures, intracranial calcifications, normal points of rarefaction such as arachnoidal granulations, and the shapes and contours of the sella turcica as well as the orbits. Appropriate consultation with a radiologist is therefore imperative. The primary physician should, however, carefully examine the scalp and soft tissues. His findings should serve to make the consultation with the radiologist more meaningful, since abnormalities may not be shown clearly on the radiographs.

Skull fractures are classified according to location (calvaria, facial structures, or base of skull) and type (penetrating fractures, depressed fractures, bending fractures, or diastatic fractures involving the sutures). They may be linear also. A linear fracture of the skull is best visualized when the side on which it exists is closest to the film, and any greater distance may obscure the detail of the fracture. To diagnose a diastatic suture requires a thorough familiarity with the variations of sutural appearances in different age groups. Unfortunately, measurements are not helpful, and only with experience can one distinguish between probable fracture and a variation of normal. Likewise, a knowledge of the vascular grooves and their appearance is vital to exclude a normal vascular groove from a linear fracture. Usually vascular grooves are sinuous and contain a thin edge of sclerotic bone along each margin.

Rapid recognition of a depressed fracture is of vital importance and usually requires special tangential views to the area of depression to measure its extent. Such fractures should be neurosurgically elevated as quickly as possible to avoid scar formation in the brain—which in turn might give rise in later times to Jacksonian epilepsy.

Healing in skull fractures is difficult to evaluate, since fibrous union occurs long before bony union. Fractures of six to twelve months' duration, for example, may still be identifiable and yet have good fibrous union.

A leak of cerebrospinal fluid from the nose may lead to the detection of a tear in the meninges, which obviously requires neurosurgical repair. If the dura is injured and is not repaired, an epidural cyst may develop and continue to impress itself on the inner table of the skull, producing a large bony defect. Some have called this the "growing fracture" of the skull. With regard to facial fractures, the otolaryngologist, who usually treats these fractures, classifies them on a scheme recommended by LeFort, depending on the extent of associated injury of the maxilla and the nasal bones. Each of these three types of fractures requires a special form of treatment.

In order to recognize minimal amounts of free air in the orbit (emphysema of the orbit), at least one of the skull films that show the orbits to good advantage, must be obtained with a horizontal beam to diagnose a fracture involving a paranasal sinus communicating with the orbit. The most frequent sites for such fractures are the lamina papyracea, the ethmoids, and the frontal sinuses. If free air is identified within the intracranial cavity, the usual routes of communication are the frontal sinuses, the roof of the orbit, and the sphenoid sinuses. Likewise the horizontal beam study may demonstrate fluid levels if they occur.

About three quarters of all fractures at the base of the skull involve the middle fossa, and even if no fracture is seen, if an air fluid level is noted on the horizontal beam study, fracture must be postulated. Likewise, if there is leakage of cerebrospinal fluid from the nose or from the ear, one must postulate that there has been an associated fracture in the skull, even though the fracture is not demonstrable on routine study. To assist in localization of such fractures, a nuclear medicine examination can be undertaken.

TRAUMA TO THE SPINAL COLUMN

Approximately 50% of the fractures of the spinal column occur as the result of traffic accidents, 40% are work related, and 10% occur around the home or during sports activities.

Injuries to the spine are classified as (1) sprains, (2) contusions, (3) fractures, (4) luxations, (5) subluxations, and (6) combined luxations and fractures. Because of radiation along nerve roots, the pain is often referred to a lower level than that of the actual injury. Here, too, close consultation with the radiologist is recommended, since technique must be perfect; positioning in the anteroposterior, lateral, and oblique views must be ideal; and occasionally special views are required, such as tomograms. Indeed, it is becoming increasingly apparent that computed tomography may reveal fractures of the spine when such are not detected on any of the conventional films, including conventional tomography.

Particular attention to a transitional zone, such as the area between the neck and the thoracic spine, is extremely difficult because of the shoulder areas obscuring two or three vertebral segments, and yet this is one of the most significant areas of injury, especially in the lower cervical region. *A cervical spine examination is not complete unless at least seven segments are identified* and the relationship of the seventh cervical segment to the first thoracic is clearly seen. Moreover, the patient with such injuries requires very special expertise in handling so that paraplegia will not result.

With regard to the cervical spine, a complete series should be obtained whenever this will not endanger the spinal cord. The routine views should consist of anteroposterior, lateral, both obliques, and special views of the odontoid process. If the seventh cervical and the first thoracic are not clearly enough identified, a special view spoken of as the "swimmer's" lateral view is obtained to show this transition zone. Occasionally, flexion and extension views of the cervical spinal are utilized, when ordered by the physician, after he has determined that this would not endanger the cervical cord.

An abbreviated classification of injuries to the neck, apart from soft tissue injuries of the vascular structures, includes (1) whiplash injury; (2) fractures of the odontoid process; (3) "explosion" injuries of the first cervical segment (Jefferson's fractures); (4) fractures of the pedicles of the second cervical segment (called the "hangman's" fracture); (5) "locked facets" in which there is a partial or complete luxation of the facets on one or both sides; (6) the "tear-drop" injury of a vertebral body; (7) the "clay-shoveler's" fracture involving the spinous process and part of the neural arch of C6; (8) luxations or subluxations of C7 with respect to T1; (9) tears of various ligaments; (10) tears of the posterior longitudinal ligament recognized especially on flexion and extension views of the cervical spine, with or without associated fractures of the spinous processes; and (11) tears of the annular ligament surrounding the odontoid process, recognized by an increased space between the anterior tubercle and the odontoid process, which in the child should not exceed 5 mm and in the adult approximately 3 mm. Stretching of this ligament may occur in the child, especially in rheumatoid arthritis.

A few pertinent comments with regard to some of these is indicated. The "whiplash" injury of the cervical spine is usually sustained when a slowly moving vehicle is hit from behind and the occupants of the vehicle in front undergo a whiplike movement of the head on the neck. Typically, no radiologic evidence of fracture is obtained in these injuries, although it is extremely important to exclude facet compression by special oblique views when this type of injury is suspected. Despite the absence of outright evidence of fracture, significant pain may result owing to ligamentous tear, and this type of injury is of great medicolegal significance.

The radiologist employs various lining techniques in the study of the lateral masses of C1 and the remainder of the spine to make certain that a Jefferson type fracture of C1 has not been sustained (Fig. 6–3A and B). Ordinarily, the lateral masses do not overhang the adjoining articulations of C2, and when they do, a Jefferson fracture involving the neural arch of C1 may be strongly suspected.

Injuries involving the first cervical segment are often difficult to interpret because of the many variations of normal that occur in the course of fusion of the six major segments of the occipital bone, the bones composing the foramen magnum, and the

odontoid process itself. Hence, consultation with a radiologist is recommended.

The odontoid process itself presents considerable problems in interpretation, both in obtaining appropriate views and in the interpretation of anomalies of fusion (os odontoideum). The fusion of the odontoid process with the body of C1 may remain incomplete on a congenital basis and present an arcuate or triangular appearance rather than the transverse appearance usually obtained with an outright fracture. Usually, such pseudoarthroses are of considerably less significance, although individuals with such anomalies may be more susceptible to injury than those without. Certainly, atlantoaxial separations must be clearly identified in this area.

The most common and dangerous injuries of the cervical spine to exclude before moving the patient off the ambulance cart are the following (Fig. 6–4):

1. Fracture of the odontoid process
2. Tear of the annular ligament, so that the normal distance between the anterior tubercle of the second cervical segment and the anterior margin of the odontoid is no greater than 5 mm in the child and 3 mm in the adult
3. Fracture of the laminae of the first cervical segment with subluxation of the lateral masses of this segment, so that they overhang the articular facets of the second segment (Jefferson fracture). (*The normal lining technique illustrated in Figure 6–3 will reveal this abnormality provided the head is not rotated when the film is obtained.*)
4. Fracture of the laminae of the second cervical segment with subluxation of C2—the so-called "hangman's fracture"
5. Comminuted fractures of the body of a midcervical segment (so-called "tear-drop" fractures)
6. Fracture of a spinous process of the seventh cervical segment (so-called "clay-shoveler's fracture")
7. Compression fractures of a vertebral body, or of an articular facet. (Oblique films of the cervical spine properly obtained are necessary to demonstrate the latter.) Compression fractures of an articular facet may be mistakenly called "whiplash injuries," where a fracture is not observed.
8. Interspinous ligamentous tears, demon-

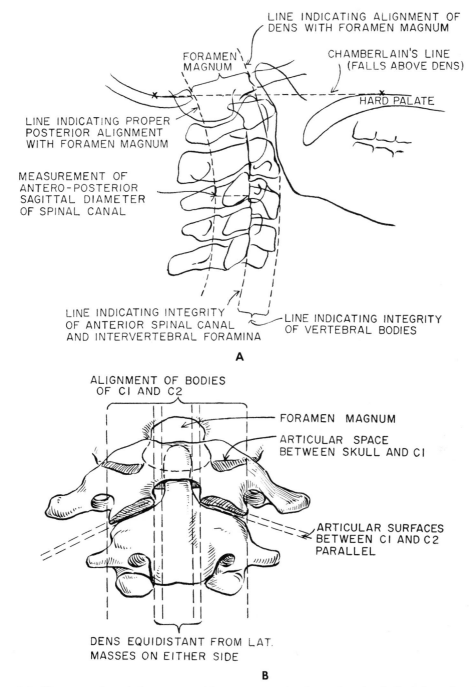

Figure 6–3. Alignment of cervical segments with respect to each other and to the skull. *A,* Lateral projection. *B,* Odontoid projection.

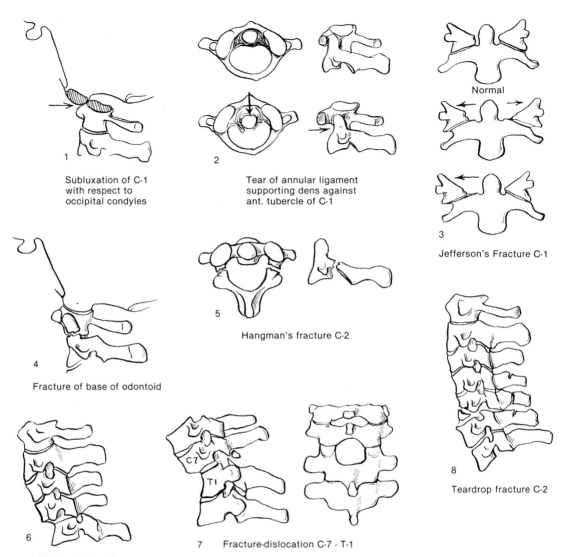

1. Subluxation of C-1 with respect to occipital condyles
2. Tear of annular ligament supporting dens against ant. tubercle of C-1
3. Jefferson's Fracture C-1
4. Fracture of base of odontoid
5. Hangman's fracture C-2
6. Bilateral locked facets
7. Fracture-dislocation C-7 - T-1
8. Teardrop fracture C-2

Normal

Figure 6–4. Diagrammatic representations of the more common injuries of the cervical spine. With a hangman's fracture there is an associated severance of the spinal cord and frequently a variable degree of anterior dislocation of C-2 on C-3. Computed tomography is useful to demonstrate associated pedicular fracture, which may occur.

strated best by film in flexion (lateral view)

9. Dislocation or subluxation of one facet with respect to another, either unilaterally or bilaterally (the so-called "locked facet")

10. Dislocation or subluxation of the seventh cervical segment anteriorly with respect to the first thoracic. *This diagnosis requires that all seven cervical segments be demonstrated in every examination of the cervical spine, even if a special view (the swimmer's view) is required to show this.*

Other injuries of cervical segments include compressions, especially at the fifth and sixth cervical segments. Another differentiation of great importance is made in a child when some narrowness of the fifth and sixth cervical segments is developmental and not the result of injury.

With regard to the thoracic and lumbar spine, the upper thoracic vertebrae are typically compressed in convulsions from any origin, whether they be epileptic or induced in the course of treatment of psychiatric conditions. The lower thoracic vertebrae are usually compressed as the result of trauma. Moreover, it is important to differentiate a pathologic fracture from that obtained purely as the result of trauma by careful analysis of the bony texture. Radionuclide studies may at times be helpful in this regard. The typical seat belt fracture is a horizontal fracture through the vertebral body and neural arch ("Chance" fracture).

Fractures of the transverse processes of the lumbar region are perhaps not in themselves clinically important, except for the extreme pain associated with them. However, they may be easily missed because of overlying gas shadows and are of significance because they indicate retroperitoneal injury, perhaps to the kidney, the pancreas, the ureter, or the spleen. Tears of the inferior vena cava may also result. Tears of the aorta may occur anywhere in its length, and more mention of this will be made in respect to crushing injuries of the thorax and abdomen.

Injuries to the coccyx are difficult to interpret, since variations of the coccyx are frequent. It is not unusual for the coccyx to form virtually a 90-degree angle with the sacrum, this being a normal variant, and fractures of this area must be interpreted with caution.

Probably half of all of the injuries to the spinal cord occur at the level of the lower thoracic and first lumbar vertebra. Only about 20% occur in the cervical region. Sometimes there are associated avulsions of nerves, which require myelograms for demonstration. The myelographic appearance is very characteristic and is carried forward by the radiologist. *Examination of the paravertebral soft tissues is most helpful in localizing injuries, since a spreading of the paravertebral ligaments usually indicates either injury or inflammation.*

Spondylolisthesis is most frequently observed in the fourth and fifth lumbar segments owing to ossification defects in the pars interarticularis of the neural arch of L4 and L5. The exact etiology of these ossification defects is unknown, but a slippage of L4 with respect to L5, or L5 with respect to S1, may result; these defects are classified according to the angle produced by such slippage: 10 degrees or less being first-degree, 11 to 20 degrees being second-degree, and 21 degrees or greater being third-degree. There would appear to be no specific association with pain, although it is recognized that individuals with such slippage are probably more susceptible to back strain than

those without. The defects in the pars interarticularis can be readily identified on oblique studies of the lumbar spine and often in the direct lateral view. At times they may even be identified in frontal perspective, and consultation with a radiologist is recommended for this identification. Usually these slippages do not progress notably in the course of many years, although occasionally this does occur.

TRAUMA TO THE PELVIS

The main sites of potential fracture of the pelvis are indicated in Figure 6–5 and these are the ilium, the wings of the sacrum, the acetabulum, and the pubis and pubic symphysis.

The "sideswiping" injury of the iliac crest is probably the most frequent cause of injury to this bone. Fractures involving the wing of the sacrum must be carefully differentiated from diastatic injuries to the sacroiliac joints, but in any case a contrecoup injury to the opposite pubis is a frequent concomitant. Gas shadows overlying the sacrum frequently interfere with an accurate detection of these. The various dislocations of the hip require accurate diagnosis for appropriate treatment. Fracture of the inferior ramus of the pubis must be carefully differentiated from the normal synchondrosis that occurs between the pubis and ischium at this level. Diastasis of the pubic symphysis is a frequent concomitant during parturition in the female, but tears and fractures at this level may result in posterior urethral injuries as well, and these frequently require urologic consultation and very careful management.

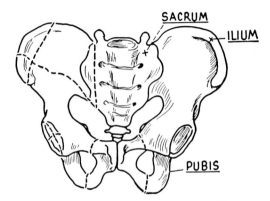

Figure 6–5. The most common sites of fracture of the pelvis.

The introduction of infection with contrast agent must certainly be avoided. Fractures of the pubic area that communicate with the perineum usually allow the free entry of air into the subperitoneal and retroperitoneal tissues in this immediate vicinity and can thereby be recognized. Further attention to this area to differentiate a retroperitoneal from an intraperitoneal injury to the urinary bladder will be described in the discussion of trauma to the abdomen.

TRAUMA TO THE THORAX

The most frequent sites of trauma to the thorax are indicated in Figure 6–1. Blunt trauma results from traffic accidents in about 58% of cases, from accidents at work in 24%, and during daily activities in 12%. The remainder occur during sports activities. The major distinctions are contusion, compression, and bruising, and, in about 5 to 6% of cases, open penetrating wounds. Approximately 7% are very serious and frequently result in death from severe injuries to the internal organs. The most frequent internal injuries involve a traumatic pneumothorax, with or without fractured ribs, blood in the thoracic cage, or both blood and air in the thorax (hematopneumothorax). There may be associated subcutaneous or mediastinal emphysema. It should be noted that for best demonstration of a pneumothorax, often a film of the chest obtained in expiration is more valuable than that in full inspiration to achieve maximum separation of the parietal and visceral pleura by the air.

Fractures involving the clavicle may be divided into those of the inner, middle, and outer thirds and are important to the following extent. The inner third fractures, including separation from the manubrium, may cause injury to the underlying glandular and/or vascular structures. Fractures of the middle third of the clavicle are the most frequent, but are important primarily because of overlapping and cosmetic distortion. For correction of this cosmetic distortion, orthopedic pinning usually is required. This may be important, particularly to the female patient. Fractures of the outer third become expressly important when the acromioclavicular joint is involved and there are tears of the ligaments of this joint or loose bodies contained within it.

Fractures of the sternum are highly variable and are best seen on the lateral view of the chest. Tomographic views may be particularly useful for demonstration of dislocations of the sternoclavicular joint, and radiologic consultation would be necessary for this special technology.

With contusions of the lung there is usually a homogeneous density in the lung substance itself at first. This may, in several days, undergo resorption of the hematoma, with cyst or pseudocyst formation giving the appearance of a thin-walled cyst. This gradually undergoes resolution to outright scar formation and a linear shadow (Fig. E–12).

Edema that is interstitial in the lungs may result from burns and the inhalation of toxic gases as well as the imbibition of household products, such as kerosene or furniture polish. In the latter instance the lung acts as an excretory organ as well as the injury resulting from direct irritation of the airway by the inhaled substance.

Rupture of the major airways may involve the trachea or tracheobronchial tree and may even be associated with tear of a major artery. Usually higher kilovoltage exposure films must be used to show the airway injury, and tomographic studies are particularly helpful under these circumstances. Computed tomography is especially helpful. When rupture of a major airway is recognized, its reconstruction is important. There may be an accompanying injury to the thoracic duct with a consequent chylothorax, which in turn is diagnosed by the character of the aspirate following removal of the fluid in the thoracic cage.

Aspiration or swallowing of foreign bodies by children and during alcoholic intoxication present special problems usually requiring consultation with the otolaryngologist. When the foreign body is opaque, it is readily recognized on the plain film of the chest. When it is nonopaque, and in a bronchus, a check-valve action will occur so that the involved lung may either be atelectatic or remain fully expanded during both inspiration and expiration. Films taken in these two modes are helpful, or this may be diagnosed by fluoroscopy. Bronchoscopic removal is essential to avoid lipid pneumonias and abscess formation. Foreign bodies, when they are swallowed, may either be blunt or sharp, opaque or nonopaque. If the foreign body is in the upper third of the esophagus and blunt, it may at times be removed by passing a balloon type catheter distal to the foreign body, inflating the balloon, and withdrawing the foreign body into the oropharynx. The otolaryngologist, however, may prefer to remove all foreign bodies by appropriate endoscopic procedures.

Perforation of the lower third of the esophagus by a foreign body usually results in free fluid within the pleural space, most frequently on the left. There may be an associated mediastinal emphysema. If the tear of the esophagus involves only the mucosa (Mallory-Weiss tear), it is usually diagnosable by endoscopy alone.

The most frequent site of aortic injury resulting from a crushing blow to the thoracic cage is at the junction of the left subclavian and descending limb of the arch of the aorta. This results not only in a tear of the aorta itself but also in a dissecting aneurysm either distal or proximal to the site of tear. If the tear is distal to the subclavian artery, plain films of the chest show an increased width of the descending thoracic aortic shadow in sequential films over a span of either a short or long time. Occasionally, chronic tears result, with spontaneous reopening of the dissection into the thoracic aorta at a lower level. If the dissection occurs proximal to the region of the coronary ostia, closure of the coronary ostia and ischemia of the myocardium usually result in death. Dissecting aneurysms or rupture of the aorta may be diagnosed with the aid of angiograms or computed tomography, with or without contrast enhancement. Crushing blows to the thoracic cage may result in tears to the right atrium particularly, with intrapericardial hemorrhage and cardiac tamponade. At times there may be combined ruptures of the aorta and tears of the right atrium which are extremely difficult to evaluate, even with contrast enhancement and angiography, and death usually ensues.

Traumatic rupture of the diaphragm is seen often with contusions of the thorax or abdomen, most often on the left. The organs most frequently herniating through the diaphragm are the colon, stomach, small intestine, spleen, liver, and omentum. Outright demonstration of the left hemidiaphragm and its tear is frequently very difficult, and computed tomography has offered the greatest advantage with respect to this diagnosis without resorting to invasive pneumoperitoneum. The latter is actually dangerous in that if the air enters the thoracic cage and a shift of the mediastinum results, the air in the thoracic cage must be quickly removed to avoid deleterious effects and even death.

Contrast investigation of the gastrointes-tinal tract may be necessary for this diagnosis.

Penetration of the thoracic cage by a bullet or similar missile may be readily visualized on plain films, and often there is a ricochet type action to other underlying organs. It is most important to evaluate possible injury to the heart or main blood vessels, and this usually requires expert consultation. An electrocardiogram may be helpful in determining injury to the heart itself. Severe chest pain and tachycardia unexplained should alert one to the distinct possibility of traumatic damage to the heart. The radiologic findings are cardiac dilatation with pulmonary congestion, enlargement and change in the contour of the heart due to small rents in the myocardium, and tamponade after bleeding into the pericardial sac.

TRAUMA TO THE ABDOMEN
(See Fig. 6–2)

Trauma to a solid organ may be readily diagnosed by insertion of a catheter into the peritoneal space, if this trauma has resulted in intraperitoneal bleeding. Hemorrhage from a hollow organ may be recognized by a catheter placed in the stomach or urinary bladder, or by recognition of blood in the urine. Blunt trauma to the abdomen usually results from traffic accidents, kicks, blows, falls, crush injuries, penetrating missiles, or, indeed, being buried alive. According to Vielberg and Schnepper,* the incidence of injury to individual organs after blunt trauma is as follows: spleen, 30%; liver, 25%; kidney, 20%; gut, 10%; omentum, 7%; urinary bladder, 3%; stomach, 2%; and pancreas, uterus, and gallbladder combined, 1%. Very often there is concomitant injury to the thorax in 28%, skull in 12%, extremities in 10%, spine in 5%, and pelvis in 4%. Often blunt trauma of the abdomen is accompanied by ileus of the bowel and injury to the abdominal wall with hematoma. If hematoperitoneum is present, it is often accompanied by displacement of organs on plain roentgenograms of the abdomen or by blood in the abdominal wall itself. Retroperitoneal hemorrhage usually results in the disappearance or widening

---

*Vielberg, H. E., and Schnepper, E. H.: Die Roentgen diagnostik stumpker bauch Traumen. Röntgen Blatter, *19*:405–424, 1976.

of the psoas shadow and possibly even displacement of the renal shadow.

Elevation of the urinary bladder from the pubic symphysis raises the suspicion of injury to the base plate of the urinary bladder. If the peritonealized portion of the urinary bladder is torn, the injection of contrast agent produces a "dog ear" appearance as the contrast agent winds its way between the overlying peritoneal loops. If the extraperitoneal portion of the urinary bladder is traumatized, contrast agent so introduced diffuses in interstitial fashion up toward the flanks and into the perineum proper. Very careful aseptic technique must be employed in such injection methodology.

Rupture of the spleen may be intracapsular or involve the internal splenic structure. The mortality is high—perhaps as high as 90%—without surgical intervention. The radiologic findings are opacification of the left upper quadrant; hematoperitoneum between the descending colon and the parietal peritoneum; displacement of the stomach; displacement of the left splenic flexure of the colon inferiorly; elevation of the left hemidiaphragm; and loss of detail of the left psoas shadow. If the hemorrhage is sufficiently severe, the kidney itself may be displaced or compressed. A measurement which is often applicable is from the tip of the spleen upward 2 cm and then horizontally 1. This measurement should not exceed 4 cm. Likewise, enlargement of the spleen for any reason is indicated by measurement from the tip of the spleen (splenic angle) to the left hemidiaphragm in supine films of the abdomen, and this should not exceed 12 cm.

Computed tomography is playing an increasing role in the diagnosis of rupture to any intra-abdominal solid organ.

Rupture of the liver has a twofold danger: internal hemorrhage and bile peritonitis. Lethality may be as high as 60%, but in recent years, with advances in surgery and diagnosis, this probably has diminished considerably. X-ray findings include (1) increase in size of the liver shadow and elevation and reduction of excursions of the right hemidiaphragm; (2) air bubbles within the liver; (3) most accurate diagnosis with angiography; and (4) with massive bleeding there is a dense opacification of the upper abdomen, most premonently on the right, with elevation of the right hemidiaphragm and lack of contour of the liver, the kidney, and psoas shadows, and downward displacement of the transverse colon and hepatic flexure.

About 80% of blunt abdominal trauma involves the small intestine. When the small intestine is involved, surgery is indicated if within 6 hours the presenting abdominal pain and tenderness do not increase. Actually, hematoma of the small bowel is frequently in the retroperitoneal part of the duodenum, with an escape of air upward to the mediastinum. This may lead ultimately to local stenosis of the duodenum, which may be documented by contrast visualization of the stomach and duodenum.

When there is rupture of a hollow viscus, even minute quantities of air may be demonstrated with a horizontal x-ray beam study if the patient's chest is elevated slightly and a coned-down film is obtained under the xiphoid process. It is anticipated that with a film vertical to the table and this view obtained, 1 or 2 cc of free air in the abdomen may be demonstrated.

Duodenal injuries are far more frequent from perforating trauma than from blunt (14 blunt as opposed to 131 open duodenal injuries).* Of the series reported by Morton and Jordan, 15 were projectile and 22 stabbing injuries. The liver was also involved in 38%; the transverse colon in 30%; the small bowel elsewhere in 29%; the pancreas in 28%; the stomach in 24%; the kidney in 21%; the vena cava in 17%; the gallbladder in 9%; and the aorta, renal arteries, and choledochal duct in 5%. If the site of the opening cannot be adequately demonstrated by surgical exploration, water-soluble contrast agent may be injected and films obtained in two planes.

Pancreatic contusion may result in hemorrhage, rupture, complete avulsion, or fragmentation, These cannot be differentiated radiologically. The main radiographic signs are opacification of the region of the pancreas on plain films of the abdomen, displacement of the body of the stomach and antrum to the right, displacement of the transverse colon downward, and pressure in the area of the left half of the transverse colon with marked dilatation of the proximal half of the transverse colon (so-called "cut-off" sign). If untreated, a pseudocyst of the pancreas can develop within days. A left lateral erect film, if possible, is most helpful, since there is an impression upon and displacement of the stomach from behind and forward.

Computed tomography of the pancreas

*Morton, J. R., and Jordan, G. L: Traumatic duodenal injuries: Review of 130 cases. J. Trauma 8:127–139, 1968.

is especially valuable [see Fig. E–74*B*(2)] in the diagnosis of pancreatic disease, as is endoscopic retrograde pancreatography (ERCP) [see Fig. E–74*B*(3) and 74*B*(4)].

Injuries to the gallbladder and bile ducts are so rare that they hardly need consideration here.

The kidney is often involved by fracture or subcapsular hematoma, particularly when there is a rapid deceleration during traffic accidents, a fall from great heights, direct contusion, projectile injury, fractures of the lower ribs, and fractures of the transverse processes of vertebral bodies. Projectile injury of the kidney may result in a mortality as high as 50%. Excretory urograms are particularly helpful if computed tomography is not available, since they show diminished function on the injured side. Retrograde pyelograms offer some information of actual damage, but renal angiography with catheterization of the renal artery may be necessary for exact description of the nature of the injury. Of equal importance in excretory urography is the demonstration of the degree of functioning of the opposite kidney, since removal of the injured kidney, if required, will necessitate dependence of the patient on the opposite "good" kidney.

As already indicated, it is important, in the case of the urinary bladder and urethra, to determine whether the injury is intraperitoneal or extraperitoneal. Sequentially, the radiologic investigations, apart from an anteroposterior view of the abdomen, are excretory urography, cytography, transurethral or suprapubic catheterization, and urethrocystography.

Injuries to the uterus, oviducts, or ovaries are rare. Radiologically, only mild signs of intraperitoneal hemorrhage result, except when the uterus is pregnant, in which case massive hemorrhage may occur.

Traumatic rupture of the large arteries or veins of the abdomen usually results in rapid death.

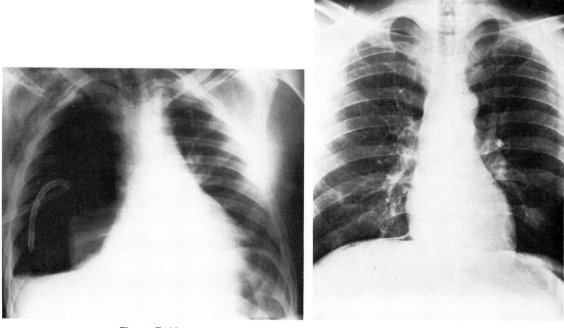

Figure E–90.

Figure E–91.

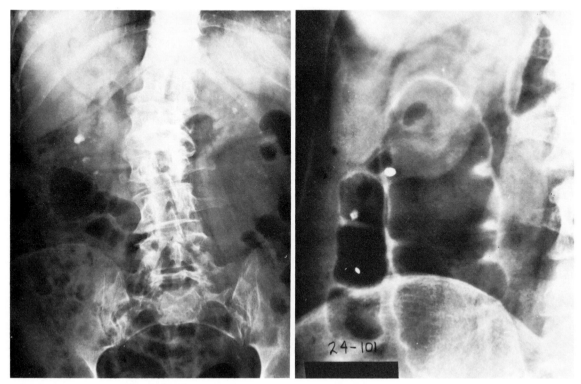

Figure E–92.

Figure E–93.

CLINICAL HISTORIES

Case 26–1 (Fig. E–90). Auto accident in which the right side of the chest sustained a very severe blow. A fragment of glass had penetrated the chest but had been removed at the time of surgery, when the intrapleural drainage tube was inserted. An anteroposterior view of the chest (above) was obtained thereafter.

Case 26–2 (Fig. E–91). Postero-anterior projection of the chest obtained in the emergency room after the patient arrived there having been awakened at night with severe diffuse abdominal pain.

Case 26–3 (Fig. E–92). The abdominal film shown is that of a patient who had experienced intermittent episodes of upper abdominal colic over a period of years, but arrived in the emergency room after a much more severe attack of upper abdominal pain, nausea and vomiting.

Cases 26–4 (Fig. E–93). The portion of the abdominal film shown is that of a patient who was undergoing sigmoidoscopy, when he experienced a severe attack of abdominal pain.

Questions

26–1. In Case 26–1, which is the MOST likely diagnosis?
A. Traumatic pneumothorax due to penetration of the lung by the fragment of glass.
B. Pneumothorax due to a fractured rib.
C. Tear of the right main stem bronchus by the glass fragment, giving rise to the pneumothorax.
D. Persistent pneumothorax after thoracotomy due to the surgery.
E. Pneumothorax persisting because of poor placement of the intrapleural drainage tube.

26–2. In Case 26–2, what is the MOST likely diagnosis?:
A. Acute coronary thrombosis.
B. Ruptured hollow viscus in the abdomen.
C. Acute biliary colic, with a gallstone ruptured out of the gallbladder.
D. Superior mesenteric thrombosis with infarcted small bowel.
E. Passage of a ureteral stone with associated tear of the ureter.

26–3. In Case 26–3, the MOST likely diagnosis is?
A. Superior mesenteric thrombosis.
B. Acute biliary colic.
C. Acute pancreatitis.
D. Rupture of a hollow viscus, probably from an upper gastrointestinal ulcer.
E. Gallstone ruptured out of the biliary tract into the gastrointestinal tract.

26–4. In Case 26–4, what is the MOST likely diagnosis?
A. Superior mesenteric thrombosis.
B. Pneumocystis intestinalis.
C. Acute biliary colic.
D. Rupture of a hollow viscus.
E. Acute pancreatitis.

Radiologic Findings. In Figure E–90 (Case 26–1), the predominant finding is the marked radiopacity of the right hemithorax with no associated pulmonary markings to suggest the presence of lung substance. In the right cardiophrenic angle there is a dense, sharply circumscribed triangular shadow fitting into this angle and separate from the cardiopericardial silhouette. There is a coiled pleural intrapleural drainage tube in situ at the right lung base. The optimum position for the uppermost end of the intrapleural tube would be higher in the chest, adjoining the posterior margin of approximately the third rib but it is not very likely that the pleural drainage tube is contributing significantly to the appearance of this chest radiograph. The mediastinum is shifted slightly to the left and the pulmonary shadows in the left lung are well within normal limits. There is no associated rib fracture.

In Case 26–2, the most remarkable roentgen finding in this postero-anterior view of the chest is evidence of free air under the right hemidiaphragm. Although it is a very small semilunate shadow of air, it is important to recognize that it contains no haustrations and does not contain the typical herringbone pattern of intramuscular air which would occur if the air were within the diaphragmatic substance proper. There is apparently no indication that the air is arising from other than the abdominal cavity. On close inspection, there is also free air beneath the left hemidiaphragm.

In Figure E–91 (Case 26–3), there is arborization of tubular free air in the distribution of the biliary tract. Moreover, *in the right upper quadrant, in the position of the gallbladder there are clusters of small and large gallstones,* faintly but partially calcified. There is evidence also of a small bowel reflex ileus. There is no indication of a colon "cut-off" sign. There is no indication of fat necrosis by the "bubbly" appearance often accompanying necrotizing pancreatitis; and there is no indication of loculated free air, such as might occur within the lesser omental bursa.

In Case 26–4, the predominant roentgen sign is the so-called "double wall sign," which indicates that there is air within the bowel substance proper and outside the wall of the large intestine resulting from free air within the abdomen. There is no indication of minimal bubbling or streaking, which is intramural in the wall of the bowel, such as occurs with pneumocystis intestinalis. There is no indication of a colon cut-off sign of reflex ileus, which is characteristic of a superior mesenteric thrombosis. And there is no indication of the bubbly appearance associated with necrotizing pancreatitis or of an increased width of the transverse mesocolon to suggest an infiltrative process in this structure arising from the pancreas or extending from the transverse colon to the pancreas.

Discussion. In Case 26–1, the marked shift of the mediastinum, flattening of the right hemidiaphragm, and collapse of the right lung into the right cardiophrenic angle are pathognomonic of a **tear of the right main stem bronchus by the glass fragment, giving rise to the pneumothorax (C).** The absence of a fractured rib, the shift of the mediastinum toward the left, and the growing pneumothorax, as indicated by the shift of the mediastinum, would suggest that the intrapleural drainage tube is not keeping pace with the amount of free air in the right hemithorax due to a free communication between the right main stem bronchus or part thereof and the intrapleural space.

In Case 26–2, the appearance is characteristic of a **ruptured hollow viscus in the abdomen (B).** The air is small in quantity but definitely does not contain haustrations to suggest an interposition of bowel between the liver and the diaphragm; nor is there a herringbone appearance of the air to suggest that the air is contained within the diaphragm musculature proper. There is no indication of free air in the biliary tree; and there are none of the roentgen signs associated with superior mesenteric thrombosis, such as: a) the colon cut-off sign; b) ileus of the small bowel as well as the proximal half of the large intestine; and c) swelling of the valves of Kerkring of the small intestine due to infarcted small bowel. Moreover there is no indication on the present chest x-ray that a communication with the outside could have occurred to account for free air beneath the right hemidiaphragm. When a ureteral stone passes down the ureter and tears the ureter, there is no release of free air unless a ureteral catheter has been introduced and the free air comes from outside the abdomen.

In Case 26–3, the most likely diagnosis is **gallstone ruptured out of the biliary tract into the gastrointestinal tract (E).** This is indicated by the free air projected over the tubular structures in the right lobe of the liver (biliary tract) and the faint but definitely visualized gallstones, which are partially calcified, in the region of the gallbladder bed. These patients will classically rupture into the gastrointestinal tract, and slowly the gallstone will move down the gastrointestinal tract, causing intermittent episodes of obstruction and colic. The gallbladder may accrete substance as it moves down the gastrointestinal tract, being too large to pass through the ileocecal valve, at which time mechanical obstruction will be observed. Unless a hollow viscus ruptured directly into the biliary tract, it would not give rise to this appearance. Superior mesenteric thrombosis and acute biliary colic alone would not account for the free air in the biliary passages, unless there was a communication between the pneumocystis intestinalis, which sometimes accompanies superior mesenteric thrombosis with the biliary passageways.

In Case 26–4, the most likely diagnosis is a **rupture of a hollow viscus with the so-called "double wall sign".** This sign indicates that there is air on the inside of the gastrointestinal tract as well as on its outside, delineating the serosa of the bowel very clearly. There is no indication of the bubbly or stripelike appearance of intramural air, such as accompanies pneumocystis intestinalis; and the findings in relation to superior mesenteric thrombosis or acute pancreatitis, as described above, are not present. This patient therefore sustained rupture of a hollow viscus during the course of the sigmoidoscopy.

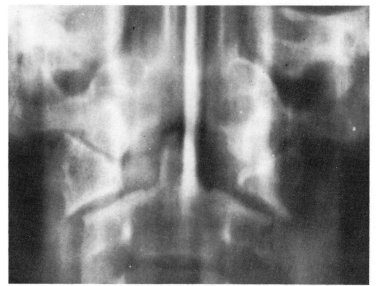

Figure E–94.

Figure E–95.

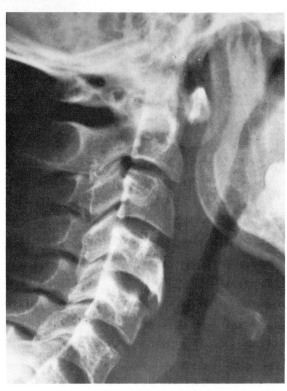

CLINICAL HISTORIES

Case 27–1. Figure E–94 is that of a patient who fell directly onto the vertex of his head, with his body straight at the time of the fall. A tomogram of C-1 is shown.

Case 27–2. Figure E–95 is that of a patient who complained of pain in the neck following a severe inflammatory process involving his throat, after which he held his neck rigidly forward.

Case 27–3. Figures E–96A and B are anteroposterior and lateral views of the cervical spine of a patient who sustained a fall directly on his head from a height of approximately 20 feet.

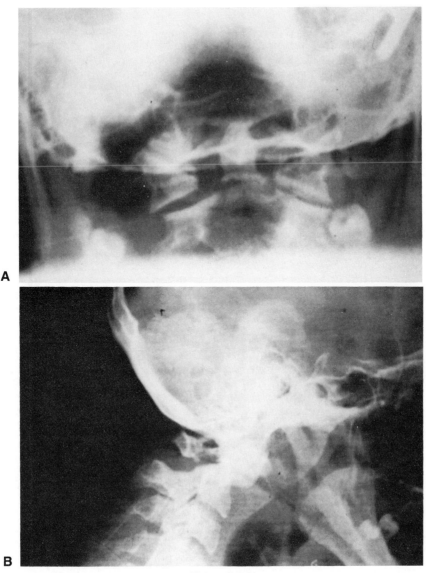

A

B

Figure E–96.

Questions

27–1. With regard to Figure E–94, which is the MOST likely diagnosis?
  A. Dislocation of the first cervical segment in respect to the second.
  B. Hangman's fracture.
  C. Dislocation of the first cervical segment with respect to the occipital condyles.
  D. Jefferson's fracture.
  E. Fracture of the dens.

27–2. With regard to Figure E–95, which is the MOST likely diagnosis?
  A. Congenital failure of ossification of the dens.
  B. Persistent terminal ossicle of the dens.

  C. Tear of the annular ligament posterior to the dens.
  D. Rheumatoid arthritis affecting the dens.
  E. Partial resorption of the dens following pharyngeal inflammation.

27–3. With regard to Figures E–96A and B, which is the MOST likely diagnosis?
  A. Failure of ossification at the base of the dens.
  B. Fracture at the base of the dens.
  C. Fracture of the dens and a "bursting" fracture of the neural arch of C-1.
  D. Normal variant.
  E. Os odontoideum.

175

Radiologic Findings. In Figure E–94 there is an overhang of the lateral masses of C-1 with respect to the lateral masses of C-2 bilaterally. Ordinarily, a straight line may be drawn vertically to marginate the outer margin of the lateral masses of both of these vertebrae, both on the outer aspect and the inner aspect. Ordinarily, the lateral masses of C-1 are equidistant from the odontoid process on both sides. (See Discussion.)

In Figure E–95, there is some resorption of the odontoid process anteriorly, with considerable soft tissue swelling of the nasopharynx and oropharynx. The atlantoaxial distance would appear to be increased. However, close inspection shows this to be due to the resorption of the anterior cortex of the dens, in that it appears irregular and its dense compact cortex is virtually lacking. The alignment of all of the vertebral bodies is otherwise intact and normal. The intervertebral joints appear well preserved with no indication of arthritis. (There is a degenerative bridging anteriorly between C-4 and C-5 due to localized cervical spondylosis.)

Figures E–95A and B are open-mouth views of the odontoid process, and lateral views of the upper cervical spine, respectively, with a sharp discontinuity shown at the base of the odontoid process; and an angulation of the dens with respect to the main body of C-2 vertebra. There is a line of separation at the base of the dens that is somewhat irregular and ragged. Incidentally, there is an overhang of the lateral mass on the right with respect to C-2.

Discussion. The correct answer for Case 27–1 (Fig. E–94) is **Jefferson's fracture.** The classic appearance of a Jefferson's fracture is the overhang of the lateral masses of C-1 with respect to C-2 in frontal perspective. One must, however, be very careful that a straight anteroposterior view is obtained. If not, with the slightest bending of the head to either side, a slight overhang of the side to which the head bends may occur normally. A hangman's fracture is a fracture through the pedicles of the second cervical segment, best visualized in the lateral view. There is dislocation of the first cervical segment in respect to the second in the region of its lateral masses due to the "bursting" type injury of the neural arch of C-1, and the dislocation is not the primary abnormality visualized. There is no indication of dislocation of the first cervical segment with respect to the occipital condyles. The tomogram shows us clearly that there is a trabecular continuity between the odontoid process and the remainder of the body of C-2, and, hence, there is no fracture of the dens.

With regard to Case 27–2 (Fig. E–95), the correct answer is **partial resorption of the dens following pharyngeal inflammation.** The resorption of the anterior margin of the odontoid process has been described, and the widening of the soft tissues in the oropharynx and nasopharynx residual from the inflammatory process of this region has been described in the clinical history. Although the atlantoaxial distance is greater than 5 mm, it is largely due to the resorption of the anterior cortex of the dens rather than to a tear of the annular ligament surrounding the dens posteriorly. This resorption is probably secondary to a synovitis caused by the pharyngitis.

There is no indication of congenital failure of ossification of the dens, which is usually manifested by an angulated resorption near the base of the dens. As indicated above, there is no indication of a tear of the annular ligament posterior to the dens, since the alignment of the cervical segments is perfectly normal. There is no indication of rheumatoid arthritis in any of the joints of the cervical spine and no associated osteoporosis to suggest its presence.

The correct answer to Case 27–3 (Figs. E–96A and B) is **fracture at the base of the dens and a Jefferson's fracture as well.** ("Bursting" fracture of C-1 is synonymous with a Jefferson's fracture.) The irregular line of radiolucency with no cortication at the margin of the lucency is pathognomonic of this finding even without associated subluxation. As indicated, when a pseudarthrosis occurs, there is increased cortication and sclerosis at the fracture margin. A pseudofracture of the dens is an appearance caused by the overlapping of certain structures over the odontoid process, such as the tongue, the posterior arch of the atlas, the upper border of the laminae of the axis, the teeth, and the remnant of the subdental synchondrosis. Although it is important to be alert to these various artefactual possibilities, there would be no suspicion in this case. The pathognomonic findings in this instance are the outright fracture at the base of the dens, the abnormal angulation in the lateral perspective of the dens with respect to the remaining portion of the body of C-2, and the overhang of the lateral mass of C-1 with respect to C-2, especially on its right aspect.

The possibility of os odontoideum was mentioned (Figs. E–97A and B). Two major types of this anomaly are due to a congenital malformation: 1) the *orthotopic* os odontoideum, which lies near the tip of the upper anterior aspect of the body of the dens and remains in this location irrespective of movement, and 2) a *dystopic* os odontoideum, which lies near the basion and may be inseparable from the basiocciput, as was the case in this patient when flexion was attempted (Fig. E–97C). This entity is not to be confused with absence or aplasia of the dens, which is an extremely rare anomaly; before making such a diagnosis, tomography should be employed to be certain that the diagnosis is not actually os odontoideum of one or the other types.

Other confusing appearances in C-1 are shown in Figures E–97C and D.

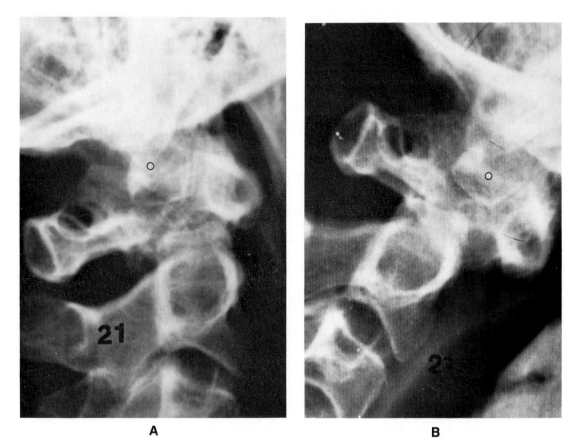

A   B

Figure E–97. Os odontoideum—not to be confused with a fracture.

Illustration continued on following page

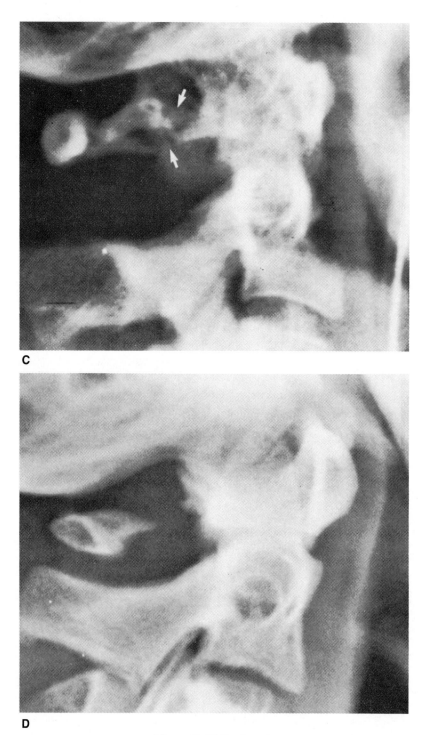

C

D

Figure E–97 *Continued.*

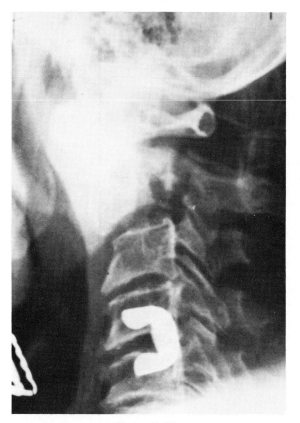

Figure E–98.

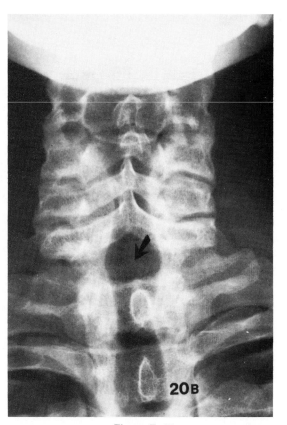

Figure E–99.

CLINICAL HISTORIES

Case 28–1 (Fig. E–98). This 52-year-old male sustained a severe hyperflexion injury of the cervical spine. Unfortunately, he died almost immediately. The above described lateral film of the cervical spine was obtained postmortem in an effort to explain what might have happened.

Case 28–2 (Fig. E–99). This is an anteroposterior radiograph of a patient who sustained a severe hyperextension injury of the cervical spine. (The arrow is shown to aid in assessing the diagnosis.)

Questions

28–1. In Case 28–1 (Fig. E–98), which of the following diagnoses is MOST likely to be accurate to explain the radiologic and clinical findings?
A. Jefferson's fracture.
B. A severe hyperflexion injury known as the "hangman's fracture."
C. Simple fracture of the neural arch of the second cervical segment.
D. A "bursting fracture" involving the second cervical segment.
E. A "teardrop fracture" of the second cervical segment.

28–2. In Case 28–2 (Fig. E–99), which of the following diagnoses is MOST accurate?
A. "Clay-shoveler's" fracture.
B. Disruption of the intervertebral disc between C-7 and T-1.
C. Compression fracture of C-7 vertebral body.
D. "Teardrop" fracture of C-7.
E. Subluxation of C-7 facets with respect to T-1 facets.

Radiologic Findings. A fracture is detected through the neural arch of the second cervical segment in Figure E–98. There is wide separation of the fragments. There is marked displacement anteriorly of C-2 with respect to C-3.

Figure E–99 is one of a series of films, and the black arrow demonstrates a rather ovoid "empty space" between the seventh cervical segment and the first thoracic segment (as indicated by the visualized inverse inclination of the transverse processes at this junctional level). It would almost appear that a spinous process is missing at the point of the arrow.

Discussion. The correct answer to Case 28–1 (Fig. E–98), is **severe hyperflexion of the second cervical segment with marked dislocation of C-2 body anteriorly,** known as the "hangman's fracture."

In *Hangman's fracture* not only is there a fracture of the neural arch of C-2 in the pedicular area as noted but also there is a tear of the annular ligament and a sufficient posterior displacement of the atlas at the moment of tear, as well as a backward displacement of the odontoid process into the neural canal to crush the spinal cord and produce a severe hemorrhage at the base of the brain surrounding the vital centers of the medulla.

A simple fracture of the neural arch of C-2, unless accompanied by these several other elements, which are not necessarily radiologically visible, is usually not particularly severe because of the large capacity of the spinal canal at this level, and because there is no associated dislocation of the apophyseal joints. There may even be a *slight* displacement of the body of the second cervical segment in some instances and still the neurologic deficit may not be conclusively severe. If there is a simple fracture of the neural arch of the second cervical segment, and if there is also a severe neurologic deficit but no injury in conjunction with the annular ligament surrounding the dens, one must look for a fracture-

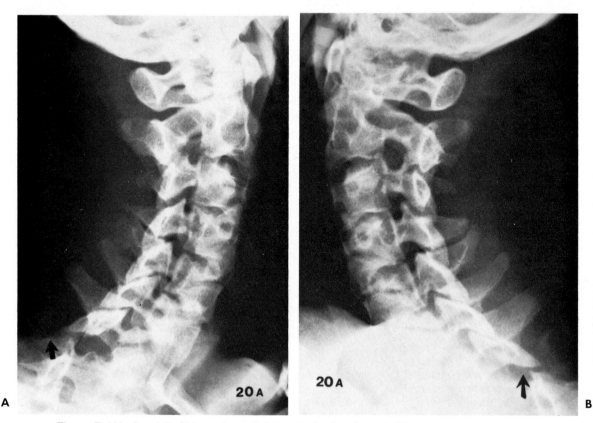

A   B

Figure E–100. *A* and *B*, Oblique views of the cervical spine shown in Figure E–99. Arrows point to the subluxation of the articular facets of C–7 and T–1.

dislocation at a lower level in the cervical spine, which was not present in this case.

Figure E–99 is a **bilateral subluxation of the facets of C-7 with respect to the superior articular facets of T-1.** This figure is virtually pathognomonic of bilateral subluxation of the inferior articular facets of the seventh cervical segment with respect to the superior articular facets of the first thoracic vertebra (Fig. E–100A and B). There may be some disruption of the posterior ligamentous structures and there may indeed be varying degrees of damage to the intervertebral discs or end-plates, but the prime injury is related morphologically to the bilateral subluxation. Ordinarily, this latter type injury responds rather readily to manipulative maneuvers; but if not, skeletal traction will usually correct it. The typical deformity in such patients is that the chin is in the midline but the patient is unable to rotate the head to either the right or left, and one can palpate a prominence of the spinous process of the first thoracic segment.

Subluxation of the facets of C-7 with respect to T-1 is best demonstrated in the right posterior oblique and left posterior oblique views, as shown in Figures E–100A and B, respectively. It should be remembered that these patients do not rotate the head, and under these circumstances it is extremely important that the oblique views be properly obtained by rotating the entire body 45 degrees to the right for the right posterior oblique, and 45 degrees to the left for the left posterior oblique. The right posterior oblique film will demonstrate the left-sided facets best; the left posterior oblique will demonstrate the right-sided facets best.

Although an intervertebral disc injury may accompany this bilateral subluxation, and it may indeed be best demonstrated by computed tomography, it is probably not the paramount injury to be corrected upon first recognition.

A "teardrop" fracture of the cervical spine is often accompanied by a subluxation of the vertebral body. It is produced by very severe hyperflexion and compression forces while the cervical spine is slightly flexed. The vertebral body involved is comminuted, and an anterior portion of the body, usually triangular in shape, is extruded anteriorly, while the posterior inferior part of the body may be driven posteriorly toward the spinal canal. If the latter occurs, the cord is compressed or very severely injured. The main component morphologically as

Table 6–1 CERVICAL SPINE INJURIES: MECHANISM OF INJURY*

A. Flexion
   1. Anterior subluxation
   2. Bilateral interfacetal dislocation
   3. Simple wedge fracture
   4. Clay-shoveler's fracture
   5. Flexion tear-drop fracture
B. Flexion-rotation
   1. Unilateral interfacetal dislocation
C. Extension-rotation
   1. Pillar fracture
D. Vertical compression
   1. Bursting fracture
     (a) Jefferson fracture of atlas
     (b) Burst fracture, lower cervical vertebrae
E. Extension
   1. Extension tear-drop fracture
   2. Posterior neural arch fracture, atlas
   3. Hangman's fracture (deceleration, hyperextension)
   4. Hyperextension fracture-dislocation

*From Harris, J. H., Jr.: The Radiology of Acute Cervical Spine Trauma. Baltimore, Williams & Wilkins Co., 1978.

Table 6–2 CERVICAL SPINE INJURIES: DEGREE OF STABILITY*

A. Stable
   1. Anterior subluxation
   2. Unilateral interfacetal dislocation
   3. Simple wedge fracture
   4. Burst fracture, lower cervical vertebrae
   5. Posterior neural arch fracture, atlas
   6. Pillar fracture
   7. Clay-shoveler's fracture
B. Unstable
   1. Bilateral interfacetal dislocation
   2. Flexion tear-drop fracture
   3. Extension tear-drop fracture (stable in flexion, unstable in extension)
   4. Hangman's fracture
   5. Jefferson fracture of atlas
   6. Hyperextension fracture-dislocation

*From Harris, J. H., Jr.: The Radiology of Acute Cervical Spine Trauma. Baltimore, Williams & Wilkins Co., 1978.

seen radiologically may be just the anterior fragment displaced forward with the posterior fragment displacement toward the neural canal being somewhat obscure. Very often the intervertebral disc is also very severely disrupted in this injury and may extrude into the vertebral body, best demonstrated by computed tomography.

A "clay-shoveler's" fracture is an avulsion fracture of the spinous process of C-6, C-7, or T1 and often a rupture of the interspinous ligament between them (Fig. E–100), depending on the extent of the *hyperflexion* injury. The clay-shoveler's fracture is stable.

Useful information for reference in respect to acute injuries of the cervical spine is given in Tables 6–1 and 6–2.

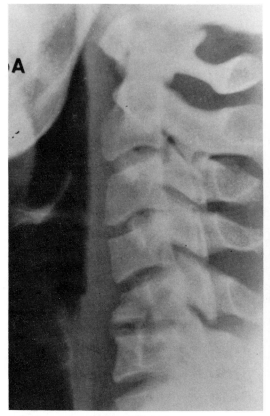

Figure E–101.

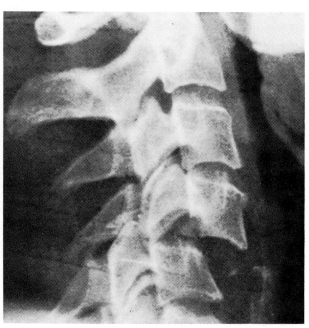

Figure E–102.

CLINICAL HISTORIES

Case 29–1. The lateral cervical spine illustrated in Figure E–101 was that of a patient who sustained a severe hyperextension and compression of his neck while apparently his neck was slightly extended.

Case 29–2. The lateral cervical spine illustrated in Figure E–102 was that of a patient who had evidence of violence on his face and forehead and apparently had sustained a severe hyperextension, compression and rotatory force applied to his head and face. (From Rogers, L. F.: Radiology of Skeletal Trauma, Vol. 11. New York, Churchill-Livingstone, 1982.)

Questions

29–1. In Case 29–1, Figure E–101, what is the MOST proper name for this injury?
A. Bursting fracture.
B. Teardrop fracture-dislocation.
C. Hyperextension fracture.
D. Posterior fracture-dislocation.
E. Rotary fracture-dislocation.

29–2. In Case 29–2, Figure E–102, what is the MOST proper name for this injury?
A. Posterior dislocation following intervertebral disc detachment.
B. Teardrop fracture-dislocation.
C. Hyperextension fracture-dislocation.
D. Posterior dislocation-fracture with "locked facets."
E. Rotary fracture-dislocation.

Radiologic Findings. In Figure E–101 there is an anterior avulsed fragment of C-5 pulled forward and a backward displacement of the posterior portion of the vertebral body. There is most likely a subluxation of the articular processes, with a disruption of the normal alignments of the segments at this level. We might postulate a disruption of the anterior ligament and a rupture of the intervertebral disc through the fractured inferior articular end-plate.

In Figure E–102, there is a fracture-dislocation of the apophyseal joints, probably bilaterally, and most likely a torn anterior longitudinal ligament. The body of C-4 is markedly anterior to the body of C-5, and there is an associated fracture from the inferior posterior margin of the vertebral body and bilateral locking of the facets. The inferior articular facets appear to have dislocated over and anterior to the superior articular facets of C-5.

Discussion. The correct answer to Case 29–1, Figure E–101, is **teardrop fracture-dislocation.** This injury is produced by a severe hyperextension compression force on the neck while it is still slightly extended, as was the case in this instance. Usually, the anterior ligament ruptures and avulses a large triangular fragment of the vertebral body and this segment is pulled forward and downward. Usually also, the intervertebral disc ruptures and extrudes through the fractures in the inferior end-plate of the vertebra involved, lying between its fragments. The posterior fragment is displaced backward, as was the case in this instance, and the posterior articulations may subluxate or even fracture, although this is not readily apparent in this instance.

By contrast, a bursting fracture of the cervical spine is produced by a severe compression force transmitted directly along the lines of the vertebral body while the cervical spine is held straight. Usually, in a bursting fracture there is a force applied directly to the vertex of the skull and directed caudally. Under these circumstances, both the anterior and posterior bony elements of the vertebral body are crushed. This force is sufficient usually to disrupt both articular end-plates of the vertebral body while the anterior and posterior ligamentous structures remain intact. With this type of injury a bone fragment frequently extrudes posteriorly, damaging the spinal cord and producing a tetraplegia.

In a hyperextension fracture usually in the presence of degenerative spurs, the ligamentum flavum bulges into the spinal canal, reducing its anteroposterior diameter, and resulting in a pinched cord. The radiograph may actually fail to show any fracture or dislocation of the vertebrae. However, the contents of the intervertebral foramina are crowded and the nerve roots are compressed. Usually, one observes osteophytes surrounding the foramina.

In a posterior fracture-dislocation of the cervical spine there is usually a unilateral or bilateral fracture-dislocation of the apophyseal joints and they appear to have dislocated over one another. This is the significant difference between Figures E–101 and E–102, where the correct answer is **posterior dislocation-fracture with locked facets.** In the latter instance, the intervertebral disc is torn from its attachment, usually from the involved vertebra, and the body of the vertebra caudad is displaced posteriorly. This is, of course, a serious injury often accompanied by neurologic damage and is unstable.

By contrast with the above, a rotary hyperextension fracture-dislocation results from a rotary force added to hyperextension compression forces such as being struck on the side of the skull. The forces are expended on the posterior bony elements on the side opposite to that to which the force was applied. The lesion usually occurs in the region of C-4, C-5, and C-6. Very often with a rotary hyperextension fracture-dislocation, the inferior articular process is fractured and displaced upward, outward and backward, and the body of the vertebra is displaced slightly forward. The fractured facet may often injure the cord, thus producing unilateral neurological damage. Neither of these cases exemplified this kind of injury.

7

Trauma to the Extremities

A method of roentgen analysis of bones is indicated in Figure 7–1. This routine of study—a systematic evaluation of the soft tissues, periosteum, compact cortex, medullary portion of bone, the joints, the alignments of fragments, the appropriate modeling of the bone, and the overall density—is applicable not only in cases of trauma but also in metabolic and other bone disease. The following salient features should be recognized:

1. Every suspected extremity being evaluated for trauma must be examined in at least anteroposterior and lateral views and, if possible, oblique views as well.
2. The technique should allow evaluation of the soft tissues as well as bones.
3. If an opaque foreign body is suspected,

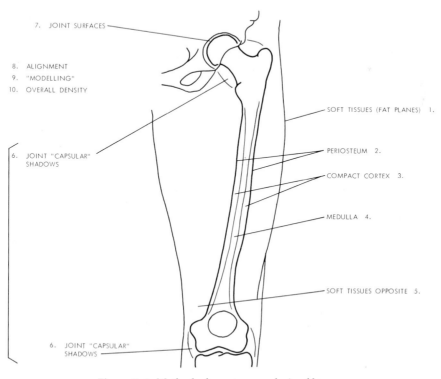

7. JOINT SURFACES

8. ALIGNMENT
9. "MODELLING"
10. OVERALL DENSITY

SOFT TISSUES (FAT PLANES) 1.

PERIOSTEUM 2.

6. JOINT "CAPSULAR" SHADOWS

COMPACT CORTEX 3.

MEDULLA 4.

SOFT TISSUES OPPOSITE 5.

6. JOINT "CAPSULAR" SHADOWS

Figure 7–1. Method of roentgen analysis of bones.

no-screen technique should be employed rather than cassettes, if the body part is not too thick.

4. In every view of an extremity, at least one joint is included, so that the apposition of fragments and alignment with respect to the joint and its appropriate biologic purpose can be adequately diagnosed.

5. Comparison studies of two comparable sides of the body should be obtained when appropriate, particularly in children, in whom epiphyseal plates and variations of normal will produce confusing appearances.

6. A complete history of the type of trauma and the physical examination with regard to the point of tenderness is most important with regard to the examination undertaken.

7. The major items for analysis of radiographs of extremities for fractures should include (a) the degree of apposition of fragments; (b) the alignment of the fragments with respect to lines of weight-bearing or movement of joints; (c) the degree of torsion of the fragments with respect to one another; and (d) the degree of shortening of the bone as a whole, which may result.

8. With regard to the soft tissues; only inferential information can be diagnosed. An evaluation should be made, if possible, regarding whether soft tissue is "caught" between the fragments, whether there is associated soft tissue injury, and how much cartilaginous or joint injury has been sustained. Some of this information obviously is not available from the radiograph, but must be carefully inferred from the history and physical findings.

9. The time intervals between the radiographic studies should minimally be the following: (a) the initial diagnostic study for diagnosis; (b) post-reduction and post-immobilization study; (c) films obtained 1 or 2 weeks later to determine whether the appropriate position has been maintained; (d) a film in approximately 6 to 8 weeks to determine whether a primary callus is occurring (primary callus is calcification in the hematoma adjoining the periosteum and bone); (e) after each plaster cast or traction change; (f) before final discharge of the patient.

10. If an injury has been sustained, or if pain persists, and no fracture is diagnosed, it is best to wait a week or two and re-examine the patient. Not infrequently a nonvisualized fracture becomes visualized after this interval because of bone resorption surrounding the fracture site.

11. Injury to major vessels is most important to exclude, and careful treatment must be given at the outset to avoid potential complications. Indeed, if a part has been amputated by the trauma and the patient has the wisdom to place the amputated part in a freezer or dry ice and bring it with him to the emergency room, a grafting procedure may be possible.

12. If vascular abnormality is strongly suspected, angiography should be performed following the injury. If such pathologic entities as arteriovenous fistulas are recognized early, systemic effects may be prevented.

13. Arthrograms are seldom performed in the acute phase following an injury for fear of introducing infection. However, arthrograms yield extremely important information regarding the status of cartilage, especially in the knee, the shoulder, the elbow, and occasionally in other joints to a lesser degree. In the case of the knee, the arthrogram is especially helpful in analysis of internal derangement in a very accurate fashion.

14. The information that must be thoroughly understood following the radiologic examination includes (a) the exact bones involved; (b) the type of fracture (Fig. 7–2); (c) the degree of apposition of the fragments as previously indicated; (d) the alignment of fragments with respect to weight-bearing or the joint action immediately adjoining the bones involved.

DEFINITION OF TYPES OF FRACTURES

The various types of fractures are summarized in Figure 7–2. *Avulsion-* or chip-type fractures are often associated with forcible tearing of the ligaments, tendons, or muscle attachments. The soft tissue injury is the most serious aspect of this type of fracture. In *oblique, spiral,* or *screwlike* fractures, soft tissue may be interposed between the fragments. These fractures are often accompanied by contrecoup fractures in an adjoin-

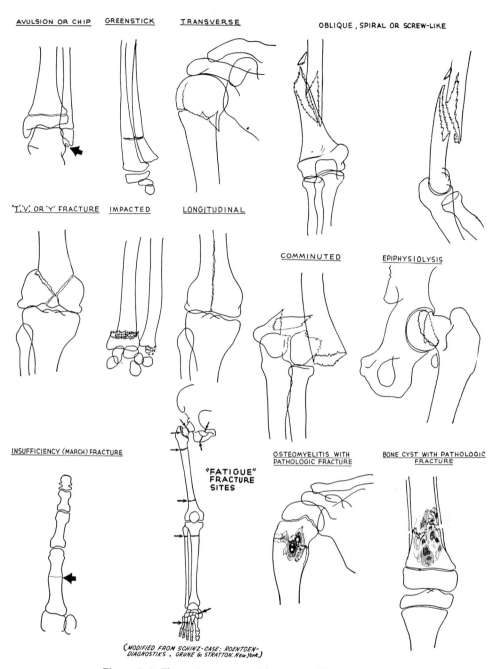

Figure 7–2. The various types of fractures of the extremities.

ing bone, such as the fibula in respect to the tibia. The examination must be sufficiently inclusive to make such diagnoses possible. If interposition of soft tissues has occurred, impairment of the healing process is very likely to ensue. *Insufficiency*, march, or stress fractures are also called "fatigue" fractures, since they practically always occur at sites of maximal strain on bone, usually in connec-

tion with a type of unaccustomed activity. The second, third, or fourth metatarsals are frequent sites for this type of fracture without any specific demonstrable trauma. Another frequent localization is the upper third of the tibia. Almost any weight-bearing bone, however, may be involved. *Pathologic* fractures may occur through a site of osteomyelitis or tumor involvement, and healing under these

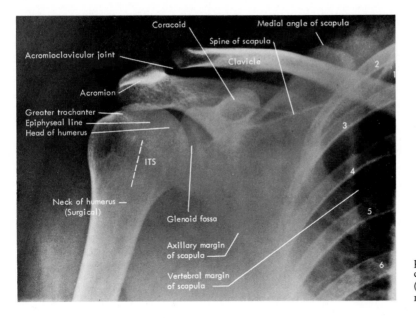

Figure 7–3. Neutral antero-posterior projection of the shoulder. (ITS) intertubercular sulcus. (The right shoulder is *viewed* in this manner also.)

Figure 7–4. Axial relationships of the wrist.

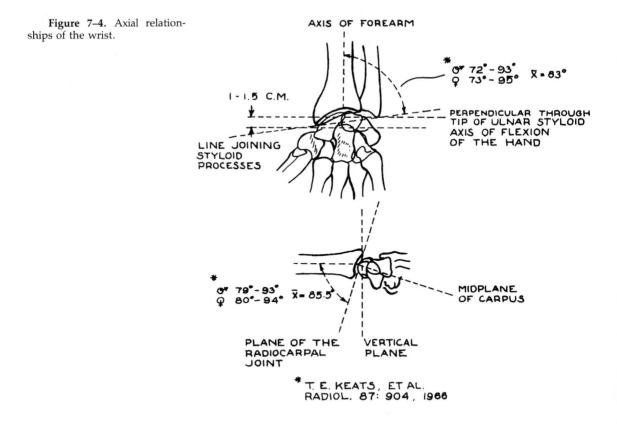

circumstances may be considerably protracted unless the underlying disease is also corrected.

FRACTURES OF THE UPPER EXTREMITY

With regard to the shoulder, the most common dislocation is the subcoracoid variety, and this is readily recognized on an anteroposterior projection. Avulsion of the greater tuberosity of the humerus may occur, however, without dislocation. Habitual dislocation of the shoulder is recognized especially by two roentgen signs: (1) an increased concavity on the superior aspect of the greater tuberosity and head of humerus (Fig. E–103), and (2) a concavity in the region of the inferior margin of the glenoid process. A film of the shoulder area should always be obtained after reduction of dislocation. The articular margin of the glenoid is always parallel to the head of the humerus, and the humerus is intact in the region of its surgical and anatomical neck (Fig. 7–3).

Dislocation of the acromioclavicular joint requires special radiographic technique in the erect position with traction or weight-bearing in the erect position and comparative studies with the opposite side. As pointed out previously, associated fractures in the outer third of the clavicle usually require open reduction. Fractures of the shoulder should always be accompanied by an evaluation of vascular or nerve injuries in the upper extremity, in view of the proximity to the brachial plexus.

In the elbow region, when dislocation occurs it is usually posteriorly. Associated avulsion fracture of the coronoid process is frequent. If a fracture of the coronoid process is recognized, it may be deduced that very likely this was preceded by dislocation with spontaneous reduction. Fragmentation of the radial head should be analyzed very carefully since (a) it may escape detection readily, (b) there may be a bone fragment within the elbow joint proper which will require open reduction and orthopedic specialized care, and (c) elbow injuries frequently accompany wrist injuries. The annular ligament surrounding the head of the radius may also be torn and is indicated radiographically only by a separation of the radial head from its appropriate location in respect to the proximal ulna. Oblique studies of the elbow should be routine. Special radiography of the

elbow is required when the patient is unable to extend the forearm; no effort should be made to diagnose injuries of this area without obtaining first an anteroposterior view of the distal humerus and thereafter an anteroposterior view of the proximal forearm.

With regard to the forearm, when both bones are involved, it is probably an indication for open reduction, since involvement of the interosseous membrane may result in healing with bridging of the interosseous membrane; and this in turn will result in interference with pronation and supination. Impairment of this type may produce lifelong disability.

Before undertaking an analysis of wrist injuries, the appropriate relationships of the styloid process of the radius and ulna in anteroposterior and lateral views should always be understood (Fig. 7–4). It will be noted that the styloid process of the radius is distal to that of the ulna, usually by 1 to 1½ cm, and the dorsal aspect of the articular surface distance, the angulation being shown in Figure 7–4. As much as possible, reduction should restore this relationship except in the very old individual or perhaps in the very young, in whom restoration will spontaneously occur during the growth process.

Likewise, in the wrist it will be noted that there are basically three joint alignments: (1) that between the radius and scaphoid and lunate; (2) that between the proximal row of carpals and the distal row of carpals; and (3) that between the distal row of carpals and the bases of the metacarpals. The close relationship of the scaphoid and lunate also must be carefully studied, since *an increase in distance on the posteroanterior projection at this joint level may be the only radiologic indication of a rotary subluxation of the scaphoid carpal bone*, which may be very disabling. The most important injuries of the wrist joint may be enumerated as follows: (1) Colles' fracture *(Fig. 7–5A, B)*, in which the metaphysis of the radius is fractured as is the styloid of the ulna usually, and there is an anterior angulation at the fracture site producing the so-called "fork" deformity; (2) the Smith fracture *(Fig. 7–6A, B)*, in which the angulation is posterior, just opposite that of the Colles' fracture, and a "garden-spade" deformity is produced; (3) lunate dislocations, in which the lunate itself is luxated out of the wrist joint and which must be differentiated from (4) a perilunate dislocation, in which the lunate remains in articulation with the radius but the rest of the wrist is dislocated either

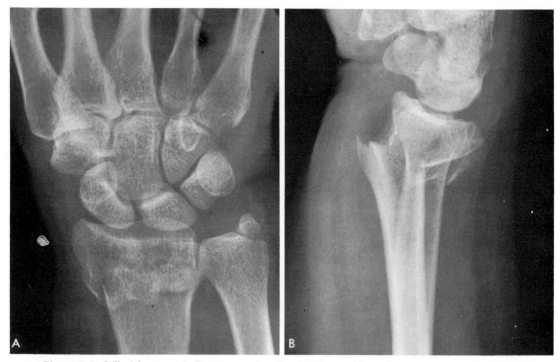

Figure 7–5. Colles' fracture. *A*, Posteroanterior view (courtesy of Dr. Allen Klein). *B*, Lateral view.

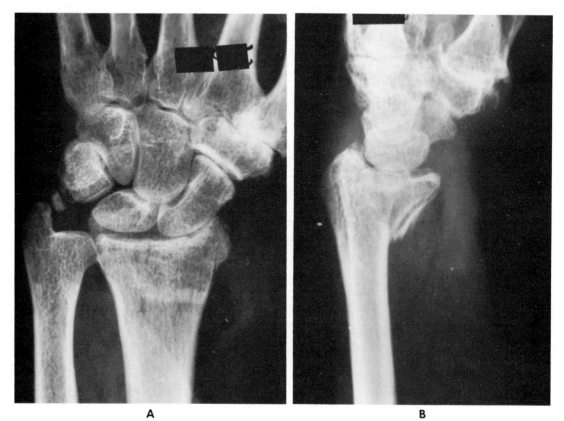

A   **B**

Figure 7–6. Radiographs illustrating the Smith fracture and the "spade" deformity. (Dorsal angulation at the fracture site.) *A*, Posteroanterior view; *B*, lateral view. (Courtesy of Dr. Allen Klein.)

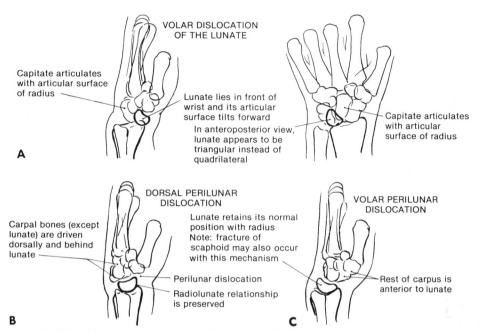

Figure 7–7. *A,* Volar dislocation of the lunate. *B,* Dorsal perilunar dislocation. *C,* Volar perilunar dislocation.

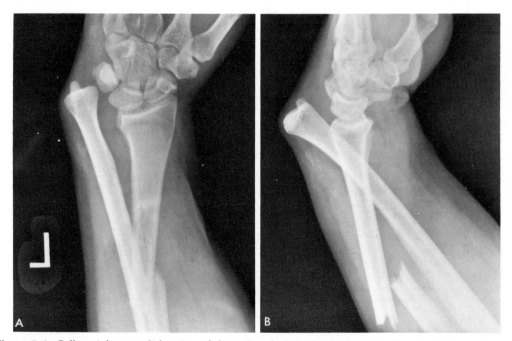

Figure 7–8. Galleazzi fracture-dislocation of the wrist. *A,* Anteroposterior view. *B,* Lateral view. (Courtesy of Dr. Allen Klein.)

Illustration continued on following page

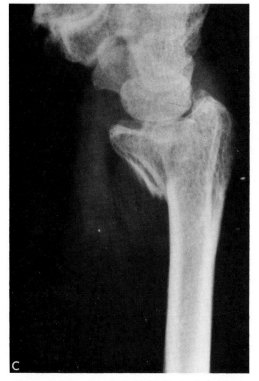

Figure 7–8 *Continued. C,* Volar Barton's fracture.

dorsally or anteriorly; dislocation may be anterior or posterior (Fig. 7–7A, B, C).

Other, less frequent, fractures of the wrist are the Galleazzi fracture (Fig. 7–8A, B), the Barton fracture (Fig. 7–8C) involving the posterior distal and dorsal margin of the radius, and the chauffeur's fracture involving a fracture of the radial styloid.

Fractures of the scaphoid bone may be divided in relation to the blood supply of this bone (Fig. 7–9). If the fracture occurs in that one-third of the bone which adjoins the wrist capsule, aseptic necrosis is far less apt to occur than if the fracture is in the inner third of this bone. A fracture occurring in the central one third of the scaphoid may or may not undergo aseptic necrosis, depending on the degree of impairment of its blood supply. A careful scrutiny of the wrist joint bones on radiographs of this area and special views of the scaphoid are frequently necessary to demonstrate fractures in this area.

Fracture-dislocations involving the first metacarpal and associated trapezium and trapezoid bones are known as Bennett's fractures, and these also must be carefully differentiated.

Text continued on page 210

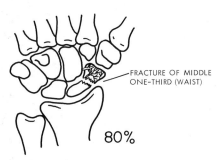

FRACTURE OF MIDDLE ONE-THIRD (WAIST)

80%

FRACTURE THROUGH THE WAIST (MIDDLE THIRD), MAY LEAD TO ASEPTIC NECROSIS PROXIMAL FRAGMENT

SOME OF THE ASSOCIATED INJURIES ARE:
   DISLOCATION OF RADIOCARPAL JOINT.
   DISLOCATION BETWEEN THE TWO ROWS OF CARPAL BONES.
   FRACTURE-DISLOCATION OF DISTAL END OF RADIUS.
   FRACTURE OF BASE OF THUMB METACARPAL (BENNETT'S FRACTURE).
   DISLOCATION OF LUNATE.

A

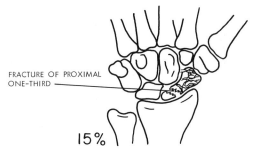

FRACTURE OF PROXIMAL ONE-THIRD

15%

FRACTURE THROUGH THE PROXIMAL THIRD

NOTE: THERE MAY BE ANY COMBINATION OF THESE AND OCCASIONALLY A SEGMENTAL FRACTURE OF SCAPHOID OCCURS

B

Figure 7–9. Classification of the most frequent fractures of the scaphoid carpal bone.

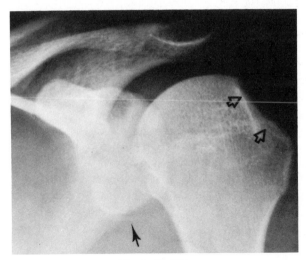

Figure E–103.

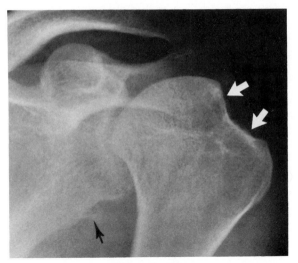

Figure E–104.

CLINICAL HISTORY

You are shown Figure E–103 and Figure E–104, which represent a similar shoulder injury.

Note the black arrows in both figures and the open arrow in Figure E–103.

Question

30–1. The MOST likely diagnosis that is applicable to both radiographs is:

A. Fracture of the neck of the glenoid process of the scapula?

B. Fracture of the neck of the glenoid and prior fractures of the greater tuberosity with resorption of same?

C. Chronic shoulder dislocation with "hatchet" deformities of both humeri?

D. Erosive changes of the humeri and the glenoid process due to recurring acute bursitis?

E. Previous shoulder cuff tear and Burkhart deformity of the glenoid due to prior dislocation.

Radiologic Findings. In both radiographs there is resorption of the superior aspect of the heads of the humeri with a concave appearance extending in toward the greater tuberosity of the humerus. The heads of the humeri are as a result deformed and somewhat flattened, demarcated by the open arrows in Figure E–103 but also present in Figure E–104.

The black arrows in each instance show evidence of avulsion and erosion of the inferior margin of the glenoid processes. In Figure E–103 there is also an ill-defined erosive change of the inferior margin of the glenoid process demarcated to some extent by zones of sclerosis.

Discussion. The correct diagnosis in this instance in both of these cases is **chronic dislocation** of the shoulder with shoulder cuff tear (and Burkhart deformity of the glenoid due to prior dislocation) and "hatchet" deformity of the head of the humerus (Hill-Sack's deformity).

The deformities indicated by the arrows are classic for this diagnosis.

The erosive changes along the inferior margin of the glenoid are well demonstrated in Figure E–103, and the periosteal elevation and calcification just below the inferior margin of the glenoid is representative of the cuff tear that has occurred in this location as the result of frequent dislocation and bony avulsion or proliferation. There is no indication of a fracture of the neck of the glenoid or a fracture of the greater tuberosity of the humerus. The erosive changes in the region of the superior aspect of the head of the humerus and the adjoining portion of the greater tuberosity are characteristic of cuff tear.

With acute bursitis one may or may not have peritendonous calcification or subacromial calcification with soft tissue swelling. One does not observe erosive changes in the bone as shown in these cases. With bursitis there may or may not be associated calcification.

Erosion of the humerus as well as the inferior margin of the glenoid is characteristic of chronic dislocation of the shoulder and represents more than a simple shoulder cuff tear.

EXERCISE

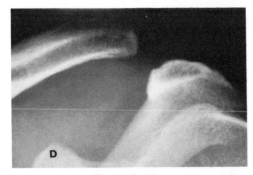

Figure E–105.

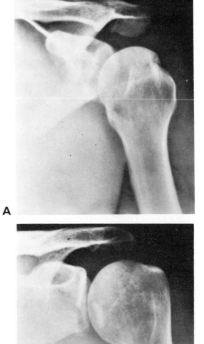

A

B

Figure E–107.

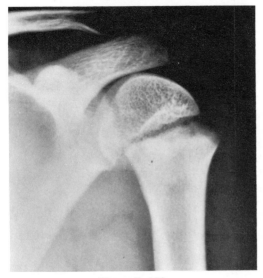

Figure E–106.

CLINICAL HISTORIES

Case 31–1 (Fig. E–105). This patient fell with his arm at his side directly onto his left shoulder so that his shoulder blade was forced downward and medially.

Case 31–2 (Fig. E–106). This 12-year-old patient also fell on his left shoulder with a marked shearing force near his upper arm.

Case 31–3 (Fig. E–107 A and B). This patient had a history of prior anterior dislocations of the shoulder. On this occasion he fell on his flexed elbow.

Questions

31–1 (Fig. E–105). The MOST ACCURATE diagnosis in this patient is:*
 A. Shoulder cuff tear.
 B. Acromioclavicular ligamentous tear.
 C. Tear of the supraspinatous ligament.
 D. Tear of the coracoclavicular ligament.
 E. Normal relaxation of the acromioclavicular joint.

31–2 (Fig. E–106). The MOST ACCURATE diagnosis in this patient is:
 A. No injury. Normal variant.
 B. Type III Salter-Harris epiphyseal injury with subluxation.
 C. Type V Salter-Harris epiphyseal injury.

 D. Type I Salter-Harris fracture of the capital epiphysis.
 E. Type II Salter-Harris fracture of the capital epiphysis.

31–3 (Fig. E–107 A and B). The MOST ACCURATE diagnosis is:
 A. Deformities related to prior anterior dislocation of the shoulder.
 B. Fresh fracture of the greater tuberosity of the humerus.
 C. Fresh fracture of the glenoid process with no other abnormalities detected.
 D. Recurrent fresh anterior dislocation.
 E. Fresh fracture of the glenoid process with deformity of the humerus due to previous dislocations.

*See page 233, Figure 8–6.

195

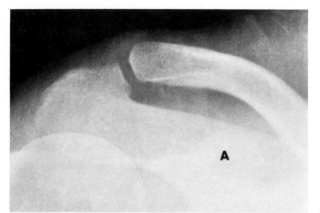

Figure E–108. Normal acromioclavicular joint.

Radiologic Findings. In Figure E–105, Case 31–1, there is an inordinate separation of the distal end of the clavicle from the acromion process of the scapula. Ordinarily, these are in close alignment with respect to one another, as is shown in Figure E–108. The space between the articular surface of the acromion process and its adjoining distal end of the clavicle is usually no more than 3 to 4 mm. We would therefore be obliged to interpret Figure E–105 as demonstrating an increased separation of the distal end of the clavicle and the acromion process. It would also appear that there is an increased separation of the clavicle from the coracoid process, lettered *D* on Figure E–105.

With regard to Case 31–2, Figure E–106, a separation of the head of the humerus through the epiphyseal plate is apparent, especially laterally. There is also a fracture through the head of the humerus vertically. There is a slight separation of the entire head of the humerus with respect to the anatomical neck of the humerus. There would appear to be no involvement of the metaphysis of the humerus proper.

In Figure E–107 *A* and *B*, Case 31–3, there is a considerable indentation between the head of the humerus and the greater tuberosity of the humerus, as noted on Figure E–107 *B* on its superolateral aspect. On Figure E–107 *A* and *B* there is an indentation and fracture of the inferior half of the glenoid process of the scapula.

Discussion. The correct answer to Case 31–1, Figure E–105, is **acromioclavicular ligamentous tear.** Alternatively, but secondary to the former problem, it would be correct to indicate that there is a **tear of the coracoclavicular ligament.** Since the tear of the coracoclavicular ligament is probably secondary to the acromioclavicular ligamentous tear, the most accurate answer would probably be the former. This injury usually results from a fall on the point of the shoulder between the greater tuberosity of the humerus and the acromion process. The scapula and the attached clavicle are forced downward and medially so that the clavicle approaches the first rib. The first rib presses upon the clavicle with a counter force and causes a rupture of the acromioclavicular ligament. In this process the coracoclavicular ligament also tears and there is a tearing of the insertions of the deltoid and trapezius muscles.

In Case 31–2, Figure E–106, the most accurate diagnosis is fracture of the capital epiphysis of the head of the humerus, with fracture also of the epiphyseal plate between the head of the humerus and the metaphysis. There is a slight subluxation of the head of the humerus with respect to the main shaft at the physis. Although this is not a classic **Type III Salter-Harris epiphyseal injury with subluxation,** this would be the most accurate diagnosis among the various possibilities given. It will be recalled that in the Type I injury, there is a separation of the epiphysis but no fracture. In the Type II, there is a separation of the epiphysis with the fracture extending into the metaphysis.

In Type III, the fracture extends through the epiphysis and there also is a fracture of the epiphyseal plate. In a Type IV, the vertical fracture of the epiphysis extends through to the metaphysis, involving a fracture of the metaphysis but no actual separation at the epiphyseal plate. In Type V, no actual disruption of the architecture of the epiphysis or metaphysis may be manifest at the time of the injury. The seriousness of the lesion becomes manifest after a period of growth and early roentgenograms give no clue to the extent of the injury. Usually, premature closure of the epiphyseal plate with loss of growth and angular deformity will result (see Fig. 8–6).

The most accurate answer to Case 31–3 (Fig. E–107 *A* and *B*) is *E*, a fresh fracture of the glenoid process (of the Bankart type) with a hatchet deformity of the glenoid process and head of the humerus due to previous dislocations (Hill-Sacks deformity).

With hyperabduction of the arm, the acromion process acts as a fulcrum that displaces the greater tuberosity of the humerus downward and outward; the inferior joint capsule is stretched and partially torn, and the head subluxates. As the head leaves the glenoid cavity, it is displaced directly downward and anteriorly, and the inferior capsule is torn, with the rotator cuff also stretched across the glenoid fossa. When this type of injury occurs frequently, an erosive process in the region of the junction of the head of the humerus and greater tuberosity results, giving rise to the Hill-Sacks deformity.

Fractures of the glenoid may be produced by direct or indirect forces. When a direct force is applied to the lateral aspect of the shoulder, a fracture of the glenoid results, with the degree of displacement of the fragments depending upon the intensity of the force (Bankart fracture). At times the fracture of the glenoid is stellate rather than purely depressed for the most part, as in the case demonstrated, in which the force undoubtedly traveled along the shaft of the humerus, since the humerus was extended at the time of the injury, and the head of the humerus forced the inferior and anterior margin of the glenoid to be fractured, as shown. Generally, fractures of the glenoid will vary depending upon position of the arm at the time of the injury. Indeed, very often with anterior dislocations of the humeral head, as this patient previously had, there is an avulsion of the anteroinferior brim of the glenoid that gives evidence of prior anteroinferior dislocations of the humeral head.

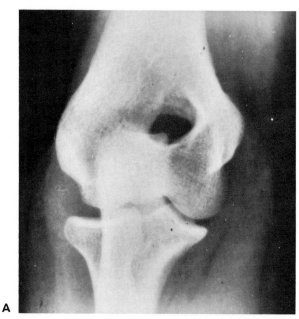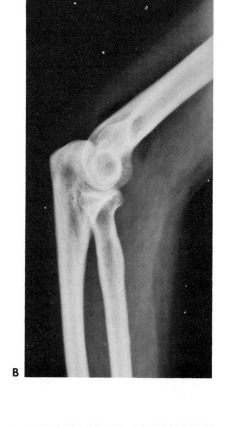

Figure E-109.

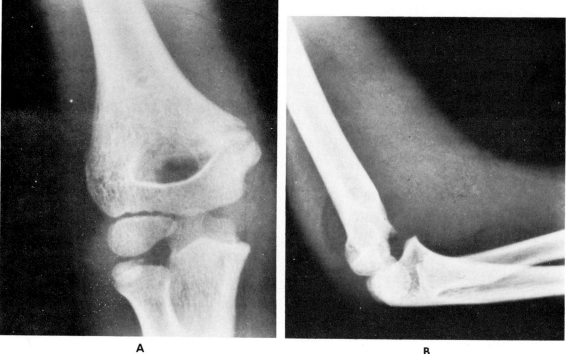

A

B

Figure E-110.

CLINICAL HISTORIES

Case 32–1 (Fig. E–109A and B). Anteroposterior view (A) (insofar as patient could straighten his elbow), and lateral (B) obtained after a fall on the outstretched hand.

Case 32–2 (Fig. E–110A and B). This child also fell on his outstretched hand and complained of pain in his elbow, which clinically showed considerable swelling.

Questions

32–1 (Fig. E–110A and B). What is the MOST accurate diagnosis in this patient?

    A. Supracondylar fracture of the humerus.

    B. Fracture of the head of the radius.

    C. Fracture of the neck of the radius.

    D. Fracture of the medial epicondyle of the humerus.

    E. Fracture of the coronoid process of the ulna.

32–2 (Fig. E–111A and B). What is the MOST accurate diagnosis in this child?

    A. Supracondylar fracture of the humerus.

    B. Intercondylar fracture of the humerus.

    C. Fracture of the distal shaft of the humerus.

    D. Tear of the annular ligament around the head of the radius.

    E. Fracture of the epiphysis of the head of the radius.

Radiologic Findings. In Case 32–1 (Fig. E–109 *A* and *B*), the angulation between the condyles of the humerus and the main shaft of the humerus is normal and there is no evidence of a discontinuity in the supracondylar portion of the distal humerus. There appears to be a small fracture line in the head of the radius with a slight outward displacement of the head of the radius, and in the lateral view (Fig. E–109*B*) the fracture appears to involve the superior aspect of the head of the radius. It does not seem to involve the neck of the radius, at least significantly. The shadowing of the medial epicondyle of the humerus is normal and there is no indication of an avulsion type injury of the coronoid process of the ulna.

In Case 32–2 (Fig. E–110*A* and *B*), there is an anterior angulation between the main shaft of the humerus and the condylar portions of the humerus, and in frontal perspective (Fig. E–110*A*) a fracture is seen in the supracondylar portion of the distal humerus. There is no overlapping of fragments in the condyles, such as might occur with an intercondylar type fracture of the humerus. The alignment of the radius and ulna appears normal and the head of the radius appears to be in normal relationship with respect to the neck and main shaft of the radius.

Discussion. The most accurate diagnosis in Case 32–1 is a **fracture of the head of the radius.** This type of injury will frequently accompany an injury to the wrist when the patient falls on his outstretched hand. Somewhat similar fractures of the head of the radius are illustrated in Figures E–111 and E–112. The injury in Figure E–112 (arrow) is considerably more severe than those of the test case as well as Figure E–111, in that there is a downward displacement of the articular surface of the head of the radius. It is important to recognize that conservative management may be feasible, *if there is no free fragment within the elbow joint proper.*

With regard to Case 32–2 (Fig. E–110*A* and *B*), the most accurate diagnosis is **supracondylar fracture of the humerus.** A somewhat similar injury is shown in Figure E–113*A* and *B*, where the fractures are more readily in evidence. There are three types of fractures in this area: the supracondylar illustrated here; the transcondylar, in which there is a medial displacement of the condyles of the distal shaft of the humerus; and an intercondylar variety, in which there is a marked displacement of the main shaft of the humerus anterior to the condyles so that the shaft abuts upon the head of the radius and the coronoid process of the ulna. The condyles in this latter instance are displaced markedly posteriorly.

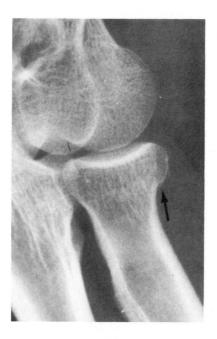

Figure E–111. Fracture of the head of the radius. (Courtesy of Dr. Alan Klein.)

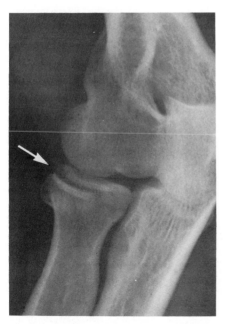

Figure E–112. Fracture of the head of the radius. (Courtesy of Dr. Alan Klein.)

The case in question is certainly not of that variety. The anterior angulation manifest with a supracondylar fracture is rather characteristic and shown in the test case as well as in Figure E–113B. It is important to recognize that reposition of fragments and correction of this angular deformity are essential if the child is to obtain normal function and normal configuration of his elbow without change in the carrying angle particularly. Actually, deformities of the elbow are quite common following the supracondylar fracture, occurring in 10 to 60 per cent of cases, with the most common deformity being a reduction of the carrying angle or varus deformity.

These fractures are associated with considerable soft tissue swelling and our test case particularly, as well as Figure E–113B, shows the marked swelling in the fat pad both anteriorly and posteriorly that should immediately alert one to the presence of this fracture. The hemorrhage and swelling indicated by this may be so severe as to cause embarrassment of the venous circulation of the forearm and even interfere with its arterial blood supply.

It is important to check the function of the median and ulnar nerves of these patients also, since they, too, may be secondarily involved later, particularly if healing with malalignment occurs. The physician must constantly check for motor and sensory deficits of the radial, median, and ulnar nerves.

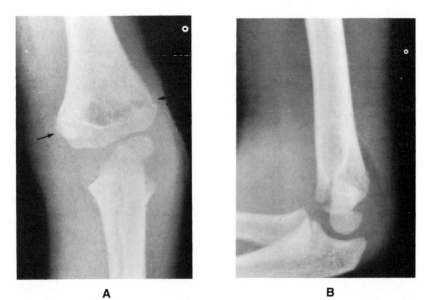

A   B

Figure E–113. *A* and *B,* Supracondylar fracture of a type similar to the exercise case. The swollen fat pad anteriorly and posteriorly is apparent. (Courtesy of Dr. Alan Klein.)

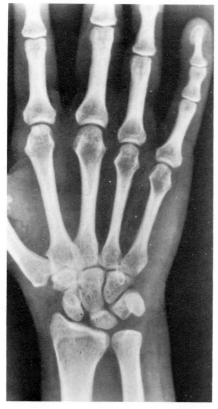
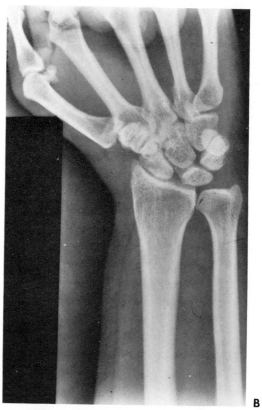

A

B

Figure E–114.

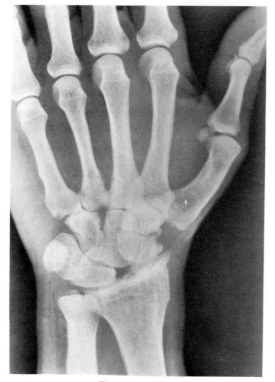

Figure E–115.

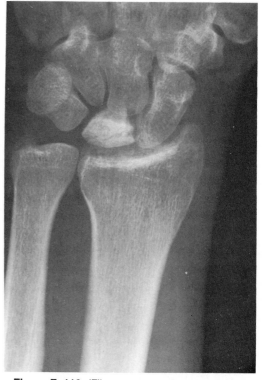

Figure E–116. (Film courtesy of Dr. Alan Klein.)

CLINICAL HISTORIES

Case 33–1 (Fig. E–114*A* and *B*) and Case 33–2 (Fig. E–115). Figures E–114*A* and *B*, and E–115 are radiographs of the wrists of two patients who fell on their outstretched hands. They exemplify similar injuries.

Case 33–3 (Fig. E–116). This patient had experienced moderate pain in his wrist for several months; however, this radiograph was obtained after a fall (which was not severe) on his outstretched hand.

Questions

33–1 and 33–2 (Figs. E–114*A* and *B* and E–115). The MOST likely diagnosis that is *common to both* is:

A. Dislocation of the lunate carpal bone.
B. Fracture of the scaphoid.
C. Rotary subluxation of the scaphoid.
D. Rotary displacement of the scaphoid with volar dislocation of the lunate.
E. Dislocation of the trapezium.

33–3 (Fig. E–116). The MOST likely diagnosis is:

A. Fracture of the scaphoid carpal bone.
B. Dislocation of the lunate.
C. Fracture of the scaphoid and lunate.
D. Fracture of the lunate with aseptic necrosis.
E. Rotary subluxation of the lunate.

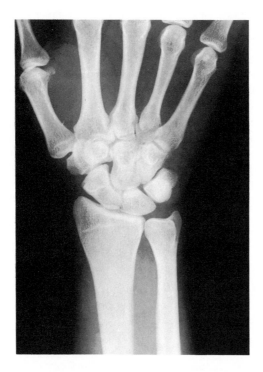

Figure E–117. Radiograph of the wrist in the PA projection. Note the close proximity of the scaphoid and the lunate normally.

Radiologic Findings. In Figure E–114*A* and *B*, it will be noted that there is an inordinate distance between the scaphoid carpal bone and the lunate. The normal appearance is illustrated in Figure E–117. There is a somewhat unusual obliquity of the scaphoid in Figure E–114*A*, in that its articulation overlaps the lateral aspect of the capitate carpal bone (again, compare with normal, Fig. E–117).

A somewhat similar appearance of separation of the scaphoid and lunate carpal bones is manifest in Figure E–115. Moreover, in the latter, the relationship of the scaphoid with the trapezium and trapezoid carpal bones is not normal and there is an inordinate space between the base of the first metacarpal and the trapezium and trapezoid bones as compared with the normal. Additionally, in Figure E–115, there is evidence of spur formation and sclerosis of bone in the distal radial articulation, with hypertrophic spurring of the adjoining trapezium and trapezoid and a small chip fracture of the styloid process of the ulna.

In Case 33–3 (Fig. E–116), the relationship of the scaphoid and lunate carpal bones shows no such increased space between them and the articulation of the scaphoid with the capitate is well within normal limits. The trapezium and trapezoid articulate appropriately with the first and second metacarpals. The outstanding feature in Figure E–116 is the marked sclerosis of the lunate carpal bone, which contains a comminuted fracture. There is some flattening of the lunate carpal bone as well. There is a minimal sclerosis of the distal articular surface of the radius, suggesting that the process is of some duration.

Discussion. The answer to Case 33–1 is *C*, **rotary subluxation of the scaphoid**. There are indeed other findings in Figure E–115, in that there is an associated subluxation of the trapezium and trapezoid and a hypertrophic arthritis of the carpus. It is important to emphasize that the only diagnosis that is in common between Cases 33–1 and 33–2 is the rotary subluxation of the scaphoid.

The scaphoid carpal bone occupies a unique position in the wrist, in that it extends obliquely from the dorsal to the volar aspect of the wrist, helping to bind the proximal row of carpals with the distal row. The carpus contains a very complex system of articulations, but basically there are two rows: the distal row articulates with the proximal surface of the metacarpal bones; and a proximal row articulates with the distal end of the radius and a triangular fibrocartilage at the distal end of the ulna. Although it would appear on posteroanterior perspective that the bones in the proximal row are arranged in a smooth arc, articulating with the radius and the fibrocartilage covering the distal end of the ulna, in lateral view it is apparent that the scaphoid occupies an oblique position from volar to posterior. In each instance there are intercarpal joints. In addition, there is (1) a radiocarpal joint, (2) a distal radioulnar joint, (3) a midcarpal joint, (4) a large carpometacarpal joint, and (5) a small carpometacarpal joint between the first metacarpal and the trapezium. The radiocarpal joint differs from the other joints in that it is not continuous with the inferior radioulnar joint and the scaphoid extends obliquely as described.

There is some independence of motion between the proximal and distal rows of carpal bones and the intercarpal joints, but most of the motion at the wrist occurs between the radius and the scaphoid and lunate. The ligamentous structures of the carpal bones are such that the proximal portion of the scaphoid and the lunate work separately and intimately in relation to the radius. On the other hand, the trapezoid, the distal portion of the scaphoid, the capitate, the hamate, and the triquetrum function as a unit and relate to the metacarpals primarily. In addition, the scaphoid has an independent rotary motion and is the only carpal bone that spans both rows. In this respect its normal relationship is important to both rows of the wrist joint, so that the latter may perform smoothly, and painlessly. With the abnormal rotary subluxation of the scaphoid demonstrated in these two cases, the latter is not possible, and frequently pain will result.

Unfortunately, injuries to the scaphoid are among the most frequently missed injuries. The scaphoid is very vulnerable to injury, its midportion is narrow, and its axis lies in both the proximal and distal rows of carpal bones. All of these factors predispose to its injury. Moreover, as pointed out in the text, the healing process depends much on the integrity of the blood supply of the scaphoid. Its blood supply is not obtained only from its own nutrient vessels but also from its association with the wrist joint capsule. The scaphoid is fractured during forceful hyperextension of the wrist, such as a fall on the outstretched hand. Frequently associated injuries are (1) dislocation of the radiocarpal joint, (2) dislocation between the two rows of the carpal bones, (3) fracture-dislocation of the distal end of the radius, (4) fracture at the base of the thumb metacarpal and possibly associated dislocation of the trapezium and trapezoid (Bennett's fracture), and (5) dislocation of the lunate. About 80 per cent of fractures occur through the midsection of the scaphoid, which is particularly vulnerable, since it is at a distance from the wrist joint capsule and its blood supply is readily severed at this point. Hence, it may undergo aseptic necrosis (Fig. 7–9).

In Case 33–3 (Fig. E–116), the most likely diagnosis is **fracture of the lunate with aseptic necrosis**. Many consider that the aseptic necrosis actually precedes the fracture, and it has been called "Kienboeck's disease." The fact that this patient had experienced pain in his wrist for a significant period of time prior to the relatively minimal trauma, would support the concept that the lunate carpal bone had been undergoing aseptic necrosis for a considerable period of time prior to the injury that resulted in the comminuted fracture. It is possible that an initiating trauma is the most common cause but, nevertheless, a superimposed trauma, as in the case presented, may bring the entire process to the attention of the patient. Actually, the fragmentation of the lunate in this instance may have in part preceded the present injury and be related to the aseptic necrosis.

None of the other distractors in this question apply in that the scaphoid is normal, and there is no indication of the rotary subluxation of the scaphoid or lunate characteristic of Cases 1 and 2 in respect to the scaphoid. Unlike the scaphoid, the lunate does not traverse the anterior and posterior aspects of the wrist and is not subject to rotary subluxation as is the scaphoid.

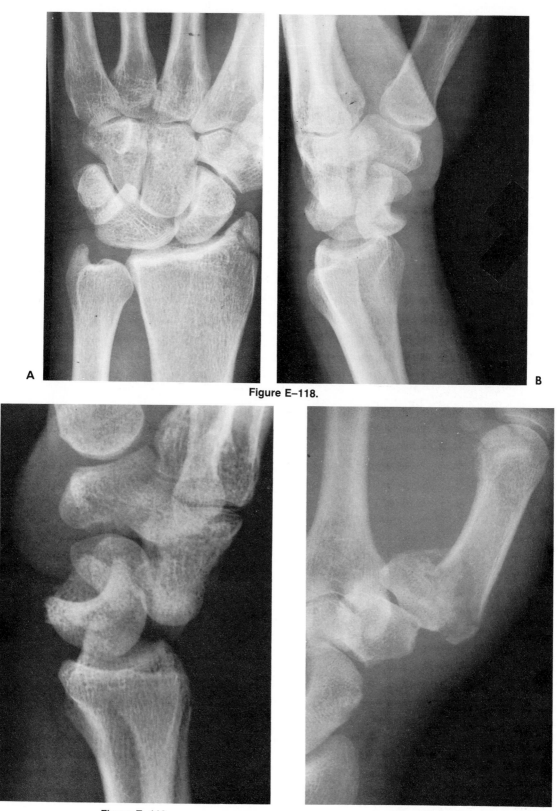

Figure E–118.

Figure E–119.

Figure E–120.

CLINICAL HISTORIES
   Case 34–1 (Fig. E–118 *A* and *B*); Case 34–2 (Fig. E–119); Case 34–3 (Fig. E–120).
All three of these patients fell on their outstretched hands (Figs. E–119 and E–120 courtesy
of Dr. Alan Klein).

Questions
   34–1. In Figure E–118 *A* and *B,* the MOST
likely diagnosis is:
   A. Dislocated lunate.
   B. Perilunate dislocation.
   C. Transcarpal fracture-dislocation.
   D. Fracture at the base of the fourth meta-
      carpal.
   E. Carpometacarpal dislocation.

   34–2. In Figure E–119, the MOST likely diag-
nosis is:
   A. Dislocated lunate.
   B. Perilunate dislocation.
   C. Transcarpal dislocation.
   D. Trapezium dislocation.
   E. Fracture of the scaphoid.

   34–3. In Figure E–120, the MOST likely diag-
nosis is:
   A. Dislocation of the trapezium.
   B. Simple comminuted fracture at the base
      of the first metacarpal.
   C. Fracture dislocation of the carpometacar-
      pal joint of the thumb (Bennett's fracture).
   D. Fracture of the scaphoid.
   E. Lunate dislocation.

Radiologic Findings. In Case 34–1 (Fig. E–118A), the lunate lies anterior to the wrist and its articular surface is tilted forward. The capitate is very faintly shown but articulates with the distal articular surface of the radius. In the oblique projection, B, the scaphoid is shown to be in normal relationship with the trapezium and trapezoid, but there is a space between the triquetrum and the scaphoid from which the lunate apparently has been dislocated. Even though this is an oblique projection, the carpometacarpal joint appears normal and there is no indication of a transcarpal fracture or fracture of any of the other bones in this area.

In contrast with Figures E–118 A and B, the lateral view of the wrist shown in Figure E–119 (Case 34–2) shows the lunate carpal bone to have retained its articulation with the distal articulation of the radius, whereas the other bones of the carpus appear to be situated on the dorsal aspect of the carpus. The capitate is "resting upon" the lunate carpal bone, and the carpometacarpal junction is normal. The important difference between Figures E–119 and E–118 A and B is the fact that in Figure E–119, the lunate has retained its articulation with the distal articulation of the radius, whereas in Figure E–118 A and B, the lunate has become dislocated from the articulation with the radius.

In Case 34–3 (Fig. E–120), there is a comminuted fracture at the base of the first metacarpal and an associated dislocation of the radial portion of its articular surface. The medial portion of the base of the first metacarpal is in relatively normal relationship with the trapezium. There is perhaps a slight widening of the joint between the fractured base of the first metacarpal and the trapezium, but the trapezium is intact and shows no evidence of fracture.

Discussion. The correct answer in Case 34–1 (Figs. E–118 and E–121) is A, a **dislocated lunate** whereas the correct answer to Case 34–2 (Fig. E–119) is **dorsal perilunate dislocation.** This latter occurs when the impact with an outstretched hand and a fall is on the palm of the hand and there is a disruption of the lunate-capitate articulation that drives the carpal bones dorsally behind the lunate. This differs from the volar dislocation of the lunate demonstrated in Figure E–118 A and B in that the latter occurs when the hand and carpus are severely hyperextended in a fall on the outstretched hand held close to the body. Under these circumstances the fingers and the metacarpal heads are the point of contact with the ground. This further forces the hand and carpus into much more severe hyperextension. Under these circumstances the capitate rolls dorsally on the lunate and the lunate is driven forward out of the joint.

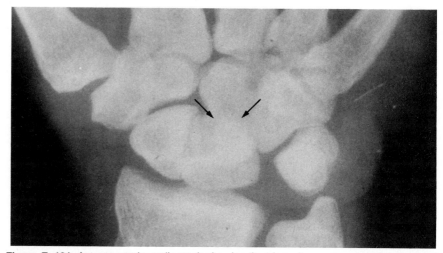

Figure E–121. Anteroposterior radiograph showing the triangular appearance of the lunate in the AP projection when dislocated.

In Figure E–120, Case 34–3, the most likely diagnosis is **fracture-disloca-tion of the carpometacarpal joint of the thumb (Bennett's fracture).** The major difference between this appearance and the usual Bennett's fracture is that the small triangular fragment at the base of the first metacarpal is usually smaller on the ulnar side than on the radial side. In this injury there is usually a disruption of the dorsal capsular structures.

In differentiation of these various entities, one must also be cognizant of the possibility of dislocation of the lunate and scaphoid together. Under these circumstances, the capitate would articulate with the radius directly. At times also there is a dorsal perilunar dislocation with fracture of the capitate, and care must be exercised to see the capitate in its entirety to exclude this possibility.

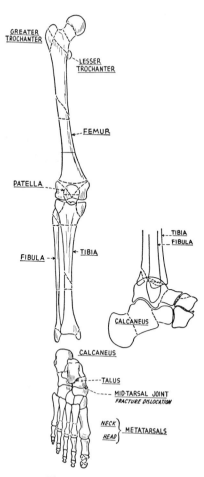

Figure 7–10. The most common sites of fractures of the lower extremity.

FRACTURES OF THE LOWER EXTREMITY

The most common sites of fractures involving the lower extremity are shown in Figure 7–10.

The varieties of hip fractures involving the neck and adjoining portions of the femur are classified as shown in Figure 7–11. This classification is of importance in respect to the vascularity of the neck and the relationship of the neck to the line of attachment of the capsule of·the hip joint. The posterior attachment of this capsule is just distal to the midcervical portion of the neck of the femur. The anterior attachment is at the level of the intertrochanteric ridge (Fig. 7–12). In view of this limited blood supply, fractures with the most favorable prognosis for healing without aseptic necrosis are those that receive a blood supply from the joint capsule additional to that which supplies the head. This, then,

would include fractures that involve the base of the neck, and those of the intertrochanteric, peritrochanteric, or subtrochanteric region.

Lining techniques are of some importance in defining fractures of the head and neck of the femur, the acetabulum, and the adjoining pubis (Fig. 7–13). These lining techniques are used most effectively on an anteroposterior view of the hip, with the foot in very slight internal rotation at the time the film is obtained. This positioning prevents foreshortening of the neck of the femur and concealment of a fracture in what otherwise might be an obscured portion of the neck of the femur. Shenton's line forms a continuous smooth curvature with the superior aspect of the obturator foramen, as shown. Skinner's line is a horizontal line from the uppermost portion of the greater trochanter and should fall below the region of the ligamentum teres, and the angulation of the neck with respect to the axis of the shaft of the femur should range from 120 to 130 degrees. Usually a fracture involving the neck of the femur reduces this angulation of the neck in respect to the axis of the shaft of the femur and is anteriorly angulated.

Fractures of the femoral shaft usually require internal fixation with a Küntchner nail or some similar device, and hence referral to an orthopedic physician is recommended.

Supracondylar or intercondylar fractures of the femur usually have articular involvement, and there is always the danger of injury of vessels or nerves in the immediate proximity. Also, internal derangement of the knee joint presents a consistent danger.

In the *knee* the following injuries are the most serious: (1) dislocations and fractures of the patella, (2) avulsion of the tibial eminence with or without tears of the cruciate ligament, (3) fractures of the tibial plateau or head of the fibula, (4) fractures of the anterior tibial tubercle with separation of the patella and the quadriceps tendon, and (5) tears of the collateral ligament, indicated by widening of the joint space on the affected side.

Internal derangement of the knee is best demonstrated radiographically by arthrography, which when properly performed is capable of a 90 to 95% accuracy in demonstrating fractures and tears of the menisci, and even tears of the cruciate ligament. Fractures of the patella may be transverse, stellate, or comminuted. A bipartite or tripartite patella must not be confused with a fracture, since

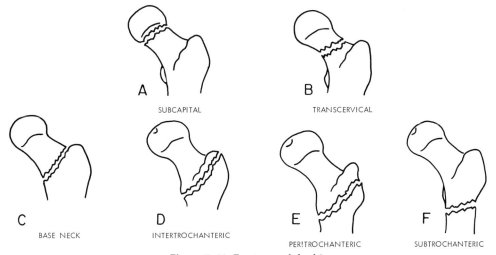

Figure 7–11. Fractures of the hip.

it is an anomalous lack of fusion without pathologic significance. The unfused portion of the patella in these instances is in the outer, upper, and inner quadrants of the patella. With fractures of the patella involving the infrapatellar fat pad, there is a release of fat as well as blood into the joint. In a film obtained with a horizontal x-ray beam and the knee outstretched as though it were being

radiographed in the anteroposterior position, the fat may be demonstrated as a layer above the blood and a diagnosis made of "lipohemoarthrosis."

Fractures of the *tibia* or *fibula*, when high on the shaft of the tibia, usually result from a strong impact at this level. They were formerly called "bumper" fractures because the bumper of a car would strike the leg in

Figure 7–12. The line of attachment of the capsule of the hip joint. The posterior attachment is just distal to the midcervical portion of the neck of the femur. The anterior attachment is at the intertrochanteric ridge. (From Perry, in Morris' Human Anatomy, New York, Blakiston, 1953.)

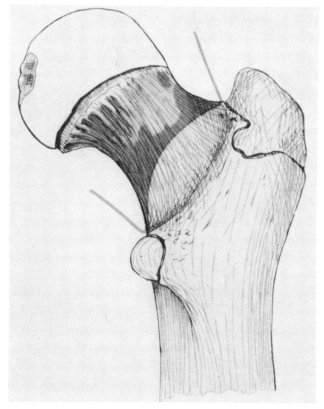

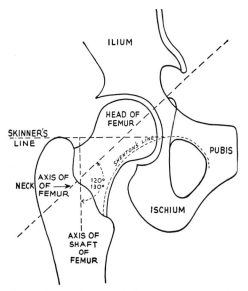

Figure 7–13. Lining techniques to demonstrate the proper axial relationships of the hip joint, for assistance in detection of fractures in the region of the hip.

ments in this regard are the medial and lateral collateral ligaments; the cruciate ligament anteriorly; the ligamentous attachment of the gastrocnemius muscle posteriorly; and the interosseous ligament between the distal shaft of the fibula and tibia. Stress x-rays may be employed to reproduce the tear of a ligament with appropriate analgesia. Fractures in this area are often classified as inversion or eversion types, and if one can reproduce the kind of stress that originally caused the fracture, the associated ligamentous injury can likewise be reproduced when one visualizes the area of the fracture. The ligamentous injuries may be far more serious than the bony injuries and may cause pain for a prolonged period. Internal fixation is often necessary (see Fig. E–125).

Fracture of the talus—especially of its neck— is most important. The critical angle of the os calcis is shown in Figure 7–14. Accessory bones of the foot must be clearly understood, and those that are seen most frequently are the os trigonum, peroneal sesamoid, and accessory navicular. These must not be misinterpreted as representing fractures.

this location. They heal with considerable difficulty and frequently result in delayed union. Fatigue fractures of the tibia are also not infrequent.

Fractures of the distal one-third of the tibia are so-called "ski-boot" fractures, and with the increasing popularity of skiing as a sport, this takes on a greater significance. These fractures ordinarily heal far better than do the "bumper" variety.

Fractures of the *ankle* occur with and without dislocation or subluxation and are among the most frequent injuries of the lower extremity. They may or may not be associated with the tearing of ligaments that support the ankle. The most important liga-

Fractures of the *foot* ordinarily cause no great problem in recognition except that fatigue fractures of the second or third metatarsals should be recognized and may not be radiographically demonstrable for a week or two. *If a patient has persistent pain in this area and the initial radiograph is negative for abnormality, the patient should be recalled in a week or two, when callus will be demonstrable and the fracture then in evidence.*

Fractures of sesamoid bones seldom occur. However, they have been described. The bipartite nature of some of the sesamoids

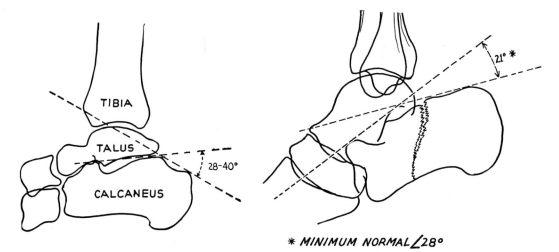

Figure 7–14. Tuber angle of the calcaneus. Normal: greater than 28 degrees and usually 35 to 40 degrees.

adjoining the first metatarsophalangeal joint is a normal variant and should not be called a fracture.

Dislocations of the toes or fractures of the tufted ends of the toes are frequently accompanied by minor bony avulsions and require careful coning, and bright light observation for detection.

PATHOLOGIC FRACTURES

A pathologic fracture is one through bone that is the site of either infection or tumor. These may include primary or metastatic tumors, osteomyelitis, syphilis of bone, storage diseases of bone, effects of radiation therapy, and even ill-defined metabolic disturbances, which are possibly the basis for fatigue fractures, as with osteomalacia. With few exceptions, it is not too difficult to diagnose a pathologic fracture. Physical examination and history are extremely important in making the diagnosis. Occasionally biopsy is necessary to confirm the diagnosis. Treatment of the underlying bone disease is as essential as treatment of the fracture. Even these fractures respond to good therapy. If radiation itself has not been responsible for the original fracture, radiation therapy is helpful in producing good healing of fractures at the site of primary or metastatic tumors.

HEALING OF FRACTURES
(Fig. 7–15)

Great importance is attached to the x-ray evaluation of the course of healing. As indicated earlier, a primary callus, representing calcium deposition within the periosteal hematoma, is ultimately resorbed and replaced by a secondary callus consisting of osseous trabeculae. In infants and children a remodeling process occurs, so that even if the deformity is fairly great at the time of healing, this may ultimately become a normal-appearing bone. This is far less likely to occur in the adult. Ultimately, complete continuity of bony trabeculae should be seen across the fracture site to establish that healing has occurred. If a radiolucency persists at the site of the fracture, it is important to analyze this closely, since dense compact bone on either side of this radiolucency would suggest that cartilage has replaced the fibrous scar tissue and nonunion of fracture is present. Otherwise the situation is called a "pseudoarthrosis," and healing may yet occur, although delayed. The radiologic examination is very helpful in this regard. For radiographic illustrations and further diagrams related to this section, the student is referred to Meschan I: *Synopsis of the Analysis of Roentgen Signs in General Radiology.* Philadelphia, W. B. Saunders Co., 1976.

Figure 7–15. *A,* Steps in the healing of fractures.

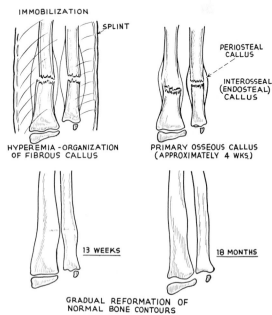

IMMOBILIZATION

SPLINT

PERIOSTEAL CALLUS

INTEROSSEAL (ENDOSTEAL) CALLUS

HEMATOMA-SOFT TISSUE SWELLING

HYPEREMIA -ORGANIZATION OF FIBROUS CALLUS

PRIMARY OSSEOUS CALLUS (APPROXIMATELY 4 WKS.)

13 WEEKS

18 MONTHS

RESORPTION OF PRIMARY CALLUS AND FORMATION OF SECONDARY CALLUS **A** (APPROXIMATELY 7 WKS.)

GRADUAL REFORMATION OF NORMAL BONE CONTOURS

Illustration continued on following page

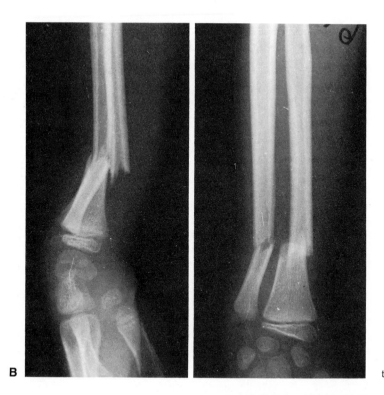

B

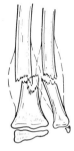

Figure 7–15 *Continued. B,* Hematoma, soft tissue swelling.

Figure 7–15 *Continued. C,* Hyperemia, organization of fibrous calculi.

IMMOBILIZATION

SPLINT

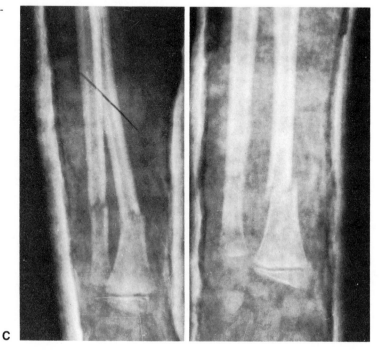

C

Illustration continued on opposite page

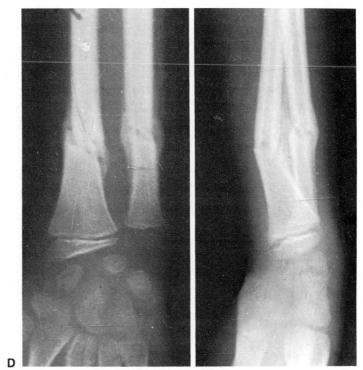

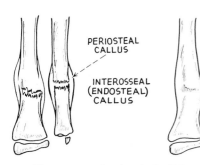

PERIOSTEAL
CALLUS

INTEROSSEAL
(ENDOSTEAL)
CALLUS

Figure 7–15 *Continued. D,* Primary osseous callus (approximately 4 weeks).

D

Figure 7–15 *Continued. E,* Gradual reformation of normal bone contours (13 weeks).

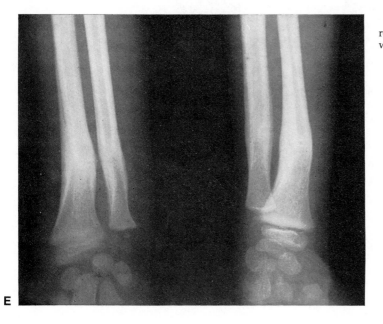

E

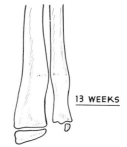

13 WEEKS

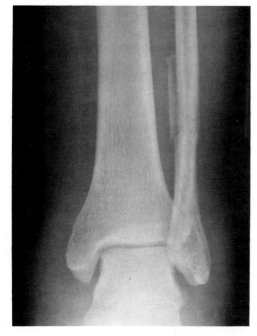

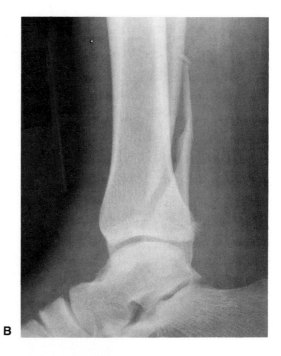

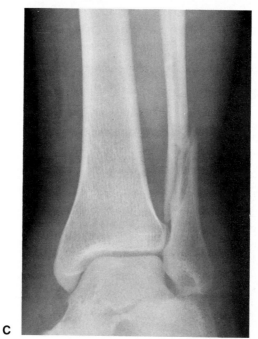

Figure E–122.

CLINICAL HISTORY

This patient is a 30-year-old female who tripped while playing basketball.

You are shown anteroposterior (Fig. E–122A), lateral (Fig. E–122B), and oblique (Fig. E–122C) films.

Question

35–1. Which of the following statements would you consider to be an accurate description of what has occurred?

A. This patient injured her ankle primarily by eversion.
B. Very likely there is an interosseous ligamentous tear.
C. The primary bony injury is a comminuted fracture of the lateral malleolus and distal fibula.
D. Very likely there is a ruptured medial collateral ligament.
E. There is probably a slight rupture of the distal tibiofibular ligament as well.

Radiologic Findings. In the anteroposterior view (Fig. E–122*A*), there is a comminuted fracture of the distal fibula extending obliquely down to the inferior adjoining margin of the tibia. There is a slight external displacement of the lateral malleolus, but the joint mortise between the tibia and talus as well as the medial malleolus are all well within normal limits. There is considerable soft tissue swelling bilaterally.

In the lateral view (Fig. E–122*B*), there is a considerable joint crevice, measuring 5 to 8 mm, in the oblique fracture of the distal fibula and probably a slight irregularity noted along the posterior margin of the distal tibia. This may represent a small avulsion.

In the oblique study (Fig. E–122*C*), somewhat similar findings are noted and there is slight separation of the tibia and fibula.

Discussion. This patient sustained an **eversion type injury of the ankle with a comminuted fracture of the distal shaft of the fibula. The slightly increased space between the talus and the medial malleolus would suggest that there was also a rupture of the medial collateral ligament.** In lateral view there is also an avulsion fracture of the posterior aspect of the medial malleolus. In the oblique projection there is a slight separation of the tibiofibular ligament, suggesting some rupture therein.

The various injuries that may occur in *eversion* injuries of the ankle are shown in Figure E–123. This is best illustrated by the midsection diagrams. (For similar analysis by diagram of *inversion* fractures of the ankle, the student is referred to Meschan, I.: *Analysis of Roentgen Signs in General Radiology.* Philadelphia, W. B. Saunders Co., 1973, pp. 156–157.

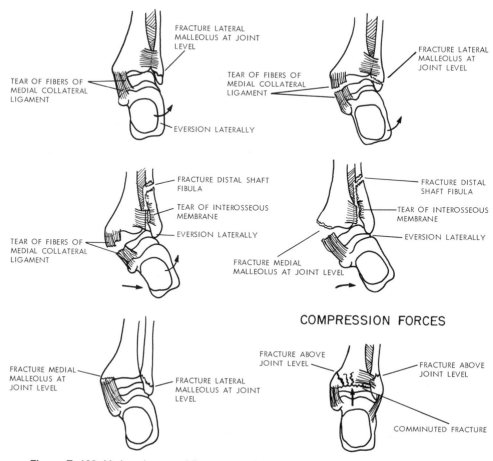

Figure E–123. Various bony and ligamentous injuries which may result with eversion fractures of the ankle. (Modified from De Palma.)

EXERCISE

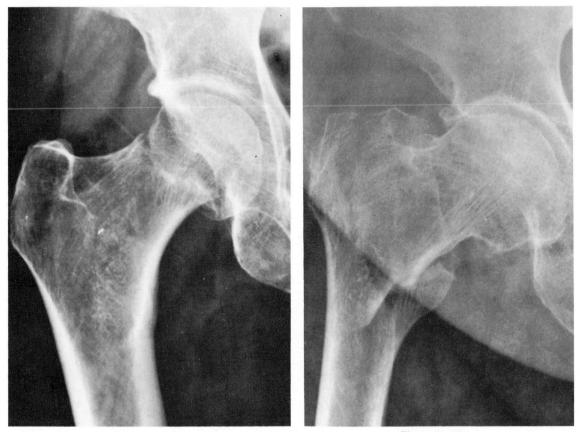

Figure E–124.

Figure E–125.

CLINICAL HISTORIES
You are shown two anteroposterior views of the hip (Figs. E–124 and E–125) representing related but not identical disorders.

In both instances the patient entered the emergency room with marked eversion of the foot (illustrations courtesy Dr. Alan Klein)

Questions
36–1. The MOST likely diagnosis in Figure E–124 is:
A. Extracapsular fracture of the neck of the femur.
B. Subcapital fracture of the neck of the femur.
C. Midcervical fracture of the neck of the femur.
D. Fracture of the neck of the femur with a fracture also in the posterior rim of the acetabulum, suggesting that some subluxation has occurred.
E. Pathologic fracture of the neck of the femur.

36–2. With regard to Figure E–125, the MOST likely diagnosis is:
A. Intertrochanteric fracture of the femur.
B. Intertrochanteric fracture and dislocation of the hip.
C. Subtrochanteric fracture of the upper shaft of the femur.
D. Intertrochanteric fracture with coxa vara deformity.
E. Midcervical fracture of the neck of the femur.

Radiologic Findings. In Figure E–124, there is a fracture immediately beneath the head of the femur. There is slight overlapping of fragments but very little deformity. Shenton's line is only minimally disturbed. Skinner's line is within normal limits, and there is no indication of a coxa vara deformity.

In Figure E–125, there is a markedly comminuted fracture extending through the intertrochanteric ridge at the base of the neck of the femur involving a fracture of the greater trochanter and probably to a lesser extent the lesser trochanter as well. There is a mild degree of foreshortening of the neck of the femur because this patient was apparently unable to completely invert the foot or keep it perfectly straight upward at the time of radiography. There is no indication of associated dislocation but there is considerable sclerosis of the subarticular bone of the acetabulum and narrowness of the joint space along the roof of the acetabulum near its junction with the head of the femur. The head of the femur is somewhat irregular in its contour, suggesting degenerative articular changes in the hip.

Discussion. In Figure E–124, the correct diagnosis is **subcapital fracture of the neck of the femur.** It is not unusual to observe a zone of radiolucency on the posterior rim of the acetabulum of this type without there having been a subluxation or adjoining fracture in the acetabulum. A fracture in this site is contained within the hip joint capsule, since the capsular attachments are either at the level of the intertrochanteric ridge or slightly cephalad near the base of the neck of the femur, but under no circumstances would the attachments be as cephalad as the fracture indicated here. Although there are zones of lucency in the neck of the femur, there is no appearance in this bone suggestive of an underlying pathologic process, such as infection or neoplasm. This was an elderly patient who had a moderate senile osteoporosis and hypertrophic arthritis of the hip as well. A midcervical fracture of the neck of the femur would be recognized about 1 cm caudad to the present fracture.

It is important to classify fractures of the neck of the femur, at least as to being *subcapital, midcervical* or *intertrochanteric,* on the basis of whether healing is likely to be complicated by aseptic necrosis. If the fracture is completely intracapsular, as in the case of a subcapital fracture or in some cases of midcervical fracture, the blood supply is received entirely from the head of the femur through the ligamentum teres and, hence, is very limited. On the other hand, if the fracture is closer to the capsular attachments (as in Fig. E–125), then ancillary blood supply may be derived from the capsule and healing will progress more favorably.

With regard to Figure E–125, the diagnosis is an **intertrochanteric fracture of the femur,** and there is no indication of a dislocation of the hip. The posterior rim of the acetabulum normally may appear slightly irregular, as is shown here, particularly in the presence of chronic hypertrophic or degenerative arthritis, which this patient had. Although there is a minimal subtrochanteric extension of this comminuted fracture, this would not be considered subtrochanteric, since most of the fracture is along the line of the intertrochanteric ridge. The deformity is definitely not a coxa vara deformity, where the angle between the neck and shaft of the femur would measure less than 120 degrees.

Most fractures of the neck of the femur are associated with anterior angulation at the fracture site. Rarely, they may be posteriorly angulated but this is so rare as not to be statistically considered probable until proven otherwise by appropriate lateral views.

With regard to potential healing, the intertrochanteric fracture receives a blood supply from the hip joint capsule as well as through the head of the femur and is more favorably situated for the healing process.

8

The Injured Child And Pediatric Emergency Radiology

In general, many of the principles that apply to trauma to the adult also have application to the injured or acutely ill child. There are, however, significant differences that the primary physician must address. Emphasis will be placed only on those factors that are important to the primary physician in his everyday practice.

MISCELLANEOUS PEDIATRIC PROBLEMS THAT PERTAIN TO THE CHEST

Special Problems Related to Pneumonia

The method of examining the normal chest in the child is similar to that in the adult. There are a few simple, but important, rules:

1. The cardiac silhouette will often appear larger in the child in comparison to the adult; relative heart volume should be determined using the table presented on page 73.
2. In the lateral view, the thymus often occupies the anterior mediastinal clear space, particularly in infants, and may be prominent in the frontal view in various ways (e.g., "batwing sign").
3. There is always an increasing radiolucency of the lateral chest film of the child as one proceeds from the cephalad to caudad aspect.
4. There may at times be shadows behind the heart which simulate air bronchograms but are of no pathologic significance

on the lateral view with outright infiltration.

5. The silhouette sign whereby a cardiac margin is obscured by a pulmonary infiltration would indicate that the infiltration in the lung is contiguous with the heart. This often particularly concerns right middle lobe pneumonias or infiltrates, especially in the medial segment, and pneumonias in the lingula on the left side.
6. Although the air bronchogram must be interpreted with great caution, behind the heart there are certain "hiding places" of pneumonia in the pediatric chest that must be mentioned: (a) *a focal pneumonia above the left hemidiaphragm* contiguous with such air bronchograms in frontal view; (b) *confluent consolidations behind the left heart*, particularly if they can be discovered in the lateral view (Fig. 8–1*A*, *B*); (c) *pneumonias concealed in the hilar regions*, if they involve the superior segment of either the right or the left lower lobe; (d) *lower lobe pneumonias that may not be visible on frontal perspective* but can be seen in the lateral view because they lie deep in the posterior costophrenic sulci; (e) pneumonias high in the upper lobe and deep in the lateral costophrenic sulcus must not be confused with normal overlying soft tissues.

Hilar and tracheobronchial adenopathy is highly significant in the child, since all lymph node bearing areas are readily enlarged in the pediatric patient in response to any inflammatory process. Bilateral involvement is especially frequent with sarcoidosis, histiocytosis X, adenopathy secondary to lymphoma or leukemia, and a "shaggy" mediastinum as may occur with inflammatory processes such as whooping cough. The lateral view of the chest is particularly helpful in detecting hilar or tracheobronchial lymphadenopathy, and familiarity with its normal appearance is important.

Pneumatoceles or air-filled cysts occur in children, and are variable in size, thin walled, fluid free, and most frequently are seen as a complication of staphylococcal pulmonary infections (Fig. 8–2). They are typically unilateral, and are often associated with pleural effusion and pneumonitis. As the child recovers from the acute illness, the pneumatocele may persist for a considerable time. These persistent cysts are usually asymptomatic, and will eventually disappear without surgical intervention.

Occasionally, pneumatoceles are seen with viral lower respiratory tract infections, with hydrocarbon pneumonias, and with

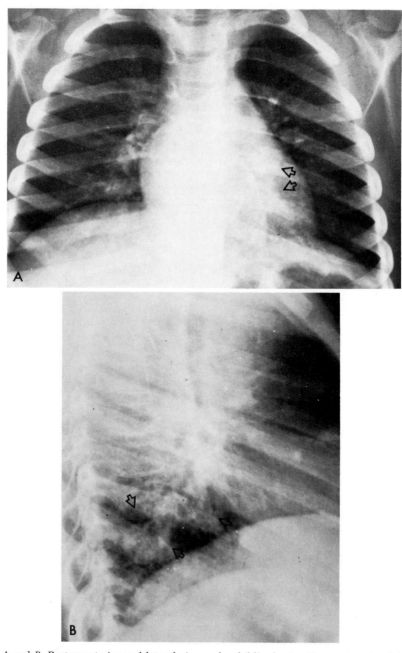

Figure 8–1. *A* and *B*, Posteroanterior and lateral views of a child's chest with pneumonia of the left lower lobe concealed on frontal perspective by the shadow of the left side of the heart.

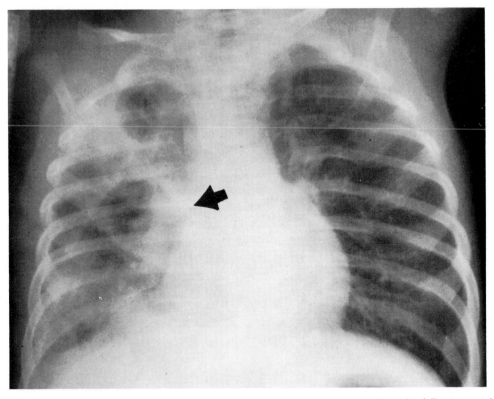

Figure 8–2. P-A view of the chest in an infant with staphylococcic pneumonia. Note the following combination of findings: (1) unilaterality; (2) pleural involvement; (3) pulmonary consolidation; (4) pneumatocele formation. The arrow points to a large pneumatocele adjoining the right side of the mediastinum.

closed or blunt chest trauma after resorption of the hematoma.

Pulmonary abscesses may be complications of either lobar or bronchopneumonia, and are readily differentiated from pneumatoceles by having air fluid levels and relatively thick walls.

Pneumomediastinal air collections occur somewhat more frequently in children than in adults, outline the various mediastinal structures, and extend upward into the soft tissues of the neck. Pneumomediastinal air can also be subpleural along the diaphragm.

Pneumomediastinum in the child may often occur, with excessive coughing, trauma, or penetration by a foreign body.

Pulmonary edema usually represents a saturation of the interstitium of the lung with fluid and may assume a "butterfly" configuration, as in the adult. However, one of the common causes of pulmonary edema in childhood is acute glomerulonephritis. No disease of the heart is demonstrated in these patients necessarily, but often the edema is related to a fluid overload. Other causes of pulmonary edema include the inhalation of irritating gases; neurogenic pulmonary

edema secondary to increased intracranial pressure, rheumatic pneumonia, collagen vascular disease, massive aspiration, fat embolism, allergic pneumonitis, and the "shock lung syndrome."

The asthmatic child often shows pulmonary overexpansion with or without chronic bronchitis. It is important to exclude associated pneumonia, pneumomediastinum, or pneumothorax. With associated bronchitis, "bronchial cuffing" and "tramline" accentuation may be present. Mucous plugs are especially common in asthmatic children and may resemble a "thumblike" extension into the lung parenchyma, as is recognized in the adult (Fig. 8–3).

The *inhalation of foreign bodies* presents a special problem in the small infant because the child may be only intermittently symptomatic, having spells of coughing, varying degrees of respiratory distress, or even cyanosis. These symptoms may subside despite the fact that the foreign body is still present. *If foreign body aspiration is suspected*, chest films must be taken in inspiration and expiration, and fluoroscopy performed. An opaque foreign body is readily detected; however, if

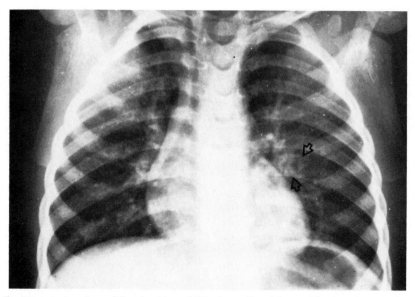

Figure 8–3. Posteroanterior view of the chest in a child who suffered from asthma with a mucous plug presenting itself radiologically on frontal view as a "thumblike" extension into the lung parenchyma (arrows).

nonopaque, the following roentgen signs are found to be helpful:

1. A persistent radiolucency of an entire lung or part of a lung in expiration.
2. The mediastinum usually shifts away from the involved lung, and the ipsilateral diaphragm remains depressed.
3. Decubitus films will ordinarily demonstrate a dependent lung as emptying itself of its air volume and becoming smaller. The obstructed lung, however, traps air, preventing it from collapsing.

The increased radiolucency following the inhalation of a foreign body is often replaced by atelectasis, and even pneumonia or bronchiectasis. Foreign bodies such as peanuts and popcorn are especially prone to produce a much more pronounced and rapidly ensuing inflammatory reaction because of their fat content.

A foreign body may also move from one location to another within the bronchial tree and produce confusing clinical and roentgenographic findings on sequential studies.

The ingestion or inhalation of hydrocarbons such as furniture polish, gasoline, kerosene, or charcoal lighter fluid presents a special problem in the child. The ensuing pneumonitis may be directly related to aspiration or result from exhalation of the hydrocarbon. Radiologic abnormalities may be absent for the first 6 or 12 hours; but because of the lipid affinity of the aspirated hydrocarbon, pulmonary surfactant is destroyed. This causes microatelectasis and problems

with gas exchange. The appearance resembles that of surfactant deficiencies which are described in the adult, where a confluent pneumonia interrupted by pneumatoceles ultimately gives way to an interstitial fibrotic appearance.

Special Problems in the Pediatric Chest Related to Penetrating and Blunt Trauma

In general, the principles regarding trauma in the adult chest apply, except that the child is more likely to incur such problems as (1) a tear of a bronchus; (2) cardiopericardial injury with pericardial effusion and myocardial contusion; (3) injury to the aorta and the great vessels; and (4) torsion of the lung about the hilus, with associated infarction.

Herniation of abdominal viscera into the thoracic cavity may occur in the child or adult—but especially in the child with normal openings of the diaphragm that are somewhat enlarged, or who has a traumatic tear of the diaphragm. Usually this requires an upper gastrointestinal study involving the small intestine as well, or a barium enema.

PEDIATRIC PROBLEMS OF THE UPPER AIRWAYS, SINUSES, AND MASTOIDS

To recognize abnormalities of this area, familiarity with the normal appearance of adenoid and tonsillar tissue, and with the retropharyngeal and laryngeal space in the child is needed. Measurements differ in children and adults and are available in standard radiology texts.

Retropharyngeal Abscess. The patient usually has fever, pain, stiffness of the neck, and dysphagia, often with associated stridor and cervical adenopathy. The retropharyngeal space as measured on lateral neck films is widened.

Sinusitis. In the infant, the paranasal sinuses are frequently not pneumatized, and are difficult to evaluate. The ethmoid sinuses are usually pneumatized by the age of two or three years but the maxillary sinuses and mastoids are not. Although frontal sinuses may never develop, they are usually pneumatized by the age of six. In contrast with adults, sinusitis in the child is often chronic, and may be associated with recurrent bouts of otitis media. In some children, proptosis may develop as the result of maxillary or ethmoid sinusitis.

Acute mastoiditis may cause actual destruction of bone with abscess formation. Bone destruction from calvarial trauma, histiocytosis X, leukemia, and lymphoma must be differentiated.

Epistaxis in the Child. This common childhood problem may result from diseases uncommon in the adult, such as angiofibromas of the nasopharynx. Foreign bodies in the nose must also be considered.

Special Pediatric Problems in the Abdomen

The radiologic examination of the abdomen in the child presents special problems because of the *relative absence of certain features* common to the adult, such as the properitoneal fat, the hepatic and splenic angles, and the gas pattern. In general, fat planes are poorly seen in infants and young children, while gas in the small intestine is not unusual in the child. With an acute abdominal problem in a child, the radiologic examination requires supine and upright views of the abdomen and frontal and lateral views of the chest. The lateral decubitus film of the abdomen may be substituted for an upright film.

Abnormal Gas Patterns

"The Airless Abdomen." After the age of 24 hours the child's abdomen should contain some air. Absence of air often results from excessive vomiting or diarrhea. Other causes include the adrenogenital syndrome in young infants, Addison's disease, and cerebral depression with diminished swallowing of air.

Air Distention in the Upper Abdomen. Air distention in the upper abdomen of the infant may be associated with esophageal stenosis where the lower portion of the esophagus communicates with the tracheobronchial tree, pyloric stenosis, or obstruction of the second, third or fourth parts of the duodenum related to atresia or webs.

Differentiation of Paralytic Ileus and Mechanical Ileus. *Paralytic ileus* is usually associated with gastroenteritis, intestinal ischemia, or systemic conditions such as sepsis, hypokalemia, and neurogenic shock. Generalized distention of the small and large intestine is typical; and air-fluid levels, although few in number, may be seen.

With *mechanical obstruction* the distended intestinal loops are more localized, and may be followed to the point of obstruction. The loops appear more orderly and stacked contiguously in the upright position. Fluid levels are more numerous.

The "Sentinel" Loop. In the adult, the "sentinel loop" usually refers to the markedly dilated transverse colon in association with such problems as carcinoma of the splenic flexure of the colon, pancreatitis, idiopathic ulcerative colitis, superior mesenteric artery thrombosis, and carcinoma of the pancreas that has extended to the splenic flexure. In the child, short segment paralytic ileus may occur in the right upper quadrant, with cholecystitis, pyelonephritis, and hepatic inflammatory or traumatic disease. In the left upper quadrant it is usually seen with pancreatitis, pyelonephritis, or splenic injury. In the right lower quadrant it occurs particularly with appendicitis or regional enteritis (and occasionally Meckel's diverticulitis). In the left lower quadrant, sentinel loops are less common but may herald the presence of salpingitis or cystitis. In the midabdomen, they may be associated with pancreatitis as in the adult.

Acute Gastric Dilatation. In the child, acute gastric dilatation may be a very serious disorder and may in turn lead to cardiorespiratory arrest as a result of a vagal response. Prompt recognition and relief by nasogastric tube decompression is imperative. It is important, however, to recognize that gastric dilatation may be less significant, such as in neglected children, especially after their first full meal or after excessive air swallowing.

Extraluminal Gas Patterns. The problems of pneumoperitoneum, retroperitoneal free air, pneumatosis cystoides intestinalis, and portal vein and biliary tract gas are much the same in the child as in the adult, except that Hirschsprung's disease is an important cause of necrotizing enterocolitis in the infant.

Appendicitis. Apart from gastroenteritis, appendicitis is probably the most common acute abdominal inflammatory problem in children. When the classic clinical and laboratory findings are present, the abdominal radiograph is probably not essential. In equivocal cases, however, certain roentgen appearances can be helpful: (1) most children with acute nonperforated appendicitis early will show diminished air in the gastrointestinal tract or localized ileus; and (2) a calcified fecalith (coprolith) in the region of the appendix virtually assures the diagnosis of acute appendicitis.

With perforated appendicitis (Fig. 8–4) there may be a widespread paralytic ileus, evidence of thickened walls of the air-containing bowel as a result of peritonitis, a suggestion of small bowel obstruction, especially in the right lower quadrant, and inflammatory mass or relative absence of gas in the right lower quadrant, and in the older child obliteration of the properitoneal fat line or hepatic angle with asymmetry in the appearance of the two flanks. Free air may be present in the region of the abscess and is recognized as different from air within the bowel, since it appears "amorphous" and remains constant in appearance on both the upright and recumbent films. A barium enema may be performed, with the full recognition that partial filling of the appendix may occur despite the fact that there is appendicitis present, with obstruction of the appendix being due to a noncalcific fecal impaction. On the other hand, an appendix filled to its very tip should be normal.

In the child, a *typhlitis occurs, particularly with leukemia,* and a mesenteric adenitis may mimic the appearance of acute appendicitis.

Acute Mechanical Problems. The acute mechanical problems particularly pertinent in children are intussusception, volvulus, hernias, and visceral torsions.

Intussusception. The clinical findings in relation to this entity include (a) crampy abdominal pain, (b) vomiting, (c) bloody stools, and (d) a palpable mass and relative emptiness on the supine films of the abdo-

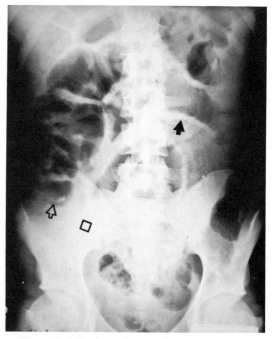

Figure 8–4. Perforated appendicitis in an adolescent with diffuse peritonitis and small and large intestinal ileus and separation of loops of bowel by peritonitis exudate. There is a relative lack of gas in the right lower quadrant, where an abscess is forming. There is a fecalith in the appendix (open arrow). (Calcified, hence a coprolith.)

men in the right flank or lower quadrant (Fig. 8–5). It is most common between the ages of 6 months to 2 years but may be seen in older children. Most cases are ileocolic. The radiographic appearances will vary depending upon the duration of the disease, but absence of gas in the right lower quadrant or flank is the most common. If the process is less than 24 hours old, it may be confirmed by a carefully administered barium enema, and the intussusception may be reduced by this procedure. Success rates vary from 45 to 80 per cent. It should be recognized, however, that, although *radiologic reduction is at times permanent,* a recurrence of the intussusception signals surgical treatment; and an intussusception of longer duration than 24 hours may indicate the presence of necrotic bowel requiring an aggressive surgical approach. During the reduction by barium enema, the head of the intussusceptum must be reduced beyond the ileocecal valve into the terminal ileum. Postevacuation and 24 hour delayed films should be obtained to verify that the intussusception has remained reduced. Recurrence rates after barium enema reduction range from 4 to 11 per cent.

Volvulus. Although volvulus of the entire small intestine is probably the most frequent type in children, volvulus of the colon, gastric volvulus, and segmental small bowel volvulus are occasionally encountered. If vascular compromise occurs, clinical signs of shock may also be evident as the bowel undergoes necrosis. Perforation and peritonitis may supervene. *A barium enema is helpful in demonstrating the exact position of the cecum because any abnormal position of the cecum is strongly suggestive of a small intestinal volvulus.*

Segmental volvulus of the small intestine is usually related to anomalous peritoneal bands, congenital mesenteric defects, internal hernias, malrotation problems, or postoperative adhesions.

Unlike the adult, volvulus of the colon is not a common problem in childhood. When it does occur, the sigmoid colon is most frequently affected.

Gastric volvulus is associated with vomiting and severe abdominal pain, is sudden in onset, and represents a surgical emergency. This may be recognized on the erect chest x-rays where two air fluid levels are seen in the chest, often partially behind the heart. If barium is administered it will stop at the gastroesophageal junction or pass into the inverted rotated stomach.

Hernias. These are subdivided into internal and external types. Over one half of internal hernias are related to herniations into the lesser omental bursa or the paraduodenal fossae. Inguinal hernias in an infant may be readily overlooked owing to the intestinal obstruction caused by the hernia. At times the incarcerated loops may be recognized in the scrotum.

Visceral Torsion. Splenic torsion is more common than that involving the liver, and occurs because the organ is poorly fixed anatomically. Acute crampy abdominal pain is usual and may be referred outside the left upper quadrant of the abdomen. The abdominal roentgenograms show an absence of the normal splenic or liver silhouette, and replacement of this space by gas-filled colon or small intestine. Radionuclide scans are particularly helpful in establishing this diagnosis.

Pediatric Abdominal Trauma. The assessment of abdominal trauma in children is similar to that in adults. One of the most commonly injured organs is the spleen. Liver injury, however, is often more serious and life-threatening. The injured liver is markedly

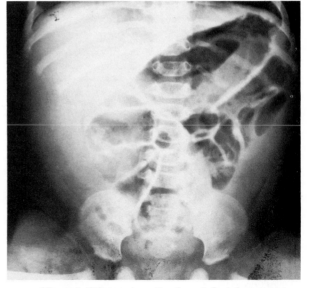

Figure 8–5. Intussusception in an infant demonstrating the ileus and relative emptiness in the abdominal film in the right lower quadrant.

enlarged, the right hemidiaphragm is displaced upward, the duodenum and stomach are medially displaced, and usually there is downward displacement of the hepatic flexure. *Pancreatic trauma* is relatively common in childhood and most often results from automobile accidents, bicycle handlebar impacts, blows of the fist to the abdomen, falls on blunt objects, and seat belt injuries, especially in older children. It is also commonly seen in the battered child syndrome. *The most helpful diagnostic imaging procedure is computed tomography*, although ultrasonography may also be useful. Usually, the pancreas is enlarged.

Injury to the other organs such as the kidney, ureter, and urinary bladder are similar to those described in the adult.

Although the *battered child syndrome* has been most frequently associated with skull fractures and intracranial injury, the abdomen must also be considered. These children with abdominal trauma may show very little evidence of skeletal injury. The pancreas is one of the most common organs involved. Small intestinal injury is probably more common in the battered child syndrome than in any other circumstance. Indeed, when a child with unexplained abdominal injury is encountered, the "battered child syndrome" must be seriously suspected.

Text continued on page 232

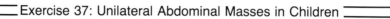

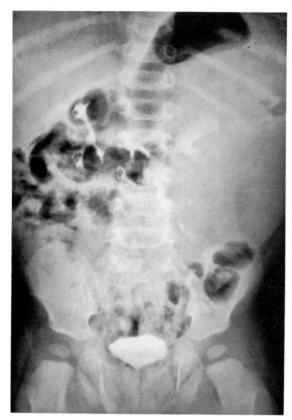

Figure E–126.

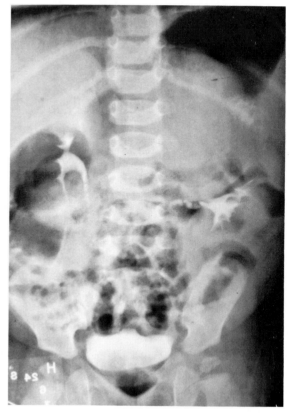

Figure E–127.

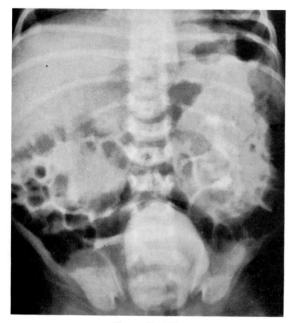

Figure E–128.

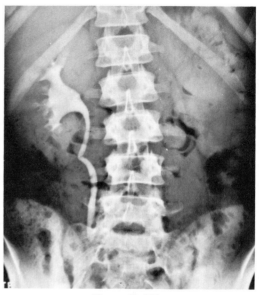

Figure E–129.

CLINICAL FINDINGS

Case 37–1 (Fig. E–126). One-year-old boy with an abdominal mass.
Case 37–2 (Fig. E–127). Six-month-old girl with an abdominal mass.
Case 37–3 (Fig. E–128). Newborn infant with an abdominal mass.
Case 37–4 (Fig. E–129). Thirteen-year-old boy with intermittent flank pain. (All figures courtesy of Dr. Thomas Sumner.)

Questions

37–1. What are the most likely diagnoses in Cases 37–1 and 37–2, respectively?
A. Wilms' tumor–neuroblastoma.
B. Wilms' tumor–adrenal hemorrhage.
C. Neuroblastoma–Wilms' tumor.
D. Neuroblastoma–adrenal hemorrhage.
E. Adrenal hemorrhage–neuroblastoma.

37–2. Which of the following is/are true?
A. Calcification is commonly seen in Wilms' tumor.
B. Calcification is rarely found in neuroblastoma.
C. Calcification is rarely found in adrenal hemorrhage.
D. Metastases from Wilms' tumor most often occur in the lungs.
E. Neuroblastoma is rarely metastatic to the bones.

37–3. What are the most likely diagnoses in Cases 37–3 and 37–4, respectively?
A. Neuroblastoma–congenital ureteropelvic junction (UPJ) obstruction.
B. Wilms' tumor–congenital absence of the kidney.
C. Multicystic kidney–congenital UPJ obstruction.
D. Congenital absence of the kidney–multicystic kidney.
E. Congenital absence of the kidney–UPJ obstruction.

37–4. Which of the following are true?
A. Multicystic kidney is the most common renal mass in the neonate.
B. Renal agenesis is likely when a kidney fails to visualize.
C. Renal ultrasound is useful in the nonvisualized kidney.
D. UPJ obstruction is usually diagnosed in older children or adults.
E. Delayed films are of no assistance in diagnosing UPJ obstruction.

Radiologic Findings. In Case 37–1, a left-sided abdominal mass is present, displacing the stomach superiorly and the colon inferiorly. Marked splaying of the left renal collecting system is evident, suggesting an intrarenal origin for the mass (Fig. E–130A). **Wilms' tumor would be the most likely consideration.** In Case 37–2, the left kidney is displaced laterally and inferiorly by a *suprarenal* mass, which contains focal calcification (Fig. E–130B). This combination of findings is most consistent with a **neuroblastoma (A is the correct answer to Question 37–2).**

In Case 37–3, the left kidney and urinary bladder are well seen; however, the right kidney is not visualized. **Multicystic kidney is the most likely consideration.** In Case 37–4, a 5-minute film from an intravenous urogram shows a normal right kidney and faint globular densities projecting over the left renal area (Fig. E–131A). At one hour, marked hydronephrosis of the left collecting system is obvious (Fig. E–131B). Congenital ureteropelvic junction (UPJ) obstruction was confirmed at surgery **(C is the correct answer to Question 37–3).**

Discussion. In a young child presenting with a unilateral abdominal mass, the main considerations are Wilms' tumor, neuroblastoma, multicystic kidney, and congenital UPJ obstruction. *In the neonate,* a rarer cause is the congenital nephroblastoma, which may be confused with a Wilms' tumor. If the unilateral mass is associated with ipsilateral renal nonvisualization, multicystic kidney and congenital hydronephrosis are the most likely considerations.

Wilms' tumor and neuroblastoma are two important neoplasms occurring in early childhood. On intravenous urography, Wilms' tumor invariably causes enlargement of the renal shadow, with separation and distortion of the collecting system, while neuroblastoma displaces and compresses the kidney. As in Case 37–2, about half of neuroblastomas arise in the suprarenal region and characteristically displace the kidney downward and outward. The remainder may arise anywhere along the sympathetic chain. Tumor calcification is rarely seen in

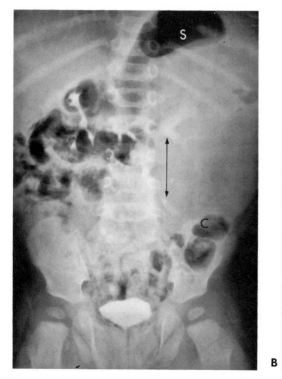
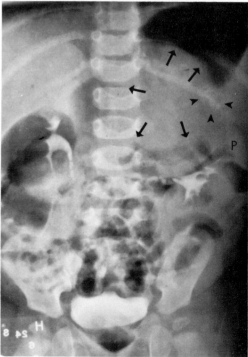

Figure E–130. *A.* Large Wilms' tumor of the left kidney displacing both the stomach (S) and the colon (C). The left collecting system is splayed (arrows) with its upper portion mildly dilated. *B.* Neuroblastoma (arrows) containing mottled calcification (arrowheads). The upper pole (P) of the left kidney is markedly displaced.

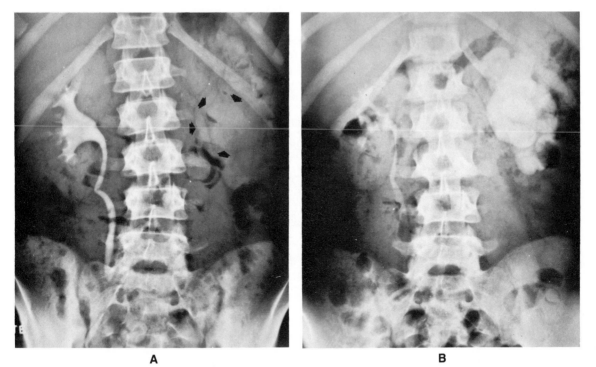

A   **B**

Figure E–131. *A.* The five minute film from the urogram showing faint opacification of the collecting system (arrows). *B.* At one hour, pelvocaliceal dilatation from congenital UPJ obstruction is obvious.

Wilms' tumor (**Question 37–2A is false**) but is typically present in neuroblastoma (**Question 37–2B is false**) and adrenal hemorrhage (**Question 37–2C is false**). Wilms' tumor most often metastasizes to the lungs (**Question 37–2D is true**), while bony metastases are a feature of neuroblastoma (**Question 37–2E is false**).

Multicystic kidney is probably the most common cause of unilateral abdominal mass presenting in the first week of life (**Question 37–4A is true**). Intravenous urography inevitably shows nonfunction on the side of the mass, even when delayed films are obtained. This combination of findings makes the diagnosis almost certain, since renal agenesis is a much rarer anomaly (**Question 37–4B is false**). Renal ultrasound is helpful not only for diagnosing multicystic kidney, but also for differentiating it from hydronephrosis (**Question 37–4C is true**). Congenital UPJ obstruction is usually discovered in the older child or young adult (**Question 37–4D is true**). Intravenous urography may show only nonfunction early, indicating the need for delayed films, which often demonstrate the presence and site of obstruction (**Question 37–4E is false**).

THE INGESTION OF FOREIGN MATERIALS BY THE INFANT OR CHILD

Corrosive Fluid Ingestion. The most frequently encountered corrosive fluid ingestion is lye. The entire esophagus may be involved, and extensive tissue necrosis with perforation occasionally occurs. This ultimately may result in stricture formation.

Ingested Foreign Bodies. Usually, ingested oval foreign bodies pass down the esophagus into the stomach and may pass through the entire intestine with little or no problem. Larger foreign bodies may become impacted at the cricopharyngeal muscle, aortic knob, or gastroesophageal junction. Opaque foreign bodies are readily detected radiographically. In the neck, however, hyoid bone ossification and laryngeal calcifications must not be mistaken for foreign bodies. Ingestion of a foreign body may be associated with stridor or even pneumonia, particularly if aspiration of food or normal secretions occurs.

PEDIATRIC EMERGENCY CONDITIONS INVOLVING THE EXTREMITIES

Important problems related to the extremities in the child that warrant discussion include subtle and frequently missed fractures, inflammatory lesions, and soft tissue and periarticular changes. Likewise, emphasis should be placed upon epiphyseal injuries, classified by Salter and Harris, as shown in Figure 8–6. The cortical or torus fractures; greenstick fractures; epiphyseal-metaphyseal fractures; and the classification of fractures by the Salter-Harris system have already been addressed.

Acute Osteomyelitis. Radiographic evidence of acute osteomyelitis frequently takes at least 10 days to two weeks to develop and may first consist of soft tissue swelling or very minimal periosteal elevation prior to bone resorption. Radionuclide bone scanning can be of considerable aid in the detection of osseous infections early because of osteoclastic and osteoblastic activity around the affected area. Indeed, radionuclide bone scans can become positive within 48 hours of injury or infection, emphasizing that the bone scan should be performed initially when the diagnosis is suspected. The radiograph is particularly helpful in follow-up studies to detect the presence particularly of sequestration and to denote appropriate treatment.

Septic arthritis, toxic synovitis, and **cellulitis** of the hip pose special problems in the child. These are afflictions of older infants and children, seldom occurring prior to the age of two years. Clinically, there is an abrupt onset of pain and limp. Although the radiographic findings may be normal at first, there is often a widening of the joint space, bulging of the gluteus medius fat pad, obliteration of the obturator fat pad, and capsular distention discernible by comparison of one side with the other. The hallmark of septic arthritis of the hip is widening of the joint space due to the lateral displacement of the femoral head.

Aseptic necrosis of the hip or slipped capital femoral epiphysis of childhood are other lesions that may present acutely.

Cellulitis of the knee is usually evident radiographically when the soft tissues anterior to the quadriceps tendon are swollen and the unossified or partially ossified cartilaginous patella appears buried within the soft tissue swelling. Although the swelling is unassociated with suprapatellar bursal distention, this may accompany the prepatellar swelling. Radionuclide bone scanning may be particularly helpful in this diagnosis.

Although overt **injuries of the lower leg** are not difficult to recognize, fracture of the tibia with an associated bending fracture of the fibula may be overlooked. In young infants, the so-called "toddler's fracture," a spiral, hairline fracture, may be barely visible on initial roentgenograms. Also, stress fractures may be most evident by their associated soft tissue swelling.

Normal Soft Tissues and Fat Pads of the Ankle. In the infant and child, three fat pads are seen in the lateral projection of the foot and ankle. The pre-Achilles fat pad is just anterior to the Achilles tendon. An anterior fat pad is located just behind the extensor tendon of the foot, and in the older child a small posterior fat pad is visible, particularly with injury, just in front of the pre-Achilles fat pad. The lateral view of the ankle is best for studying joint effusions, seen as an increased soft tissue density over the ankle and outward displacement of the fat pads.

Injuries of the Ankle Particularly Frequent in Children. In the young infant, a *cortical buckle* (torus) fracture through the distal tibia and fibula is very common. In the older child, the more common injury involves the epiphysis and/or metaphysis, as described by the Salter-Harris classification.

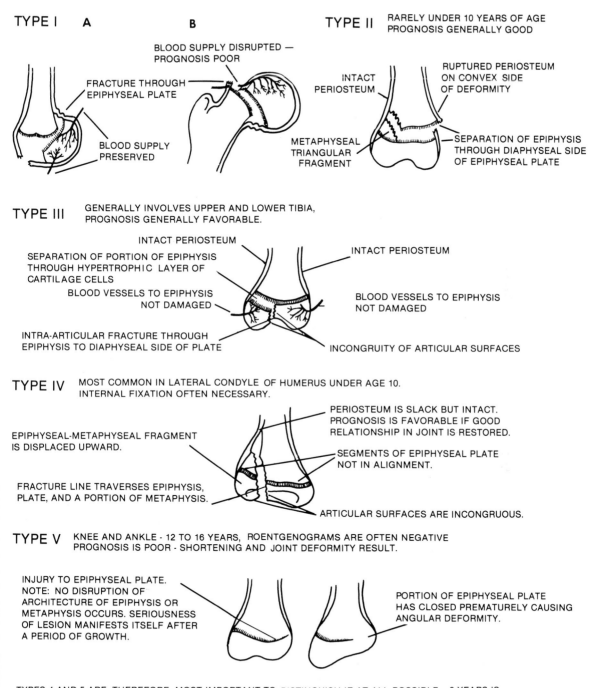

TYPE I   **A**   **B**   **TYPE II**   RARELY UNDER 10 YEARS OF AGE
                                                         PROGNOSIS GENERALLY GOOD

BLOOD SUPPLY DISRUPTED —
PROGNOSIS POOR

FRACTURE THROUGH
EPIPHYSEAL PLATE

INTACT
PERIOSTEUM

RUPTURED PERIOSTEUM
ON CONVEX SIDE
OF DEFORMITY

BLOOD SUPPLY
PRESERVED

METAPHYSEAL
TRIANGULAR
FRAGMENT

SEPARATION OF EPIPHYSIS
THROUGH DIAPHYSEAL SIDE
OF EPIPHYSEAL PLATE

TYPE III   GENERALLY INVOLVES UPPER AND LOWER TIBIA,
              PROGNOSIS GENERALLY FAVORABLE.

INTACT PERIOSTEUM

SEPARATION OF PORTION OF EPIPHYSIS
THROUGH HYPERTROPHIC LAYER OF
CARTILAGE CELLS

BLOOD VESSELS TO EPIPHYSIS
NOT DAMAGED

INTACT PERIOSTEUM

BLOOD VESSELS TO EPIPHYSIS
NOT DAMAGED

INTRA-ARTICULAR FRACTURE THROUGH
EPIPHYSIS TO DIAPHYSEAL SIDE OF PLATE

INCONGRUITY OF ARTICULAR SURFACES

TYPE IV   MOST COMMON IN LATERAL CONDYLE OF HUMERUS UNDER AGE 10.
             INTERNAL FIXATION OFTEN NECESSARY.

PERIOSTEUM IS SLACK BUT INTACT.
PROGNOSIS IS FAVORABLE IF GOOD
RELATIONSHIP IN JOINT IS RESTORED.

EPIPHYSEAL-METAPHYSEAL FRAGMENT
IS DISPLACED UPWARD.

SEGMENTS OF EPIPHYSEAL PLATE
NOT IN ALIGNMENT.

FRACTURE LINE TRAVERSES EPIPHYSIS,
PLATE, AND A PORTION OF METAPHYSIS.

ARTICULAR SURFACES ARE INCONGRUOUS.

TYPE V   KNEE AND ANKLE - 12 TO 16 YEARS, ROENTGENOGRAMS ARE OFTEN NEGATIVE
            PROGNOSIS IS POOR - SHORTENING AND JOINT DEFORMITY RESULT.

INJURY TO EPIPHYSEAL PLATE.
NOTE: NO DISRUPTION OF
ARCHITECTURE OF EPIPHYSIS OR
METAPHYSIS OCCURS. SERIOUSNESS
OF LESION MANIFESTS ITSELF AFTER
A PERIOD OF GROWTH.

PORTION OF EPIPHYSEAL PLATE
HAS CLOSED PREMATURELY CAUSING
ANGULAR DEFORMITY.

TYPES 4 AND 5 ARE, THEREFORE, MOST IMPORTANT TO DISTINGUISH IF AT ALL POSSIBLE.   2 YEARS IS
CONSIDERED MINIMUM BEFORE ONE CAN EXCLUDE THE POSSIBILITY OF SHORTENING AND DEFORMITY.
RADIOGRAPHIC RE-EVALUATION SHOULD BE PERFORMED AT 2 TO 6 MONTH INTERVALS, INCLUDING COMPARISON
VIEWS WITH THE OPPOSITE EXTREMITY.

Figure 8–6. Salter-Harris classification of epiphyseal injuries. Modified from DePalma AF: The Management of
Fractures and Dislocations. Philadelphia, W. B. Saunders, 1959.

Inversion-rotation and eversion injuries of the ankle are also common in children, the ankle mortise in the latter often seriously disturbed with posterior malleolar fractures of the Salter-Harris type II. Some of these ankle fractures are visualized only in the lateral projection.

THE BATTERED CHILD SYNDROME

Introduction. This is a *very important medical and sociological emergency*, and it is important to suspect this injury if (a) the radiologic manifestations of injury are more extensive than clinically suspected; (b) the clinical history is poorly correlated with the radiographic findings; and (c) multiple injuries are sustained that are unsuspected. Calvarial injuries are common with underlying subdural hematomas. The most characteristic lesion, however, is the epiphyseal-metaphyseal fracture, usually of the Salter-Harris types I and II.

These fractures are usually multiple and in different stages of healing. Often, the child presents with soft tissue injuries, and fractures are not clinically suspected. A complete bone survey should be obtained. Other types of injuries include pancreatitis, duodenal injuries, and involvement of other intra-abdominal organs.

PEDIATRIC HEAD PROBLEMS

Clinical Findings that Would Allow Obtaining Skull Roentgenograms in Cases of Head Injury. X-rays of the skull are frequently overdone and are often obtained for medical/legal purposes only. Skull roentgenograms are indicated, however, if there is a *history of unconsciousness, amnesia, or vomiting*; if there is a *palpable bony malalignment* following injury; if there is a *discharge, especially bloody, from the ear*, or *from the nose*; or if there is an *eardrum discoloration*. Other clinical indications include stupor, coma, positive Babinsky reflex, cranial nerve abnormality, and serious head injury with suspected depressed skull fracture. Otherwise the skull roentgenogram is of limited value. Probably, when head injury is seriously suspected, *computed tomography would be more helpful* since injury to the brain or its meninges is usually more important than the calvarial fracture, if present.

It is most important to detect depressed fractures, because a depressed fragment may give rise to convulsive seizures, particularly of the Jacksonian type. A familiarity of normal sutural anatomy at various ages is important, since diastasis of the sutures may be the only indication of cranial injury.

Regarding serial films, the mere presence of a linear fracture does not dictate a need for a follow-up radiograph. However, if there is a diastasis of sutures or fractures, repeat radiographs should be obtained a few weeks or months later, to check for the development of a *post-traumatic leptomeningeal cyst.*

Other aspects of fractures of the skull such as differentiation of basal skull fractures, differentiation of the normal lines and sutures of the skull, occipital region fractures and pseudofractures, and differentiation of multiplicity of Wormian bones, are similar to those of the adult, as also are fractures of the face.

THE SPINE AND SPINAL CORD

Special Interpretive Problems in Children. *Physiologic displacement of the body of C2 on the body of C3 is a common phenomenon in childhood and is not pathologic.* These patients may demonstrate a flattening of the antero-superior aspect of the body of C3, and at times of C4.

Injuries of the atlas and axis must be very carefully interpreted in light of the many anomalies that may occur with respect to the odontoid process. It should be remembered, however, that the predental distance is normally wider in children than in adults and it is not unusual for this distance to measure up to 4 or 5 mm in contrast with a maximum normal of 3 mm in the adult.

Extension Injuries of the Lower Cervical Spine. The fracture occurs in the articular facets and posterior elements, with little in the way of vertebral body compression. The "tear-drop" fracture is one of the most significant of hyperextension injuries, and is usually associated with significant ligamentous injury and an unstable spine. Prevertebral soft tissue swelling is often present. The ligamentum flavum may buckle during hyperextension, causing a focal compression of the spinal cord. This may result in serious injury to the spinal cord, even though the cervical spine films may appear normal.

Extension Injuries of the Atlas and Axis.

These are quite common in the infant, and among the most common are those through the posterior arch of C1, the fractures of the dens, and the classic hangman's fracture of C2 described in relation to the adult. These fractures usually cause narrow defects through the posterior arch of C1 and may thereby be differentiated from a congenital defect of the arch.

Lateral Flexion Injuries of the Cervical Spine. Lateral flexion injuries in the child may cause contralateral widening and disruption of the joints of Luschka. If such widening occurs at every spinal level, it is probably normal; however, if disparity is localized, underlying ligamentous tear and potential instability of the cervical spine must be suspected.

Rotation Injuries of the Cervical Spine. These occur in either the upper or lower cervical spine, may be associated with flexion or extension injuries, and may result in a unilateral "locked" or "jumped" facet.

CERVICAL CORD AND NERVE ROOT INJURIES

Brachial Plexus Injuries. Brachial plexus injuries are usually of the avulsion type, resulting from excessive lateral flexion and rotation of the spine or from excessive posterior stretching of the arm. A paralysis of the affected limb occurs. With C5 to C7 injuries, a Duchenne-Erb's paralysis of the shoulder and upper arm results, while a Klumpke's paralysis of the hand results from C8 to T1 injuries. The typical myelographic findings include extravasation of the contrast material along the nerve routes and formation of traumatic meningoceles or cysts.

The Central Cord Syndrome. In the central cord syndrome, spinal radiographs may be normal despite a severe injury to the cervical spinal cord with neurological deficit.

This injury results from pinching and squeezing of the cord between the anterior and posterior walls of the spinal canal secondary to buckling of the ligamentum flavum during hyperextension.

Anomalies of the Base of C1 and the Base of the Skull Causing Problems. The most important of these varied anomalies is the hypoplastic dens associated with an os odontoideum. The appearance suggests a fractured dens, but actually the os odontoideum is an overgrown os terminale and the dens itself is hypoplastic. By adolescence it becomes fused with the dens. The lesion is unstable and frequently requires surgical stabilization.

Thoracolumbar Spine Trauma Peculiar to Children. These consist of flexion, extension, lateral flexion, rotation, and axial compression type injuries. The seat-belt injury is termed the Chance fracture and can be readily detected by its horizontal configuration on the frontal view.

Miscellaneous Problems of the Spine in Children. Infections of the spine, extending along the psoas musculature, pathologic features, and intervertebral disc herniations do occur in the child but do not differ significantly from those in the adult. On the other hand, a calcified intervertebral disc in the adult is usually of no significance, but in the child it probably is of pathologic significance, even though its etiology may be unknown.

The normal variations in the thoracolumbar region which may cause problems in the child are the lack of ossification of the ring epiphysis of the vertebral body; the extra-epiphysis along the anterior/superior aspect of a vertebral body simulating a teardrop fracture and the bipartite transverse process or rudimentary rib of a lumbar vertebra which may be misinterpreted as a fracture. Likewise, the accessory ossicle of the transverse process must not be misinterpreted.

Urinary Tract

A supine film (Fig. 4–2A and B) study of the abdomen (KUB) is first obtained (a preliminary plain film study should always first be obtained prior to the introduction of contrast agents, if at all possible). As was described previously, the nine basic roentgen signs are applied to this preliminary film prior to the introduction of any contrast agent (see Chapter 4).

If there is any question regarding calculi contained within the kidney or abnormalities of size or contour with respect to the kidney or the KUB film, nephrotomograms are obtained of the kidney areas usually at four different levels: the 8 cm level is probably the average mid-kidney level in most individuals, and when this is studied, appropriate tomographic levels are chosen for best visualization of the entire kidney regions bilaterally.

Thereafter, a suitable iodinated water-soluble contrast agent is injected as rapidly as possible in large bolus, obtaining the first film of the kidney areas within one minute. Hopefully, of at least 100 ml (in the adult) of 50 to 60% of the water-soluble iodinated contrast agent will have been injected by that time. A low to intermediate kilovoltage is employed during suspended respiration.

IODINATED WATER-SOLUBLE CONTRAST AGENTS

The most frequently utilized iodinated water-soluble intravenous contrast agents used are sodium, meglumine (methyglucamine), or a combination of the two as the radiolucent cations, and diatrizoate, iothalamate, or metrizoate as the radiopaque anion. Theoretically, the sodium agents are preferable to the meglumine, since they are less viscous and less likely to lead to intense diuresis, allowing for an easier injection of a large bolus and diluting the pyelogram less. Irrespective of the contrast agent employed, most uroradiologists now use a minimum dose of 300 mg of iodine per kilogram of body weight for the standard adult with normal renal function. In renal failure, this dose may be doubled, *provided the patient is hydrated prior to the introduction of the contrast agent.* These water-soluble iodinated contrast agents are excreted primarily by the glomeruli of the kidney and find great usefulness not only in examinations of the urinary tract but also in angiography, arthrography, and neuroradiologic angiography, although generally the meglumine products are preferred for angiography. At the one-minute interval, the film obtained is the *nephrogram* (Fig. 9–1A and B), since there is a diffuse opacification of the entire kidney. Useful films for the study of renovascular hypertension may be obtained by further films at one-minute intervals for 4 or 5 minutes. Normally, the collecting system should be visualized at least by three minutes. Delay in appearance time is one of the roentgen signs of renovascular hypertension. Opacification of the gallbladder may occur even in the presence of normal renal function, but it becomes especially apparent when one kidney is suddenly obstructed, as in the case of a ureteral calculus. There is no contraindication to intravenous urography performed in this manner, except in cases of impaired renal function, when the patient must be hydrated prior to the study; the same is true in cases of myeloma and in infants.

REACTIONS TO CONTRAST MEDIA

Unfortunately, adverse reactions to these intravenous contrast agents may be

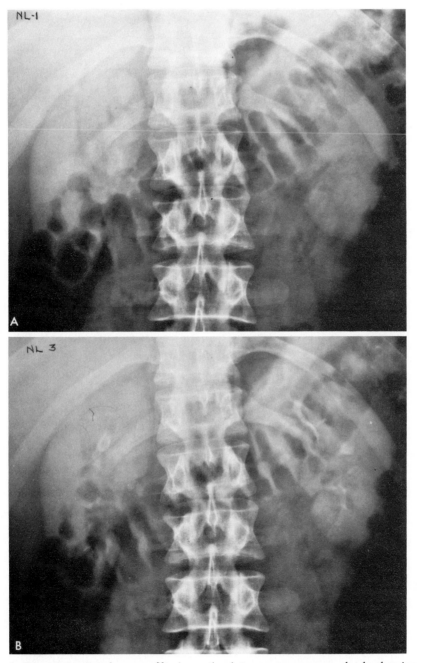

Figure 9–1. *A,* One minute "nephrogram film in routine intravenous urogram, clearly showing renal outlines. *B,* Ten minute film in the same patient. The renal outlines are not seen as well.

quite severe or even lethal on rare occasions; hence they must be used cautiously and with very careful attention and indication (Table 9–1). There is, unfortunately, no simple method for anticipating adverse reactions. Injection into the eye for corneal response, skin tests, and any test except for the actual intravenous use of the agent is of no avail. The minimal reactions, which consist of a feeling of warmth, sensation of flushing, nausea, vomiting, and even urticaria, are not contraindications to the procedure. They may be treated with antihistamines if desired. The major reactions, as indicated in Table 9–1, may require emergency treatment—even cardiopulmonary resuscitation. Therefore, anyone who would perform an excretory urogram must be prepared to deal with severe

Table 9–1 MAJOR REACTIONS TO CONTRAST MEDIA, COMPLICATIONS THEREFROM, AND THEIR TREATMENT

Type	Complication	Treatment
Cardiovascular system	Cardiac arrest	Sharp blow to precordium
	Asystole	External cardiac massage, etc.
	Ventricular fibrillation	External defibrillation immediately
	Hypotension, syncope	Posture, vasopressor drugs, etc.
	Pulmonary edema	Aminophylline, Demerol, Lasix, phlebotomy, oxygen, morphine
Respiratory system	Respiratory arrest (or obstruction)	Maintain airway (by natural or artificial means)
		Pulmonary ventilation
Central nervous system	Toxic convulsions	Nembutal or diazepam IV
	Coma	Solu-Cortef IV
Allergic reaction	Angioneurotic edema	Adrenaline, Solu-Cortef
	Bronchoplasm	Aminophylline, Benadryl

Modified after Weigen and Thomas and ACR Bulletin on Reactions to Contrast Media. (Weigen, J. F., and Thomas, S. F.: Reactions to intravenous organic iodide compounds and their immediate treatment. Radiology 71:21, 1958.)

contrast medium reactions. As a precaution, steroids may be injected 24 hours prior to the actual test, and in no instance in which this has been done has a death been reported. However, studies along these lines are still premature, and although prior injection of steroids may be of some avail, this is not certain.

The best pyelograms for demonstrating caliceal detail require abdominal compression (Fig. 9–2A and B). The compression is released when optimum visualization of the ureters and urinary bladder is desired. Nephrotomography is employed during the collecting system phase of the appearance of the contrast agent (5 to 10 minutes following the intravenous injection) for optimum visualization (Fig. 9–3A and B). If the ureters are not seen in their entirety, following release of the abdominal compression, oblique films of the abdomen and even prone films may be employed (Fig. 9–4A and B).

When the urinary bladder is fully distended it may be desirable to obtain both oblique views of the urinary bladder; a voiding cystourethrogram may also be obtained following this sequence in the oblique projection to see the urethra in its entirety. For optimum cysturethrography, retrograde examination is desirable (Fig. 9–5A, B, C).

Following voiding, another KUB film is obtained in order to see if there is any retention in the upper urinary tract and to study the degree of emptying of the urinary bladder. Normally, approximately 100 ml of contrast agent remains in the urinary bladder following voiding.

In general, the intravenous urogram is "hand tailored" to the clinical problem at hand; and with 90-second development of each film, the subsequent film is chosen at the optimum interval. If obstruction is encountered, delayed films even as long as 24 to 48 hours may be useful.

INTRAVENOUS UROGRAPHY IN CHILDREN

Dehydration is contraindicated in infants and is undesirable in young children. In general, a dose of 1 to 2 ml of the contrast agent is employed on a body weight basis. A short exposure time and protection of the gonads are routine. If a voiding cystourethrogram is desired, it is performed following the excretory urogram.

RETROGRADE PYELOGRAMS

These are obtained only if the visualization by excretory urography is inconclusive. The study is best performed by the urologist under fluoroscopic control and may be done in one of two ways: (1) by gently wedging a bulb catheter in the lower ureter at the time the contrast medium is injected, or (2) by introducing a catheter into the upper urinary tract *via* the ureter with subsequent injection of the contrast agent. The latter requires cystoscopy and the insertion of ureters into each ureteral orifice, passing the ureters as far as the renal pelves bilaterally. If the ure-

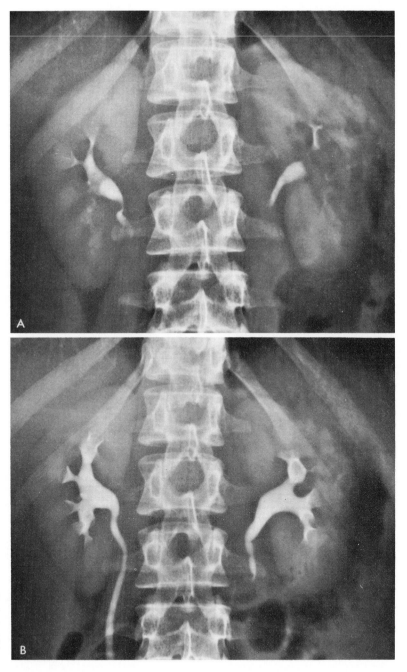

Figure 9–2. *A*, Five minute film from routine urogram showing poor pelvicaliceal distention. *B*, Following ureteral compression, better distention and definition of the collecting system are evident.

A

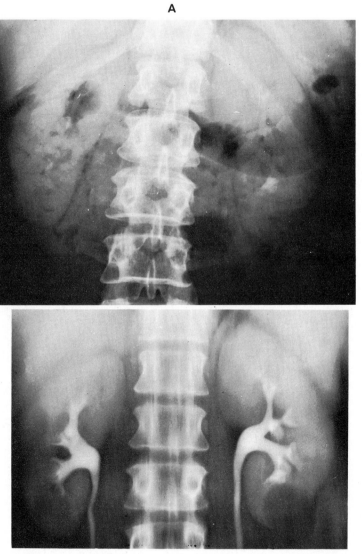

B

Figure 9–3. Value of drip-infusion urogram with tomogram. *A,* Routine low dose excretory urogram showing poor visualization of renal pelvis and calices. *B,* Drip-infusion urogram with tomogram. Excellent visualization of renal parenchyma and collecting system. Previously unsuspected mass (simple cyst) is present in lower pole of left kidney. (From Emmett, J. E., and Witten, D. M.: Clinical Urography. 3rd ed., Vol. 1, Philadelphia, W. B. Saunders Co., 1971.)

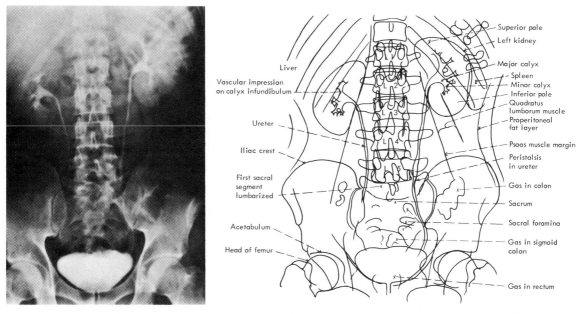

Figure 9–4. Representative excretory urogram (also called intravenous pyelogram) obtained 15 minutes after the intravenous injection of a suitable contrast agent. *A,* Radiograph. *B,* Labeled tracing.

Figure 9–5. *A,* Normal cystogram, antero-posterior view. *B,* Normal retrograde cystoure-throgram.

Illustration continued on following page

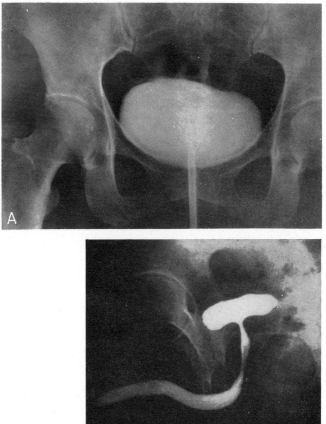

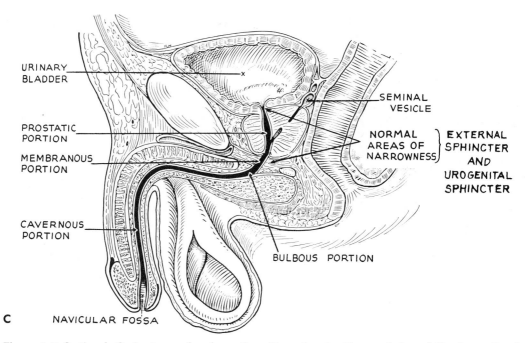

Figure 9-5 *Continued. C*, Anatomy of male urethra. (Reproduced with permission of Goodyear, Beard, and Weens, and Publishers of Southern Medical Journal.)

teral pelves are not visualized at this time, it is assumed that obstruction has been encountered. A further film is obtained while the catheters are being removed and contrast agent injected. Artefactual air bubbles must be avoided.

As the technique for excretory urography has improved, the need for retrograde studies has diminished sharply.

LOOPOGRAM

When the urinary bladder has been surgically removed, usually in treatment of carcinoma or some similar involvement of the urinary bladder, an ileal loop is constructed for anastomosis with the ureters bilaterally. The kidneys, kidney calices, pelves, and ureters, as well as the ileal loop, may be studied by excretory urography or by retrograde injection through the ileal loop. Occasionally, leakage of contrast agent is demonstrated at the sites of anastomosis. There is often reflux from the ileal loop to the upper urinary tracts with infection supervening, often causing hydronephrosis and hydroureter. The

determination of the extent of this occurrence is the main purpose for this examination.

NEPHROSTOMOGRAM

If there is a nephrostomy tube in place, or if contrast agent is to be injected directly into the renal pelvis under fluoroscopic or ultrasound control with a long narrow calibered needle, the diatrizoate or iothalamate is injected through these tubes, with distention of the collecting system and visualization of the collecting system down to the area of potential obstruction. Such a film can demonstrate the extent of ureteral obstruction, when present.

ULTRASONOGRAM
(Fig. 9-6)

Ultrasound has proved enormously important in the investigation of the kidney for abnormalities in its contour and for the differentiation of solid and cystic lesions of the kidney. Space-occupying lesions within the kidney substance or obstruction that may be inferred from a dilated pelvicaliceal system

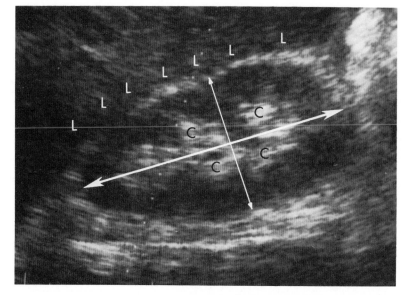

Figure 9–6. Longitudinal ultrasonic scan of a normal right kidney (long interconnected arrow = interpolar length; short interconnected arrow = anteroposterior dimension). Central echoes represent the pelvicaliceal complex (C). The renal parenchyma is relatively sonolucent. (L = interface with liver.)

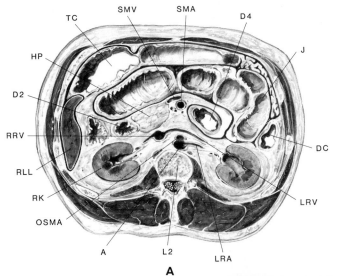

A

Figure 9–7. *A,* Cross-sectional diagram of abdomen at L2 level. *B,* Corresponding computed tomograph obtained approximately at this level. A = aorta; OSMA = origin of superior mesenteric artery; RK = right kidney; RLL = right lobe of liver; RRV = right renal vein; D2 = 2nd part of duodenum; HP = head of pancreas; TC = transverse colon; SMV = superior mesenteric vein; SMA = superior mesenteric artery; D4 = fourth part of duodenum; J = jejunum; DC = descending colon; LRV = left renal vein; LRA = left renal artery.

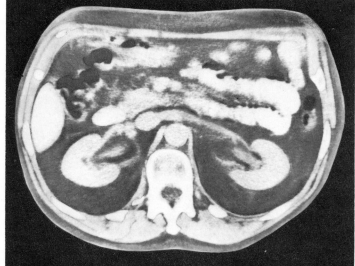

B

may readily be determined. This entire technology will be more adequately described subsequently.

COMPUTED TOMOGRAPHY
(Fig. 9–7A and B)

The application of this specialized technique will be separately described subsequently.

SEMINAL VESICULOGRAPHY

Direct injections into the vas deferens in the scrotum or cannulation of the prostatic utricle have been performed in the past with the injection of diatrizoate into these structures under local or general anesthesia. This procedure is rarely performed since the advent of computed tomography, because significant information regarding the seminal vesicles (and perforate) particularly can be obtained with the aid of this more recent procedure.

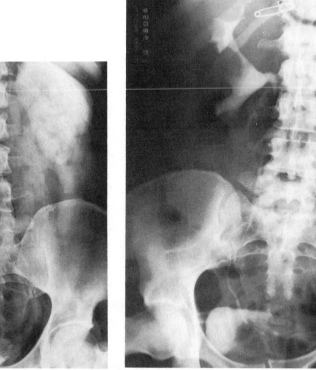

Figure E–132.

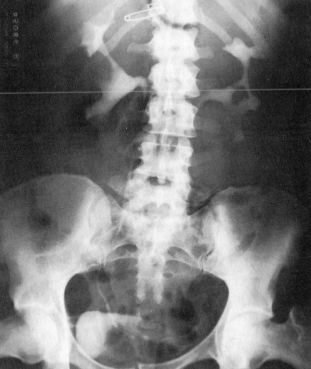

Figure E–133.

CLINICAL FINDINGS

Case 38–1 (Fig. E–132) is a 25-year-old man with microscopic hematuria.

Case 38–2 (Fig. E–133) is a 45-year-old woman with hypertension and uremia.

Questions

38–1. The enlarged, dense left kidney in Case 38–1 is explained BEST by?

A. Renal vein thrombosis.

B. Compensatory hypertrophy.

C. Duplex kidney.

D. Acute urate nephropathy.

E. Obstructive uropathy.

38–2. In Case 38–2, which of the following is LEAST likely?

A. Adult polycystic disease.

B. Acute tubular necrosis.

C. Leukemic infiltration.

D. Hodgkin's disease.

E. Tuberous sclerosis.

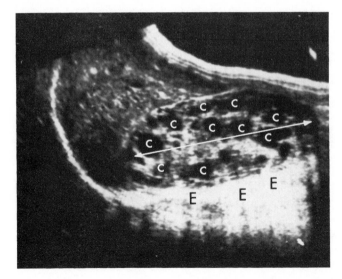

Figure E–134. Longitudinal ultrasonic scan of a markedly enlarged polycystic right kidney (arrows). Multiple sonolucent cysts (C) are seen within the kidney associated with increased transmission of sound through the organ (E). (Courtesy of Dr. Neil Wolfman.)

Radiologic Findings. In Case 38–1, the left kidney is enlarged and densely opacified due to calculus obstruction at the ureterovesical junction. (**E is the correct answer to question 38–1**). The persistently dense nephrogram results from accumulation of contrast material within the renal tubular system, and is a common feature of obstructive uropathy. Acute urate nephropathy also produces a dense, persistent nephrogram, but invariably affects both kidneys. In renal vein thrombosis, the nephrogram is usually faint or poorly seen.

In Case 38–2, both kidneys are markedly enlarged, with stretching and distortion of the pelvicaliceal systems. In view of the clinical history, this appearance would be most consistent with adult polycystic disease, as was true in this patient. Lymphoma, leukemia, or tuberous sclerosis could appear similarly. Acute tubular necrosis, however, produces bilaterally dense and persistent nephrograms, comparable to the appearance of urate nephropathy (**B is the correct answer to question 38–2**). Intravenous urography is usually diagnostic for polycystic disease, except in its early development, when abdominal ultrasound or computed tomography may be more sensitive (Fig. E–134).

Discussion. Diffuse enlargement of one or both kidneys can result from many different causes (Tables E–2 and E–3). Usually, the causes of unilateral renal enlargement differ from those producing bilateral enlargement. In several disorders, such as obstructive uropathy or renal vein thrombosis, either one or

Table E–2. CAUSES OF UNILATERAL ENLARGEMENT OF THE KIDNEY

Compensatory hypertrophy	Renal vein thrombosis*
Duplicated pelvicaliceal system*	Acute arterial infarction
Multicystic kidney	Acute pyelonephritis
Obstructive uropathy*	Xanthogranulomatous pyelonephritis

*These disorders will occasionally affect both kidneys.

Table E–3. CAUSES OF BILATERAL ENLARGEMENT OF BOTH KIDNEYS

Adult polycystic disease	Acute glomerulonephritis
Tuberous sclerosis (hamartomas)	Nephromegaly (cirrhosis/acromegaly)
Sickle cell anemia	Diabetic glomerulosclerosis
Leukemia/lymphoma	Systemic lupus erythematosus
Multiple myeloma/amyloidosis	Polyarteritis nodosa
Acute tubular/cortical necrosis	Miscellaneous proliferative disorders
Acute urate nephropathy	Other necrotizing disorders
Acute interstitial nephritis	

both kidneys may be enlarged. In addition to clinical history and number of kidneys involved, other radiographic features are important in differentiating between the various disorders. In both compensatory hypertrophy and pelvicaliceal duplication, an increased renal length is present in an otherwise normal kidney (Fig. E–135). However, the opposite kidney will be diseased or absent in compensatory renal enlargement and normal or duplex if duplication is present.

The functional status of the kidney and the appearance of the renal contour and pelvicaliceal system are also helpful in differential diagnosis. In obstructive uropathy, urate nephropathy, and acute tubular necrosis, a dense and persistent nephrogram is typically seen, while in disorders such as renal vein thrombosis and acute arterial infarction the kidney fails to opacify. Depending on the severity of involvement, many of the diseases that affect the kidneys bilaterally may show both a poor nephrogram and faint visualization of the collecting system.

Evaluating the contour of the kidney for smoothness or irregularity is important. Although most diseases that enlarge the kidney also preserve its relatively smooth contour, the presence of irregularity is more suggestive of polycystic disease, lymphoma, xanthogranulomatous pyelonephritis, or tuberous sclerosis. Stretching of the pelvicaliceal system is a common occurrence in a pathologically enlarged kidney; however, distortion of the collecting system is more often seen in those disorders that also cause irregularity of the renal contour.

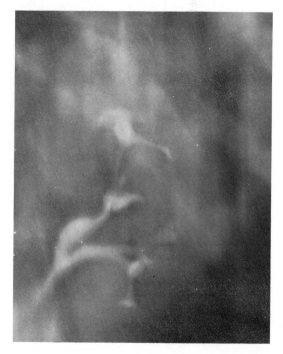

Figure E–135. The left kidney measured 2.5 cm longer than the right. The discrepancy in renal length is explained best by duplication of the collecting system.

Exercise 39: Solitary Renal Masses

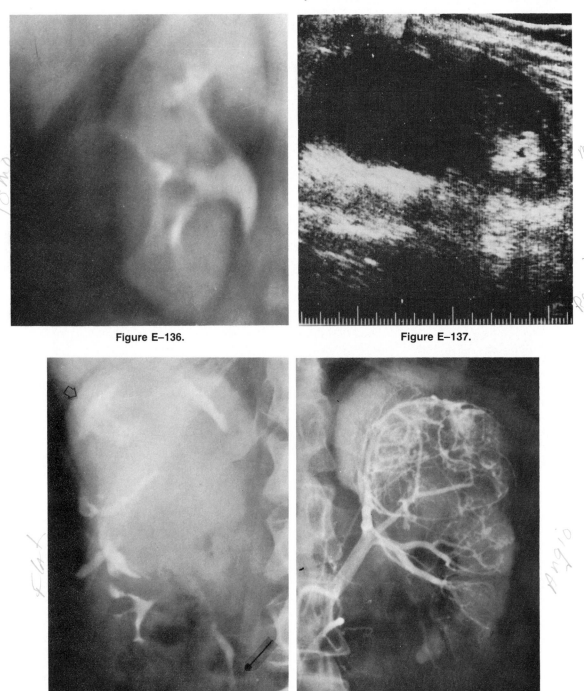

Figure E–136.

Figure E–137.

A

B

Figure E–138.

248

CLINICAL FINDINGS
    Case 39–1 (Fig. E–136). Forty-five-year-old with a focal renal mass.
    Case 39–2 (Fig. E–137). Sixty-year-old woman with a renal mass examined by longitudinal ultrasound. (Courtesy of Dr. Neil Wolfman).
    Case 39–3 (Fig. E–138A). Fifty-year-old woman with large right renal mass.
    Case 39–4 (Fig. E–138B). Renal mass examined by angiography. (Courtesy of Dr. Thomas Hunt).

Questions
    39–1. In Case 39–1, what urographic feature is NOT present?
    A. Sharp transition between the mass and normal kidney.
    B. Presence of a "beak sign" and thin outer wall.
    C. Caliceal destruction and amputation.
    D. Relative lucency of the mass compared to normal kidney.
    E. Normal appearing pelvicaliceal system.

    39–2. In Case 39–2, what ultrasonic feature is NOT present?
    A. Paucity of echoes off the back wall of the mass.
    B. Significant transmission of sound through the mass.
    C. Sharply defined anterior border of the mass.
    D. Sharply defined posterior border of the mass.
    E. Absence of internal echoes within the mass.

    39–3. In Case 39–3, what urographic feature is NOT present?
    A. Caliceal distortion and displacement.
    B. Homogeneous lucency throughout the mass.
    C. Focal caliceal dilatation.
    D. Poorly defined borders of the mass.
    E. Absence of the "beak sign" and thin wall.

    39–4. In Case 39–4, what is the LEAST likely angiographic diagnosis?
    A. Angiomyolipoma (hamartoma).
    B. Large renal abscess.
    C. Renal cell carcinoma.
    D. Renal cell adenoma.
    E. Simple renal cyst.

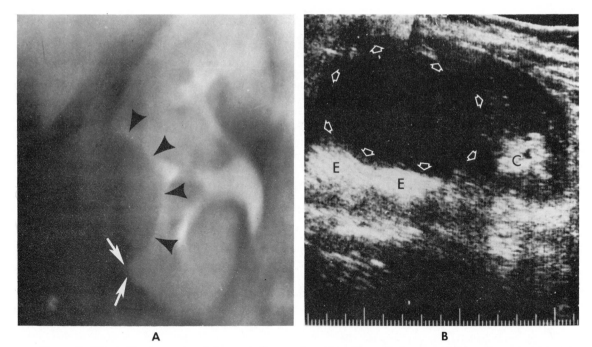

Figure E–139. *A,* Simple renal cyst demonstrating an abrupt transition with the normal kidney (arrowheads) and a triangular "beak sign" inferiorly (arrows). *B,* Sonolucent renal mass (arrows) involving the upper half of the kidney. Marked accentuation of echoes (E) along the back wall of the cyst. The echo complex inferiorly represents the lower pole caliceal complex (C).

Radiologic Findings. Case 39–1 demonstrates the urographic features of a simple renal cyst. The lesion appears homogeneously lucent compared to the contrast-opacified normal renal parenchyma. The outer wall of the cyst is thin, while its borders with the normal kidney are sharply demarcated and "beaked" (Fig. E–139*A*). The pelvocaliceal system appears normal **(C is the correct answer to Question 39–1)**.

Case 39–2 shows the ultrasonic features of a large simple renal cyst. The lesion is sonolucent (i.e., absence of internal echoes), indicating significant transmission of sound through the mass (Fig. E–139*B*). The borders are sharply defined with accentuation of echoes off the back wall **(A is the correct answer to Question 39–2)**.

Case 39–3 represents a carcinoma of the upper pole of the right kidney. The calices are displaced, distorted, and dilated. The borders of the mass are poorly defined. The carcinoma opacifies similar to the normal parenchyma, indicating a noncystic lesion **(B is the correct answer to Question 39–3)**.

Case 39–4 illustrates the typical angiographic features of a renal cell carcinoma. These include tumor neovascularity, contrast puddling, and early venous filling due to arteriovenous shunting. Renal abscess, hamartoma, and adenoma may appear as vascular lesions angiographically; however, the simple renal cyst would be avascular **(E is the correct answer to Question 39–4)**.

Discussion. These cases illustrate the urographic, ultrasonic, and angiographic features of two important causes of a focal renal mass. On intravenous urography, the simple renal cyst appears as a homogeneously lucent mass. It is sharply demarcated, often demonstrating a characteristic "beaking" at its junctions with the normal kidney. The outer wall of a simple cyst is thin in contrast to the occasional thick wall seen in necrotic carcinoma or in renal abscess. The caliceal system may appear normal or displaced by a renal cyst, but will not be invaded or amputated.

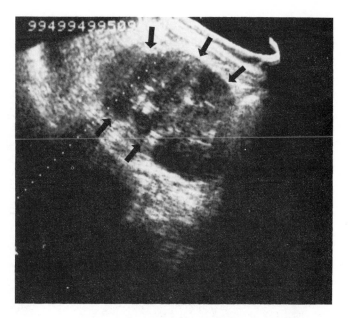

Figure E–140. Renal cell carcinoma (arrows) shown on longitudinal ultrasound. Numerous internal echoes are present, contrasting to the sonolucency of a renal cyst. (Courtesy of Dr. Neil Wolfman.)

On the other hand, renal cell carcinoma may have variable urographic appearances depending on the size of the tumor, the extent of neoplastic invasion, and the degree of necrosis within the lesion. They generally present, however, as poorly defined masses infiltrating the adjacent renal parenchyma. Vascular renal carcinomas opacify urographically, usually having a density similar to that of the normal kidney. At times, irregular opacification of the tumor is seen, owing to the presence of necrosis. Completely necrotic carcinomas may appear relatively lucent, and then simulate a simple renal cyst. Invasion or amputation of the caliceal system by a renal mass suggests carcinoma.

Other methods for imaging renal masses include ultrasound, computed tomography, and angiography. The ultrasonic features of a simple renal cyst include sharply defined borders, absence of internal echoes, and accentuation of back wall echoes due to significant sound transmission through the cyst, while renal carcinoma typically shows internal echoes, poor sonic transmission, and a paucity of back wall echoes (Fig. E–140). The computed tomographic features mirror the urographic findings, particularly for simple renal cyst. Angiographically, renal cysts are typically avascular and lucent.

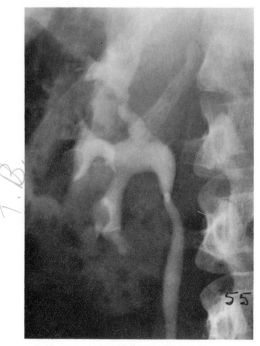

Figure E–141.

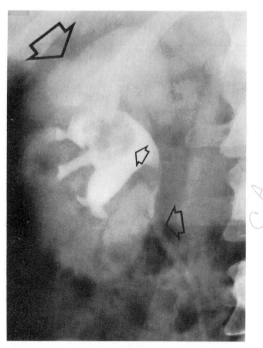

Figure E–142.

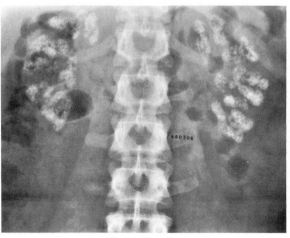

Figure E–143.

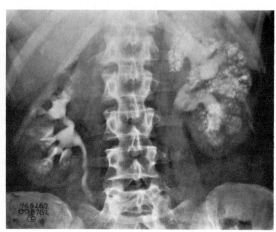

Figure E–144.

CLINICAL FINDINGS

Case 40–1 (Fig. E–141). Forty-five-year-old woman with back pain and hematuria.
Case 40–2 (Fig. E–142). Fifty-five-year-old man with gross hematuria.
Case 40–3 (Fig. E–143). Forty-year-old woman with renal colic.
Case 40–4 (Fig. E–144). Sixty-year-old man with hematuria.

Questions

40–1. In Case 40–1, which of the following would be the LEAST likely?
A. Caliceal diverticulum.
B. Renal tuberculosis.
C. Papillary necrosis.
D. Analgesic nephropathy.
E. Transitional cell carcinoma.

40–2. In Case 40–2, what is the MOST likely consideration?
A. Renal papillary necrosis.
B. Urate calculus.
C. Cystine calculus.
D. Transitional cell carcinoma.
E. Renal cell carcinoma.

40–3. In Case 40–3, the MOST appropriate description of this appearance is?
A. Nephrolithiasis.
B. Urolithiasis.
C. Nephrocalcinosis.
D. Dystrophic calcification.
E. Tuberculous calcification.

40–4. What would be the MOST likely cause for the appearance in Case 40–4?
A. Medullary sponge kidney.
B. Hyperoxaluria.
C. Hyperparathyroidism.
D. Renal tubular acidosis.
E. Hypervitaminosis D.

Table E–4. DISORDERS ASSOCIATED WITH RENAL PAPILLARY NECROSIS

Analgesic abuse	Renal vein thrombosis
Urinary tract infection	Renal transplant rejection
Urinary tract obstruction	Renal tuberculosis
Diabetes mellitus	Hypotension/shock
S-hemoglobinopathy	Dehydration/sepsis

Radiologic Findings. In Case 40–1, the lower pole calices are irregular and an oval collection of contrast medium projects within the renal medulla (Fig. E–145A). This patient was an analgesic abuser and developed renal papillary necrosis. Caliceal diverticulum and tuberculosis are the other considerations when small contrast collections are seen near the pelvicaliceal junction **(E is the correct answer to Question 40–1)**.

In Case 40–2, a large filling defect is present in the upper portion of the renal pelvis and is associated with nonvisualization of the superior pole calices. The combination of caliceal destruction and a pelvic filling defect is most suggestive of transitional cell carcinoma **(D is the correct answer to Question 40–2)**.

In Case 40–3, innumerable calcifications are present throughout the kidneys. The large number of calcifications and their distribution suggest a parenchymal location. Thus, nephrocalcinosis would be the most appropriate description for this appearance **(C is the correct answer to Question 40–3)**.

In Case 40–4, many of the collecting ducts of both kidneys are dilated, although the left kidney is more severely affected. The plain film showed multiple renal calcifications. This case represents nephrocalcinosis due to medullary sponge kidney **(A is the correct answer to Question 40–4)**.

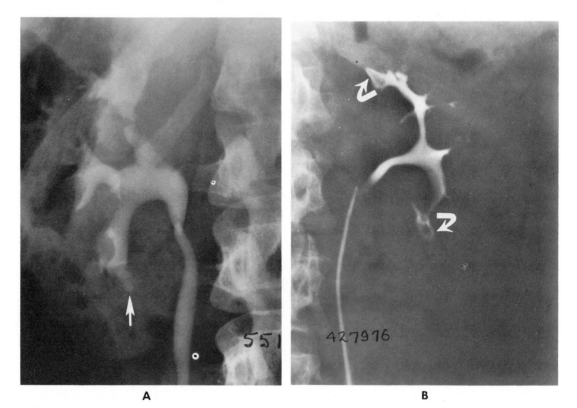

A   B

Figure E–145. *A,* Contrast collection (arrow) projecting off the deformed lower pole calix. This has been called the "egg-in-the-cup" deformity and represents the cavity left by the vacated papilla. *B,* Retrograde pyelogram showing multiple ring shadows (arrows). The triangular lucencies within the rings are the necrotic papillae.

Table E–5. CAUSES OF LUCENT DEFECTS WITHIN THE PELVICALICEAL SYSTEM

Nonopaque calculus	Fungus ball
Uroepithelial neoplasm	Gas/air bubble
Renal neoplasm	Vascular impression
Blood clot	Aberrant papilla
Pyelitis cystica	Incomplete filling

Discussion. Renal papillary necrosis can result from many different causes (Table E–4), and presents with a variety of urographic appearances. The necrotic papillae may calcify and be seen on plain film, or they may enter the collecting system, causing filling defects or renal colic from ureteral obstruction. The cavity left by the vacant papilla creates the so-called "egg-in-the-cup" deformity, as in Case 40–1. If the necrotic papilla remains in situ, however, it may be partially or completely encircled by contrast medium (Fig. E–145*B*). Analgesic abuse (i.e., analgesic nephropathy) is the most common cause of renal papillary necrosis.

Filling defects within the pelvicaliceal system can be due to many causes (Table E–5). Nonopaque calculi, blood clots, and uroepithelial tumors are the most common. The uroepithelial tumors present variously as subtle caliceal irregularity, as focal infiltration of the renal parenchyma, or as large filling defects within the collecting system.

The causes of calcification of the kidney fall into three general categories: (1) dystrophic calcification; (2) nephrolithiasis; and (3) nephrocalcinosis. Dystrophic calcification occurs within focal inflammatory or neoplastic lesions of the kidney, such as renal abscess, tuberculosis, or carcinoma. Nephrolithiasis refers to the presence of calculi within the renal collecting system, rarely appearing as innumerable densities scattered symmetrically throughout both kidneys. Conversely, nephrocalcinosis applies to widely distributed renal parenchymal calcification, and results from many underlying causes (Table E–6).

Cases 40–3 and 40–4 are examples of nephrocalcinosis due to medullary sponge kidney. In this disorder, saccular dilatation of the papillary ducts promotes urinary stasis and the development of multiple intraparenchymal stones. These stones may remain in situ or pass into the collecting system, leading to the usual complications of stones in that location. Along with medullary sponge kidney, renal tubular acidosis and hyperparathyroidism make up the most common causes of nephrocalcinosis.

Table E–6. UNDERLYING CAUSES OF NEPHROCALCINOSIS

Primary hyperparathyroidism	Hypervitaminosis D
Medullary sponge kidney	Sarcoidosis
Renal tubular acidosis	Cortical/tubular necrosis
Primary hyperoxaluria	Other hypercalcemic states
Milk-alkali syndrome	Idiopathic

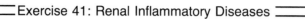

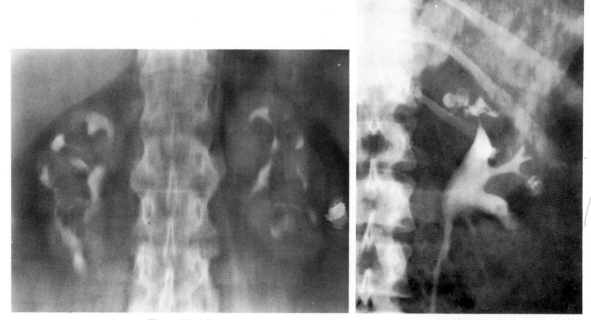

Figure E–146.

Figure E–147.

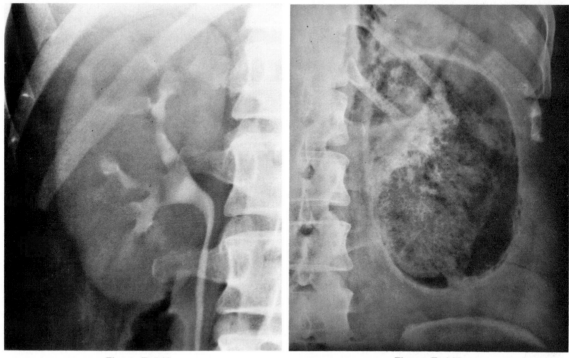

Figure E–148.

Figure E–149.

CLINICAL FINDINGS

Case 41–1 (Fig. E–146). Fifty-year-old woman with mild uremia.
Case 41–2 (Fig. E–147). Thirty-five-year-old man with sterile pyuria.
Case 41–3 (Fig. E–148). Forty-five-year-old woman with diabetes mellitus and fever.
Case 41–4 (Fig. E–149). Fifty-year-old diabetic with fever and flank pain.

Questions

41–1. In Case 41–1, both kidneys show the following changes EXCEPT?
A. Focal parenchymal scarring.
B. Blunting of the calices.
C. Loss of renal parenchyma.
D. Enlargement of both kidneys.
E. Renal sinus lipomatosis.

41–2. In Case 41–2, the caliceal abnormalities are MOST likely due to?
A. Chronic atrophic pyelonephritis.
B. Transitional cell carcinoma.
C. Renal tuberculosis.
D. Papillary necrosis.
E. Acute pyelonephritis.

41–3. The MOST likely cause for the upper pole lucency in Case 41–3 is?
A. Renal abscess.
B. Transitional cell carcinoma.
C. Renal cyst.
D. Renal cell carcinoma.
E. Renal adenoma.

41–4. Plain film of the abdomen in Case 41–4 suggests WHICH OF THE FOLLOW-
ING?
A. Perinephric abscess.
B. Atrophic pyelonephritis.
C. Xanthogranulomatosis pyelonephritis.
D. Tuberculous pyelonephritis.
E. Acute pyelonephritis.

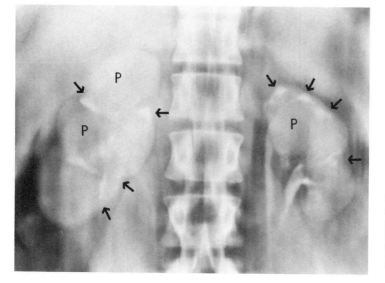

Figure E–150. Patient with chronic atrophic pyelonephritis. The kidneys are small, particularly on the left. Multiple parenchymal scars overlie blunted calices (arrows). Focal areas of compensatory hypertrophy simulate renal masses, a resemblance given the name "pseudotumor" (P).

Radiologic Findings. In Case 41–1, both kidneys are reduced in size. Multiple focal parenchymal scars overlie blunted calices (Fig. E–150). The peripelvicaliceal lucency represents renal sinus fat (i.e., lipomatosis), a common finding in renal atrophy **(D is the correct answer to Question 41–1).** This appearance is typical of chronic atrophic pyelonephritis.

In Case 41–2, stricturing of the upper and mid-polar infundibula is associated with caliceal distortion and dilatation. These findings are most consistent with renal tuberculosis **(C is the correct answer to Question 41–2).** Papillary necrosis and chronic atrophic pyelonephritis can cause ballooning of the calices but are rarely associated with infundibular stricturing, a finding also atypical for acute pyelonephritis. Conversely, transitional cell carcinoma may produce focal narrowing of the collecting system; however, involvement at multiple sites would be unusual.

Case 41–3 shows a lucent lesion in the upper pole of the kidney, minimally distorting the adjacent calices. Renal masses that may appear lucent urographically include simple renal cyst, necrotic renal cell carcinoma, and renal abscess. Transitional cell carcinoma usually infiltrates the pelvocaliceal system, while renal adenoma is a solid lesion. The indistinct upper margin and thick outer wall of the mass excludes simple renal cyst. The clinical history is most suggestive of renal abscess, which was proven by needle aspiration **(A is the correct answer to Question 41–3).**

Case 41–4 shows an oval lucency in the expected vicinity of the left kidney. Mottled and streaky lucencies are also present within the kidney (Fig. E–151). In view of the clinical history and the focal collection of gas surrounding the kidney, perinephric abscess would be the most likely diagnosis **(A is the correct answer to Question 41–4).** The other possibilities listed are almost never associated with this appearance.

Discussion. Chronic atrophic pyelonephritis is an important cause of renal failure in adults. It is also known as reflux nephropathy because of its relationship to vesicoureteral reflux in early childhood. Typically, the kidneys are small and irregularly scarred, with the major differential consideration being multifocal renal infarction.

The gamut of radiographic findings in tuberculosis of the urinary tract is broad. Plain films may show focal or diffuse urinary tract calcification (Fig. E–152A), while urographic changes range from subtle caliceal-papillary abnormalities through infundibular stenosis and finally to autonephrectomy.

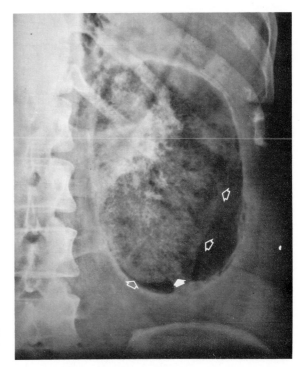

Figure E–151. The renal outline (arrows) is seen within the large oval lucency. Streaky and mottled lucencies are present in the kidney.

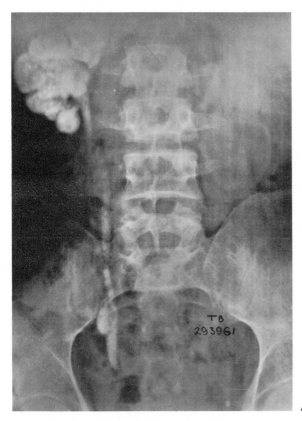

A

Figure E–152. *A*, Plain film of abdomen in tuberculosis of the urinary tract. The right kidney and ureter are diffusely calcified. The kidney did not function as a result of tuberculous autonephrectomy.

Illustration continued on following page.

Renal and perinephric abscesses occur with increased incidence in the diabetic patient. Perinephric abscesses are most often due to urinary tract infection but may arise elsewhere in the retroperitoneum or from a hematogenous source. Clinical and radiographic correlation, along with needle aspiration, is usually necessary for proper diagnosis.

A summary diagram of urinary tract changes in urinary tract tuberculosis is shown in Figure E–152B.

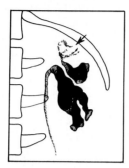
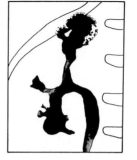
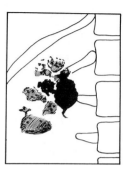

IRREGULAR FILLING OF CALYX

CORTICAL DESTRUCTION, ABSCESS CALCIFICATION, CICATRIX FORMATION.

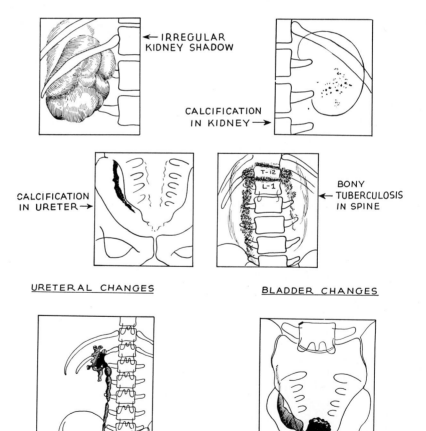

←IRREGULAR KIDNEY SHADOW

CALCIFICATION IN KIDNEY→

CALCIFICATION IN URETER→

BONY TUBERCULOSIS IN SPINE

T-12
L-1

URETERAL CHANGES

BLADDER CHANGES

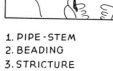

1. PIPE-STEM
2. BEADING
3. STRICTURE

BLADDER IS SMALL IRREGULAR AND CONTRACTED.

B

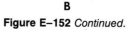

Figure E–152 Continued.

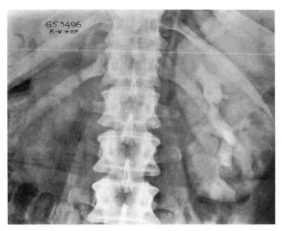

Figure E–153.

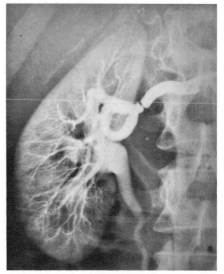

Figure E–154.

A

CLINICAL FINDINGS

Case 42–1 (Fig. E–153). Forty-five-year-old man with high blood pressure. Film at 5 minutes from a hypertensive urogram.

Case 42–2 (Fig. E–154A). Thirty-year-old woman with hypertension evaluated angiographically. (Courtesy of Dr. Thomas Hunt.)

Questions

42–1. In Case 42–1, what urographic finding MOST reliably suggests renovascular stenosis?

A. Delayed caliceal appearance time.
B. Normal appearing collecting system.
C. Hyperconcentration of the contrast medium.
D. Smooth, small kidney from atrophy.
E. Irregular, small kidney from scarring.

42–2. In Case 42–2, what is the MOST likely cause for the renal artery stenosis?

A. Atherosclerosis.
B. Fibromuscular dysplasia.
C. Renal artery aneurysm.
D. Arteriovenous fistula.
E. Neurofibromatosis.

Radiologic Findings. In Case 42–1, the right kidney is small and its collecting system has not yet opacified. Later filming showed a normal pelvocaliceal system, suggesting the presence of renovascular stenosis as the cause of delayed caliceal appearance time **(A is the correct answer to Question 42–1).**

In Case 42–2, focal stenosis affects the main renal artery near the bifurcation of its ventral and dorsal branches. The location of the narrowing and age of the patient make fibromuscular dysplasia the most likely cause of the stenosis **(B is the correct answer to Question 42–2).**

Discussion. Renovascular disease as a cause of hypertension is uncommon, occurring in less than 5% of cases. Atherosclerosis and fibromuscular dysplasia account for most cases of renovascular hypertension. Atherosclerosis is responsible in nearly two thirds of patients, and typically involves the orifice of the renal artery. Fibromuscular disease affects about one third of patients, and usually spares the renal artery orifice. Radiologic evaluation of the patient with hypertension has primarily involved the use of intravenous urography, radionuclide renography, and renal angiography with renal vein renin sampling. The urogram and renogram have served as screening modalities, while angiography has been used for more definitive evaluation.

The hypertensive urogram differs in part from the routine urogram. Following the preliminary films, a rapid bolus (usually 50 ml) of contrast medium is given intravenously followed by serial filming of the kidneys at one minute intervals for 4 to 5 minutes. After 5 minutes, additional filming is done in the standard manner. The urographic findings suggesting the presence of a renovascular lesion include (1) disparity in renal size with a small, smooth kidney representing ischemic atrophy; (2) delayed appearance of the contrast medium in the collecting system; (3) increased concentration of the contrast medium; and (4) ureteral notching due to collateral circulation. The most specific sign, however, is delayed caliceal appearance time.

When the clinical history or positive screening tests suggest the presence of renovascular disease, angiography is used to diagnose the type of lesion and assess its hemodynamic significance. Unfortunately, angiography does not always accurately predict hemodynamic significance. Bilateral renal vein catheterization and comparison of renal vein renin values on the two sides is most helpful. The ultimate proof that a renovascular lesion is causally related is relief of hypertension following transluminal angioplasty or surgical correction. The types of renovascular lesions that may produce hypertension are many; however, atherosclerosis or fibromuscular disease are by far the most common (Table E–7).

In recent years, the limitations of the hypertensive urogram have become apparent. The false negative rate has been 15 to 20%, while the false positive rate has been about 10%. However, due to the low prevalence of renovascular disease among all hypertensive patients, the predictive accuracy of a positive urogram is less than 50%. The error rates for the radionuclide renogram are similar, and its predictive accuracy is probably also poor. Considering their cost, the standard radiologic screening methods for hypertension are relatively ineffective in detecting the small percentage of patients with clinically important renovascular disease.

The physiologic basis for renovascular hypertension producing "loss flow" and "hyperconcentration" is indicated in Figure E–154B.

Table E–7. RENOVASCULAR LESIONS THAT MAY CAUSE HYPERTENSION

Common causes	Uncommon causes
Atherosclerosis	Renal artery aneurysm
Fibromuscular dysplasia	Arteriovenous fistula
	Thrombosis/embolism
	Arteritis (various types)
	Neurofibromatosis
	Traumatic narrowing

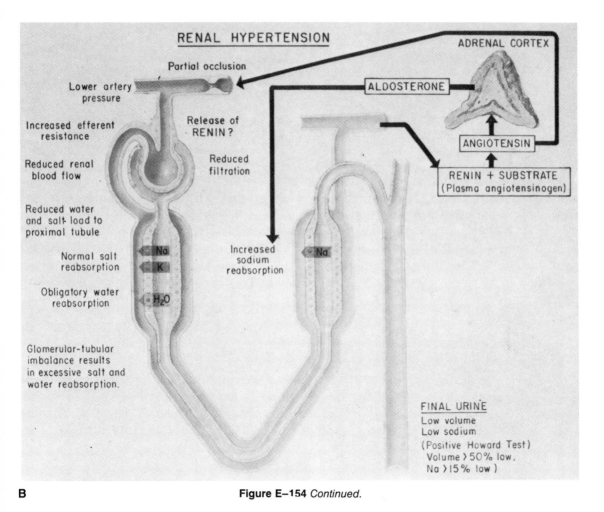

B

Figure E–154 *Continued.*

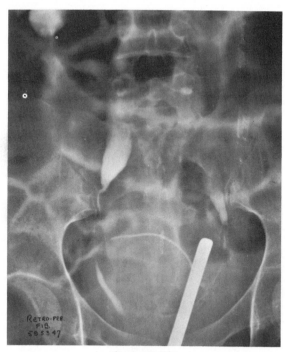

Figure E–155.

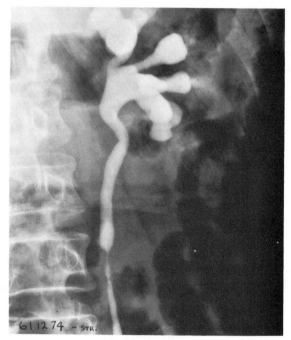

Figure E–156.

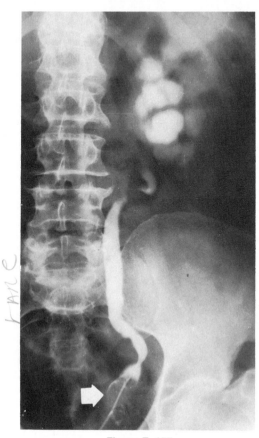

Figure E–157.

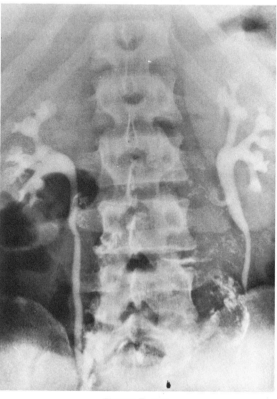

Figure E–158.

CLINICAL FINDINGS
  Case 43–1 (Fig. E–155). Forty-five-year-old woman with migraine headaches.
  Case 43–2 (Fig. E–156). Fifty-year-old man with microscopic hematuria.
  Case 43–3 (Fig. E–157). Sixty-five-year-old woman with flank pain and hematuria.
  Case 43–4 (Fig. E–158). Thirty-five-year-old man with fever and lymphadenopathy.

Questions
  43–1. In Case 43–1, the focal narrowing of both ureters at the pelvic brim suggests?
  A. Iatrogenic trauma.
  B. Cervical carcinoma.
  C. Retroperitoneal fibrosis.
  D. Retroperitoneal metastases.
  E. Ureteral carcinomas.

  43–2. In Case 43–2, the LEAST likely cause of the midureteral stricture would be?
  A. Congenital origin.
  B. Tuberculous ureteritis.
  C. Carcinoma of the ureter.
  D. Metastasis to the ureter.
  E. Iatrogenic trauma.

  43–3. In Case 43–3, the MOST likely diagnosis would be?
  A. Congenital stricture.
  B. Iatrogenic stricture.
  C. Intraluminal blood clot.
  D. Metastatic carcinoma.
  E. Transitional cell carcinoma.

  43–4. In Case 43–4, the appearance of the left ureter is BEST explained by?
  A. Tuberculous ureteritis.
  B. Aortic aneurysm.
  C. Ureteral carcinoma.
  D. Extrinsic neoplasm.
  E. Retroperitoneal fibrosis.

Radiologic Findings. In Case 43–1, both lower ureters show focal narrowing at the level of the sacral promontory. Although cervical carcinoma is an important cause of ureteral obstruction, the ureters are involved more typically near the bladder base. Furthermore, the bilateral and symmetric ureteral involvement would be unusual not only for cervical carcinoma but also for retroperitoneal metastases and iatrogenic trauma. Transitional cell carcinoma may be multicentric; however, synchronous carcinomas at a similar level in both ureters would be unlikely. Thus, retroperitoneal fibrosis is the most likely diagnosis **(C is the correct answer to Question 43–1).** The patient had been treated for migraine headaches with Sansert, a well known cause of retroperitoneal fibrosis.

In Case 43–2, the focal stricture of the midureter could result from a variety of causes. Stricture following a difficult stone passage or iatrogenic intervention would be most common and was the cause in this case. Ureteral tuberculosis, metastasis, or carcinoma could have a similar appearance (Fig. E–159). On the other hand, a congenital stricture in this location would be unlikely **(A is the correct answer to Question 43–2).** Nearly all congenital narrowings of the ureter occur at the ureteropelvic junction, ureterovesical junction, or lower end of an ectopic ureter.

In Case 43–3, the lower ureter shows saccular dilatation due to an intraluminal filling process with associated ureteral obstruction. Ureteral filling defects that expand its lumen are most often caused by intrinsic tumor or stone. Calcification within the lesion on plain film is virtually diagnostic of a stone. Although a blood clot can present as a filling defect, its soft consistency will not expand the ureter. In this case, transitional cell carcinoma was found surgically. **(E is the correct answer to Question 43–3).**

In Case 43–4, the left ureter is displaced laterally and mildly dilated. The densities near the deviated ureter represent lymphangiographic contrast medium within abnormally enlarged retroperitoneal nodes. In view of the history and

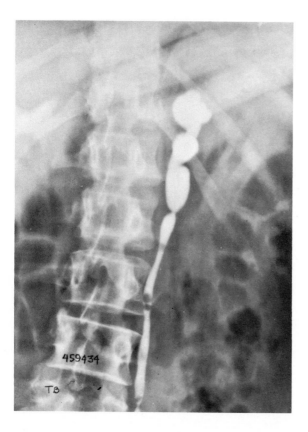

Figure E–159. Left retrograde pyelogram in a patient with tuberculous autonephrectomy. Multiple strictures involve the upper ureter and renal pelvis.

Table E–8. CAUSES OF URETERAL OBSTRUCTION

Intraluminal impaction	Tuberculous ureteritis
Calculus	Simple ureterocele
Blood clot	Schistosomiasis
Necrotic papilla	Extrinsic causes
Fungus ball	Pelvic neoplasms
Intrinsic causes	Retroperitoneal neoplasms
Congenital origin	Ovarian vein syndrome
Functional disorders	Retroperitoneal fibrosis
Post-calculus stricture	Lymphocele/urinoma
Traumatic injury	Crohn's disease
Ureteral neoplasms	

urographic findings, ureteral involvement from extrinsic neoplasm would be the most likely consideration **(D is the correct answer to Question 43–4).** Hodgkin's disease was diagnosed on lymph node biopsy.

Discussion. Clinical suspicion of ureteral obstruction is a common indication for intravenous urography. Ureteral obstruction can occur at any level and may result from many different causes (Table E–8). These causes can conveniently be divided into intraluminal impactions, intrinsic ureteral problems, and extrinsic processes secondarily involving the ureter. The most common causes of ureteral obstruction, however, are stone impaction, extrinsic neoplasms, and trauma, particularly iatrogenic injury.

If the urographic examination is inconclusive, retrograde pyelography can often delineate the lower level of obstruction and define its nature. Abdominal ultrasound, computed tomography, and lymphangiography may also be useful, particularly for clarifying extrinsic causes, such as lymphoma.

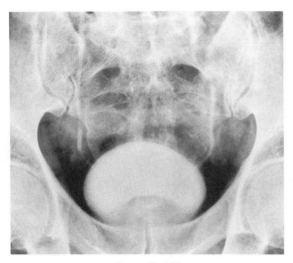

Figure E–160.

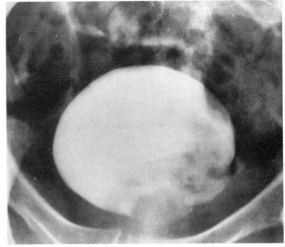

Figure E–161.

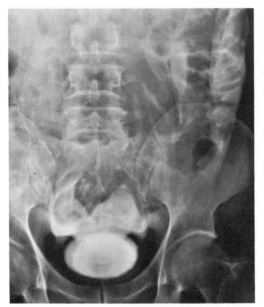

Figure E–162.

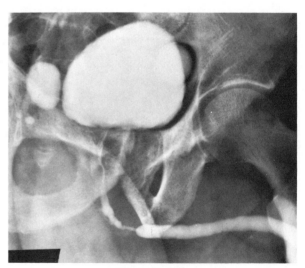

Figure E–163.

CLINICAL FINDINGS

Case 44–1 (Fig. E–160). Sixty-year-old man with urinary hesitancy.
Case 44–2 (Fig. E–161). Sixty-five-year-old woman with gross hematuria.
Case 44–3 (Fig. E–162). Thirty-five-year-old man after blunt abdominal trauma.
Case 44–4 (Fig. E–163). Forty-five-year-old man with dysuria.

Questions

44–1. In Case 44–1, the MOST likely cause for the bladder base impression is?
A. Ectopic ureterocele.
B. Bladder carcinoma.
C. Bladder calculus.
D. Prostate enlargement.
E. Urethral diverticulum.

44–2. In Case 44–2, the MOST likely cause for distortion of the bladder base is?
A. Carcinoma of the bladder.
B. Invasive cervical carcinoma.
C. Invasive vaginal carcinoma.
D. Invasive rectal carcinoma.
E. Large urethral diverticulum.

44–3. In Case 44–3, the cystogram is DIAGNOSTIC of?
A. Perforated bladder carcinoma.
B. Multiple bladder diverticula.
C. Intraperitoneal bladder rupture.
D. Extraperitoneal bladder rupture.
E. Rupture of the posterior urethra.

44–4. In Case 44–4, retrograde urethrogram shows ALL the following EXCEPT?
A. Urethral stricture.
B. Urethral diverticulum.
C. Multiple bladder diverticula.
D. Irregular bladder wall.
E. Thickened bladder wall.

Radiologic Findings. In Case 44–1, a symmetrically smooth impression is present at the base of the bladder. In a man, this appearance is nearly always due to benign enlargement of the prostate **(D is the correct answer to Question 44–1).** Prostatic carcinoma invading the bladder and carcinoma of the bladder more typically cause an irregular and asymmetric deformity. In a woman, a symmetric impression at the bladder base can be due to the levator ani muscle, cystocele repair, or chronic urethral syndrome.

On the other hand, Case 44–2 demonstrates irregular deformity at the bladder base, with greater involvement along the left wall. The lesion appears intrinsic to the bladder making carcinoma the most likely possibility **(A is the correct answer to Question 44–2).** Although the bladder can be invaded by rectal, cervical, or vaginal carcinoma, such invasion should be associated with an evident extrinsic mass.

In Case 44–3, earlike puddles of contrast medium project superiorly off the dome of the bladder, extending up the left paracolic gutter and outlining the colon. These findings indicate bladder perforation. Localization of contrast medium to the peritoneal cavity is diagnostic of intraperitoneal rupture **(C is the correct answer to Question 44–3).** This type of injury is typically associated with blunt trauma to the abdomen, usually in the presence of a distended bladder. Extra-peritoneal bladder rupture more commonly occurs with bony injury to the pelvis, and is often associated with trauma to the posterior urethra.

In Case 44–4, irregular narrowing of the bulbous urethra represents urethral stricture. The bladder contour is mildly irregular, indicating trabeculation from muscular wall thickening. Two well-defined saccular diverticula project off the bladder wall **(B is the correct answer to Question 44–4).** These bladder changes indicate chronic outlet obstruction caused by the urethral stricture. The bulbous urethra is the most common site in the male for stricture formation. The most frequent causes relate to injury from instrumentation or catheterization, or to gonococcal infection, as in this case.

Discussion. Many methods are available to evaluate the lower urinary tract radiologically (Table E–9). The urinary bladder is evaluated as part of the intravenous urogram (i.e., antegrade cystogram) or by direct catheter injection of contrast medium into the bladder (i.e., retrograde cystogram). In the latter case, the density of the contrast medium used is paramount, since lesions can be obscured if the medium is too dense. In recent years, ultrasound and computed tomography have emerged as important techniques to evaluate the urinary bladder.

The urethra can also be evaluated with antegrade or retrograde techniques. The posterior urethra is best demonstrated with an antegrade method, while the anterior urethra can be well shown with retrograde urethrography. In women, however, special techniques may be needed, depending on the clinical situation. To detect optimally diverticula of the female urethra, a special catheter, which occludes both ends of the urethra, is often used. Evaluation of urinary incontinence may be facilitated by inserting a chain of tiny metal balls into the female urethra. This permits measurements to be made between the urethra, bladder base, and bony pelvis.

Table E–9. RADIOLOGIC EVALUATION OF THE LOWER URINARY TRACT

Evaluation of the bladder	Evaluation of the urethra
Antegrade cystography	Antegrade urethrography
Retrograde cystography	Retrograde urethrography
Percutaneous cystography	Chain urethrogram (women)
Chain cystogram (women)	Diverticula techniques (women)
Radionuclide cystography	
Pelvic ultrasound	
Computed tomography	

10

Alimentary Tract

Barium sulfate in colloidal rather than particulate suspension is probably the most commonly used contrast agent in diagnostic radiology, particularly in the alimentary tract. It is innocuous and inert; it does not modify the normal function of the gastrointestinal tract; and even if it is aspirated, it is usually coughed up for the most part. If any remains in the lungs, it is almost completely removed by the macrophages in the course of time. If a leakage from the gastrointestinal tract into the peritoneal space occurs, a minimal granulomatous process and adhesions may result.

The newer barium sulfate compounds are adapted for special use in the alimentary tract so that the mucosa is coated without the additional adjunct of double contrast with a gaseous medium. Alternatively, after coating the mucosa with a high-density barium sulfate suspension, a gaseous medium may be introduced, usually as a powder, producing the so-called "double-contrast studies." Double-contrast studies are particularly useful for demonstrating small polypoid lesions in the gastrointestinal tract which otherwise might escape detection, especially if they are less than 1 cm in diameter. To enhance this detection, most radiologists use various relaxants, the most popular in this country being glucagon in very small doses intravenously just before the study begins. Glucagon in 0.5-mg doses intravenously is sufficient for examination of the colon, although the dose may be increased to 1 mg if desired. For upper gastrointestinal tract studies, as little as 0.2 mg of glucagon may be used to allow a greater time for visualization of the mucosa of the stomach and to slow down entry into the duodenum, which may obscure the mucosal relief of the stomach. In many parts of Europe, Buscopan, a vagoparalytic drug, is utilized and is less expensive, accomplishing the same result.

PREPARATION OF THE PATIENT

For contrast studies of the alimentary tract, the preparation of the patient varies with the part being examined.

In examination of the upper gastrointestinal tract, the patient is instructed not to eat or drink after midnight of the previous day, so that the stomach and small intestine are empty at the time of the study the next morning.

In the case of the colon, the cleansing of the colon is paramount for a successful examination. In some institutions, two- and three-day preparations are required. A one-day preparation has been sufficient in most instances if the following procedure is carried out aciduously.

The patient has a liquid meal at noon the day before the examination. At approximately 4:00 PM, 12 ounces of magnesium citrate and, 2 hours thereafter, 4 ounces of Neoloid (or 2 ounces of castor oil) are administered. The patient is instructed to have a minimum of 12 glasses (8-oz) of water thereafter between the administration of the magnesium citrate and midnight preceding the day of examination. This, in essence, gives the patient an "internal water enema." Nothing by mouth is permitted after a 6:00 PM liquid meal except water until midnight. The patient appears in the x-ray office or department at 8:00 AM the following morning, where an enema is given by a nurse or attendant, rolling the patient about at the time of the cleansing enema and utilizing two quarts of water warmed to body temperature. This enema may be repeated two or three times until returns are absolutely clear. Afterward the patient is required to wait for approximately one hour until the colon is thoroughly "dried out," since the high-density barium employed, particularly for the double-contrast study, requires that the mucosa be dry for best visualization of its surface. The so-called "full column barium enema," without the introduction of air, may be carried out immediately after the cleansing enema, since the barium employed in this procedure admixes with the small amount of water that may adhere to the mucosa in the colon after the cleansing enema.

ESOPHAGRAM
(Figs. 10–1A, B,
10–2A, B, and 10–3)

Although every examination of the upper alimentary tract includes an examination of the esophagus, the concentrated examination of the esophagus requires somewhat more time and greater care. Particular attention is paid to the swallowing function, which occurs so rapidly that it often requires video replay for optimum detail.

First the vocal cords are studied for their mobility and the piriform sinuses for their

distensibility and flexibility. Thereafter, anteroposterior and lateral views of the neck and upper portion of the esophagus are obtained, videotaping the procedure preceding and during the film studies with the patient in the erect position. The full length of the barium-filled esophagus is thereafter studied, having been carefully examined prior to the introduction of the contrast agent. After the videotaping, the column of barium is observed as it travels the whole length of the esophagus until it passes through the gastroesophageal junction. At least four films are obtained. The full esophagus is then examined for its rugal pattern, double-contrast air being combined with barium visualization, and special notice is made of the upper half of the esophagus including the larynx. The patient is then placed in the prone position in the right anterior oblique, where these various studies are once again repeated: videotaping first, and thereafter peristalsis of the esophagus with a full column of barium, rugal pattern studies, double-contrast studies, and a special study of

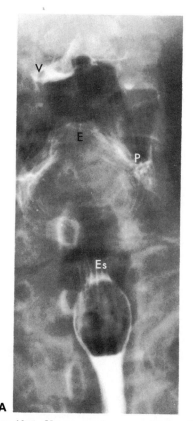

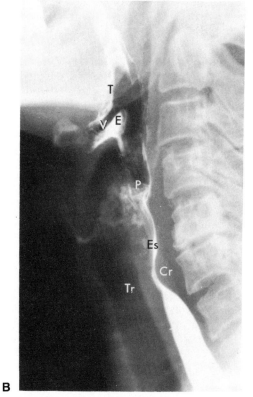

A   B

Figure 10–1. Upper esophagus and hypopharynx. A, Anteroposterior projection. B, Lateral projection. V = vallecula; E = epiglottis; P = pyriform sinuses; Es = esophagus; T = tongue; Cr = cricopharyngeus muscle indentation on esophagus; Tr = trachea.

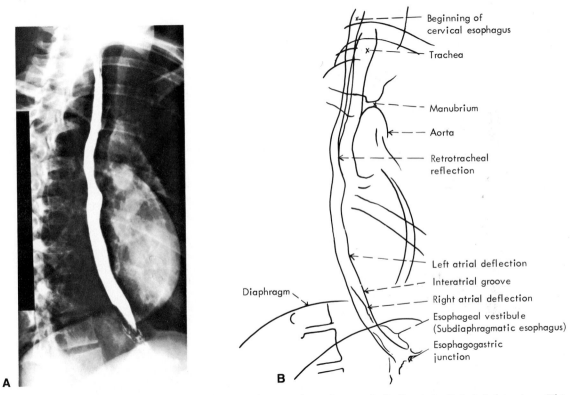

Figure 10–2. Right posteroanterior oblique projection of esophagus. *A,* Radiograph. *B,* Labeled tracing. (This same projection is frequently taken in the recumbent position as well.)

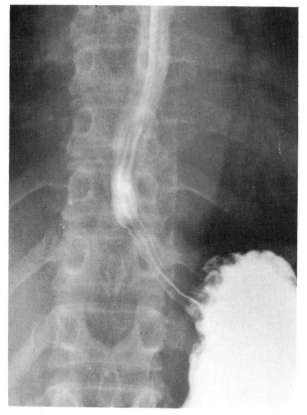

Figure 10–3. Rugal pattern of the collapsed esophagus.

the upper esophagus immediately after swallowing.

With the patient erect the esophagus is emptied largely by gravity; however, when the patient is recumbent, emptying of the esophagus occurs primarily as the result of its peristalsis. Diseases such as scleroderma, in which peristalsis may be lacking, may then be identified. The various peristaltic waves of the esophagus are carefully evaluated: (1) a primary wave, (2) a secondary superimposed smaller peristaltic wave, and (3) tertiary contractions which occasionally occur dividing the esophagus into large beadlike appearances. The latter may be evaluated only after tonometric determinations are performed, since usually they are of no pathologic significance. They occur particularly frequently in the elderly (presbyesophagus).

The esophageal gastric junction is carefully studied for hiatal hernia and gastroesophageal reflux.

Three forms of hiatal hernia may occur: (1) the truly *shortened esophagus,* either congenital or acquired from longstanding inflammation such as may occur with scleroderma; (2) a *sliding* type, in which the fundus of the

stomach is in its normal location beneath the diaphragm but under certain circumstances slides through the esophageal hiatus above the diaphragm; and (3) a paraesophageal type, in which a portion of the fundus of the stomach slides through the esophageal hiatus of the diaphragm and is covered by a complete peritoneal coating. It is this last form of hiatal hernia that probably is more frequently associated with a burning sensation since, in the recumbent position, its acid content may be related to ulceration. With the advent of double-contrast studies, the demonstration of ulcerations within hiatal hernias has become very accurate. Nevertheless, it is advisable to corroborate the presence or absence of ulceration with endoscopy.

In the presence of hiatal hernia, it is important to note the size of the gastroesophageal junction and the presence or absence of gastroesophageal reflux. If the size of the gastroesophageal junction is 13 mm or greater it is probable that there is no true esophageal stenosis at this level. However, Schatzki has demonstrated that if the diameter of this ring is 12 mm or less, this area acts as a stricture and represents an associated esophagitis and very likely is important in symptomatology. Esophagitis without stricture formation often requires endoscopy for corroboration, although a careful examination of the rugal pattern of the lower esophagus often reveals irregularities, widening, thickening, shallow ulceration, or a "bubbly" pattern. The radiologic imaging of the lower esophagus is relatively inaccurate except in the presence of outright stricture formation. To assist in the demonstration of esophageal varices a smooth muscle relaxant, such as propantheline (Probanthine) is of some advantage.

Text continued on page 281

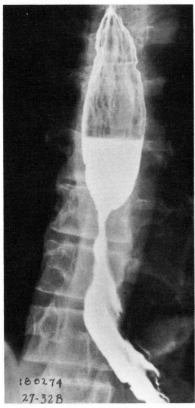

Figure E–164.

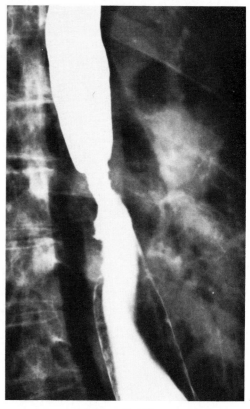

Figure E–165.

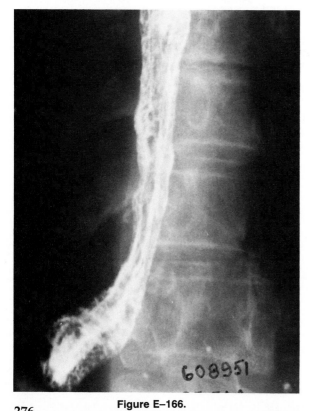

Figure E–166.

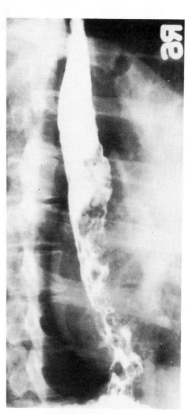

Figure E–167.

CLINICAL FINDINGS

  Case 45–1 (Fig. E–164). Thirty-five-year-old woman with dysphagia.
  Case 45–2 (Fig. E–165). Fifty-five-year-old man with dysphagia.
  Case 45–3 (Fig. E–166). Forty-five-year-old woman with leukemia.
  Case 45–4 (Fig. E–167). Fifty-year-old man with cirrhosis.

Questions

  45–1. In Cases 45–1 and 45–2, the MOST LIKELY DIAGNOSES respectively are?
  A. Peptic stricture–squamous cell carcinoma.
  B. Peptic stricture–adenocarcinoma.
  C. Scirrhous carcinoma–peptic stricture.
  D. Esophageal ring–peptic stricture.
  E. Esophageal ring–adenocarcinoma.

  45–2. Which is the LEAST characteristic feature of peptic stricture?
  A. Usually associated with hiatal hernia.
  B. Located above the esophageal hiatus.
  C. Typically located in the lower esophagus.
  D. Usually appears as a tapered narrowing.
  E. Often confused with an esophageal ring.

  45–3. In Cases 45–3 and 45–4, the MOST LIKELY DIAGNOSES respectively are?
  A. Caustic esophagitis–esophageal carcinoma.
  B. Herpetic esophagitis–esophageal carcinoma.
  C. Candida esophagitis–esophageal varices.
  D. Reflux esophagitis–esophageal varices.
  E. Reflux esophagitis–esophageal carcinoma.

  45–4. Which of the following statements are TRUE?
  A. Caustic esophagitis most often produces a focal stricture.
  B. Herpetic esophagitis can be seen in normal persons.
  C. Candida esophagitis is invariably associated with oral thrush.
  D. Reflux esophagitis is a common symptom-producing esophageal malady.
  E. Reflux esophagitis cannot be diagnosed radiographically.

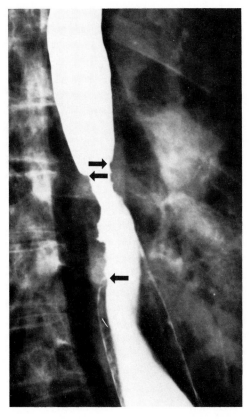

Figure E–168. An abrupt transition in caliber (arrows) identifies the junction between the malignancy and the normal esophagus.

Figure E–169. Another patient with peptic esophageal stricture. The contour of the stricture is smooth with gradual tapering to the level of maximal stenosis. Hiatal hernia (HH) is also present.

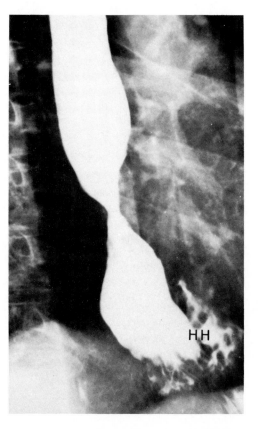

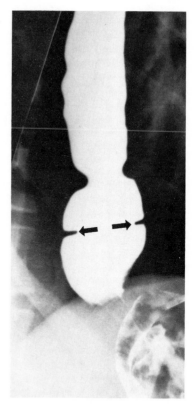

Figure E–170. A lower esophageal mucosal ring is present (arrows). This structure demarcates the lower end of the esophagus and is seen only when it lies above the level of the esophageal hiatus.

Radiologic Findings. In Case 45–1, a tapered narrowing involves the lower esophagus in association with partial obstruction, as evidenced by esophageal dilatation and a barium-air level above the constriction. In Case 45–2, however, the narrowing is abrupt and the margins are irregular (Fig. E–168). These represent respectively peptic esophageal stricture in a young woman and squamous cell carcinoma in an older man **(A is the correct answer to Question 45–1).**

In Case 45–3, fine irregularity is present throughout the lower half of the esophagus. This appearance in a leukemic patient with dysphagia strongly suggests infectious esophagitis, particularly due to candidiasis. In Case 45–4, nodular irregularity involves the lower half of the esophagus. In view of the clinical history for cirrhosis, esophageal varices would be the most likely consideration **(C is the correct answer to Question 45–3).** Esophageal varices appear as multiple, changeable filling defects in the lower esophagus, having a characteristically nodular and linear configuration.

Discussion. Peptic stricture results from severe reflux esophagitis and typically occurs in the lower esophagus, associated with hiatal hernia. A smooth, tapered narrowing is characteristic of benign stricture (Fig. E–169), while an irregular narrowing with an abrupt transition in caliber suggests malignancy. Peptic strictures are rarely confused with the various lower esophageal rings **(E is the correct answer to Question 45–2).** The mucosal ring is the most common, and appears as a thin, smooth annular constriction at the lower end of the esophagus (Fig. E–170). When the caliber of the mucosal ring is under 13 mm., it becomes an important consideration in the patient with dysphagia.

Esophagitis has many different causes (Table E–10). Long stricturing is typical of caustic esophagitis, and distinguishes it from the other types **(Question 45–4A is false).** Infectious esophagitis is most commonly due to *Candida albicans* or less likely to herpes simplex virus. Herpetic esophagitis has been reported in otherwise healthy individuals as an acute, self-limiting disease

Table E–10. CAUSES OF ESOPHAGITIS

Commoner Causes	Rarer causes
Reflux esophagitis	Crohn's disease
Infectious esophagitis	Bullous skin disorders
Caustic esophagitis	Ulcerative colitis
Radiation esophagitis	Behçet's disease
	Thermal injury
	Medications

(Question 45–4B is true). However, esophagitis from infection is most often seen in the immunocompromised patient. In such patients with dysphagia, candida esophagitis is always a consideration, and often occurs in the absence of oral thrush **(Question 45–4C is false).** Reflux esophagitis is certainly the most common symptom-producing malady of the esophagus **(Question 45–4D is true).** Although the mild form of reflux esophagitis is rarely detected radiographically, the moderate and severe forms are often diagnosed **(Question 45–4E is false).**

UPPER GASTROINTESTINAL
SERIES
(Figs. 10–4A, B, 10–5A, B,
and 10–6A–D)

The examination of the esophagus is routinely included, but not to the detailed extent previously described. The two main techniques employed for examination of the stomach and duodenum, as in the case of the colon, are (1) those employing the single full-column barium technique and (2) the double-contrast technique with a high-density barium coating the gastric mucosa followed by the administration of gas-emitting powder. As in the case of the colon, the demonstration of polypoid lesions 10 mm or less in diameter is enhanced by the double-contrast technique. It is probable that the demonstration of ulcers is equally accurate

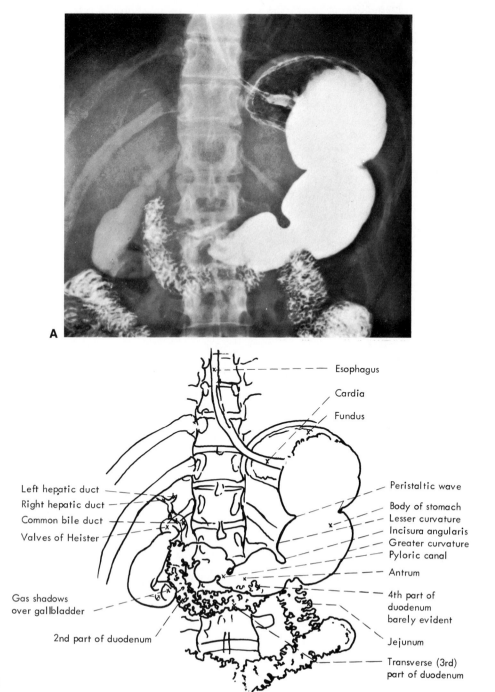

A

B

Esophagus
Cardia
Fundus

Left hepatic duct
Right hepatic duct
Common bile duct
Valves of Heister

Gas shadows
over gallbladder

2nd part of duodenum

Peristaltic wave

Body of stomach
Lesser curvature
Incisura angularis
Greater curvature
Pyloric canal

Antrum

4th part of
duodenum
barely evident

Jejunum

Transverse (3rd)
part of duodenum

Figure 10–4. Recumbent posteroanterior projection of stomach and duodenum (an oral cholecystogram was also at this time in the film illustrated). A, Radiograph. B, Labeled tracing.

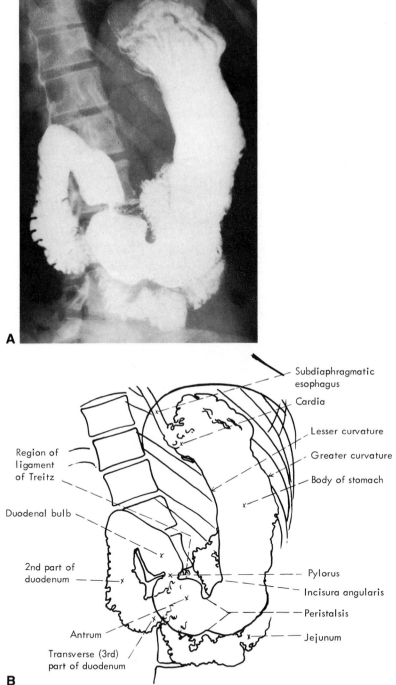

A

B

Subdiaphragmatic
esophagus

Cardia

Lesser curvature

Greater curvature

Body of stomach

Region of
ligament
of Treitz

Duodenal bulb

2nd part of
duodenum

Pylorus

Incisura angularis

Peristalsis

Jejunum

Antrum

Transverse (3rd)
part of duodenum

Figure 10–5. Right posteroanterior oblique prone projection of stomach and duodenum. *A,* Radiograph. *B,* Labeled tracing.

by either technology. In each instance a careful examination of the mucosal pattern is carried out before the full amount of barium is utilized and, in the case of the double-contrast technique, before the gas-emitting powders are administered. In each of the two techniques a thorough examination of the stomach requires complete coating of the stomach and examination of the patient in the supine position with both obliques and in the prone position with both obliques. Even with the full column study, when no additional gas is administered, a double-contrast evaluation of the duodenal bulb is routinely obtained in the left posterior oblique position, with the patient supine.

In hypotonic duodenography, marked distention of the duodenum is utilized to enhance visualization of filling defects contained within the second, third, and fourth parts of the duodenum either from intrinsic lesions of the duodenum or from pressure of an enlarged or diseased pancreas. For hypotonic duodenography, Pro-Banthine, 15 to 30

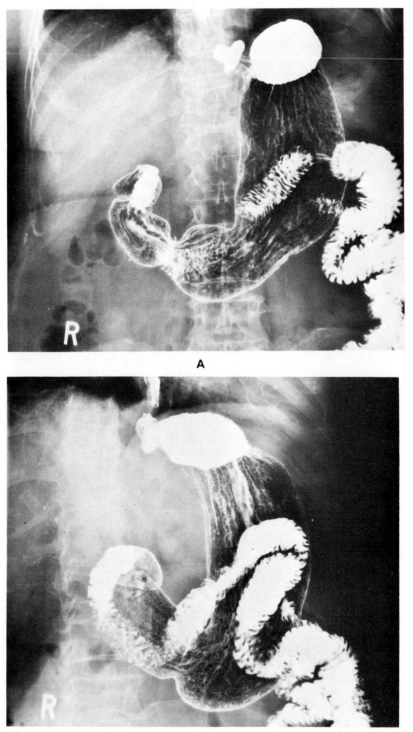

A

B

Figure 10–6. Examples of double-contrast high density barium-air studies of the stomach. *A,* In the posteroanterior projection. *B,* In the right anterior oblique projection.

Illustration continued on following page

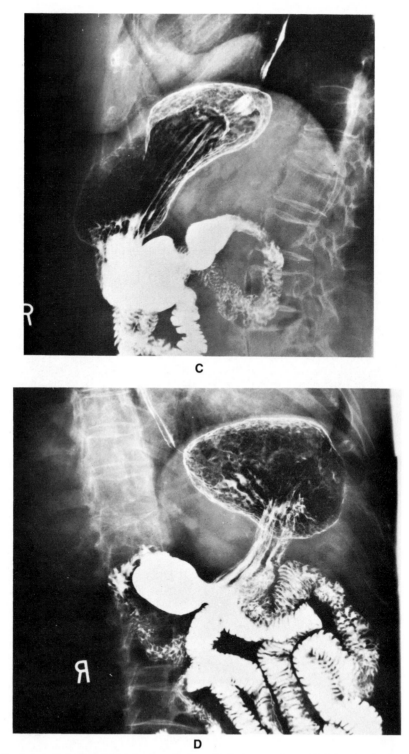

Figure 10–6 *Continued. C,* In the right lateral projection. *D,* Patient supine with left side elevated and right side lower, angulation approximately 30 degrees.

mg intravenously, or glucagon, 0.5 to 1 mg intravenously, is employed when no contraindications, particularly for the Pro-Banthine, are present. Although the dilating agent wears off very quickly, the Pro-Ban-

thine is certainly contraindicated in patients with cardiovascular disease, glaucoma, or renal disease. Glucagon is employed sparingly when severe diabetes is known to be present.

Text continued on page 300

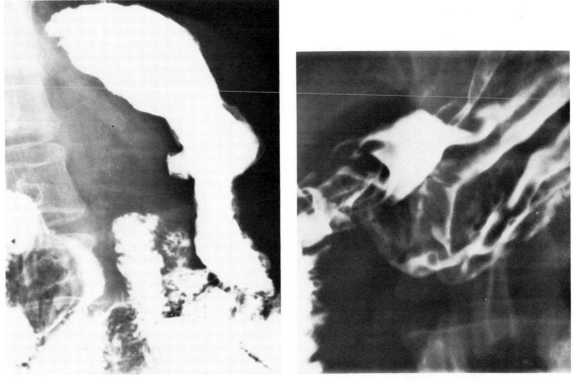

Figure E–171. **Figure E–172.**

CLINICAL FINDINGS

Case 46–1 (Fig. E–171). Forty-eight-year-old woman with epigastric pain.
Case 46–2 (Fig. E–172). Fifty-eight-year-old man with weight loss and anemia.

Questions

46–1. What feature of the lesser curvature ulcer in Case 46–1 is MOST suggestive
of a benign process?
A. Actual size of the ulcer.
B. Rectangular shape of the ulcer.
C. Location along the lesser curvature.
D. Penetration into the gastric wall.
E. Presence of only one ulcer.

46–2. What feature of the antral ulcer in Case 46–2 is MOST indicative of a malignant
process?
A. Actual size of the ulcer.
B. Stellate shape of the ulcer.
C. Antral location of the ulcer.
D. Presence of only one ulcer.
E. Irregular rugal pattern near ulcer.

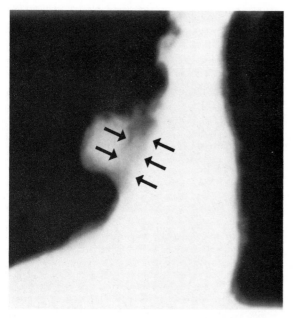

Figure E–173. The ulcer collar (arrows) is seen as a relatively lucent band between the ulcer and the gastric lumen.

Radiologic Findings. In Case 46–1, the ulcer penetrates into the gastric wall without an associated luminal mass **(D is the correct answer to Question 46–1)**. Tangential view of the ulcer reveals a thick edematous collar at its junction with the gastric lumen (Fig. E–173). The combination of these signs indicates a benign peptic process (Table E–11).

Case 46–2 represents an ulcerating adenocarcinoma of the stomach. Although the stellate shape and shallowness of the ulcer favor a malignant process, the adjacent thickened and nodular rugal pattern is ominous (Fig. E–174A), and strongly suggests the presence of carcinoma **(E is the correct answer to Question 46–2)**. Malignancy must always be suspected when a gastric ulcer shows features not typical for a benign lesion (Table E–12).

Discussion. The vast majority of gastric ulcers are benign peptic processes. The size, shape, and location of a gastric ulcer are of little value in differentiating between a benign or malignant etiology. The more important radiographic features include (1) the presence or absence of penetration into the gastric wall; (2) the appearance of the surrounding gastric mucosa; (3) the changes at the junction between the ulcer neck and the gastric lumen; and (4) the temporal response of the ulcer to treatment.

A benign ulcer typically penetrates into the gastric wall, whereas a malignant ulcer usually projects partially into the lumen, and is often associated with an irregular mass. The mucosal surface adjacent to an ulcer will appear normal if the lesion is benign, or distorted if malignancy is present. The ulcer collar is due to edematous swelling at the neck of the ulcer. A thinner, Hampton's line may be seen in the same location with less swelling. Both of these are reliable signs of

Table E–11. RADIOGRAPHIC SIGNS OF BENIGN GASTRIC ULCER

Penetration into the gastric wall
Symmetrically radiating mucosal folds
Margin signs at the ulcer neck
   Thin Hampton's line
   Thicker ulcer collar
   Smooth ulcer mound
Complete and permanent healing

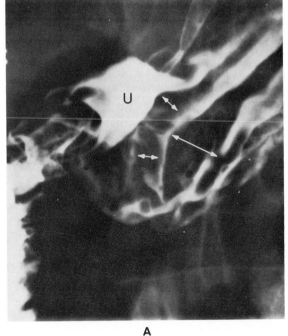

Figure E–174. *A,* The rugal folds become thickened and nodular (arrows) as they approach the ulcer (U), indicating an adjacent infiltrating process, highly suggestive for malignancy. *B,* The appearance of a gastric benign ulcer that has almost completely healed. The concentration of the rugae toward the spot of barium (open arrow) still demonstrates where the ulcer had been, but the ulcer was many times larger than this, and an ulcer mound could be readily demonstrated originally. The ulcer in this instance is almost completely healed and is represented only by a pit where the scar is still present.

A

B

Table E–12. RADIOGRAPHIC SIGNS OF MALIGNANT GASTRIC ULCER

Intraluminal location of an ulcer
Distorted or absent mucosal folds
Ulcer within a suspicious mass
Eccentric, shallow ulcer
Nodular surface of the mass
Abrupt margin of the mass
Carman-Kirklin meniscus complex

benign ulcer. The response of the ulcer to treatment is also important. If a gastric ulcer shows complete and permanent healing, it represents a benign process. Partial or incomplete disappearance, however, may be observed with either a benign or a malignant ulcer.

Rarely, an ulcerating malignancy of the stomach may appear as an intraluminal meniscoid collection of barium partially encircled by an irregular lucency of nodular tumor. This combination has been called the Carman-Kirklin meniscus complex, after the original investigators (Fig. E–174B).

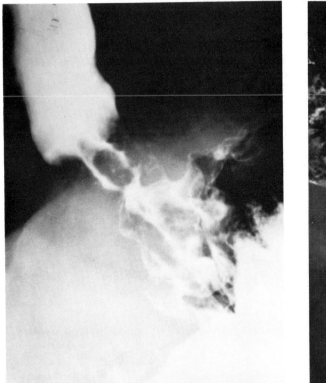

Figure E–175.

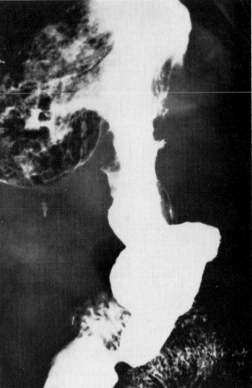

Figure E–176.

CLINICAL FINDINGS

Case 47–1 (Fig. E–175). Fifty-four-year-old man with progressive dysphagia.
Case 47–2 (Fig. E–176). Sixty-year-old woman with epigastric pain.

Questions

47–1. In Case 47–1, the MOST likely diagnosis is?
A. Gastric adenocarcinoma invading the esophagus.
B. Gastric lymphoma invading the esophagus.
C. Esophageal squamous carcinoma invading the stomach.
D. Esophageal adenocarcinoma invading the stomach.
E. Esophageal lymphoma invading the stomach.

47–2. In Case 47–2, the MOST likely cause for the gastric narrowing is?
A. Adenocarcinoma of the stomach.
B. Hodgkin's disease of the stomach.
C. Lymphocytic lymphoma of the stomach.
D. Leiomyosarcoma of the stomach.
E. Neurofibrosarcoma of the stomach.

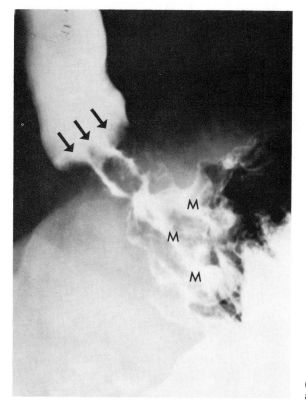

Figure E–177. Irregular mass (M) arising from the gastric cardia and invading the esophagus (arrows).

Radiologic Findings. In Case 47–1, a fungating mass is present in the gastric cardia and invades the lower end of the esophagus (Fig. E–177). The most likely cause for this appearance is gastric adenocarcinoma with esophageal involvement **(A is the correct answer to Question 47–1).** Squamous cell carcinoma of the esophagus presenting as a large mass in the gastric cardia and primary adenocarcinoma of the esophagus are both unlikely. Lymphoma involving the esophagogastric region occurs only rarely.

In Case 47–2, irregular narrowing affects the mid-body of the stomach. The larger spiculations are due to neoplastic ulceration. In view of its frequency among primary gastric malignancies, gastric adenocarcinoma is the most likely cause of this appearance **(A is the correct answer to Question 47–2).** Lymphoma would be a possibility, but is less likely statistically.

Discussion. Adenocarcinoma accounts for 95% of all primary malignancies of the stomach, while lymphoma and leiomyosarcoma are responsible for most of the remainder. Of the various lymphomas, Hodgkin's disease least often involves the stomach. The different morphologic types of gastric adenocarcinoma that have been described include the superficial, ulcerative, polypoid, fungating, infiltrative, and scirrhous varieties. A carcinoma of the stomach will often show a combination of these features. The differential considerations in gastric carcinoma depend in part on the morphologic presentation. For example, an ulcerative carcinoma must be distinguished from a benign gastric ulcer, a polypoid carcinoma from an adenomatous polyp or leiomyoma, and a fungating carcinoma from lymphoma or leiomyosarcoma.

Invasion of the esophagus by gastric adenocarcinoma is not uncommon. Under this circumstance, the development of dysphagia or odynophagia suggests secondary esophageal involvement. Various esophageal motility disturbances may be seen radiographically as a result of carcinomatous invasion of the esophagus. Occasionally, esophageal symptoms are the most prominent complaint of the patient with this type of gastric carcinoma. Thus, this possibility

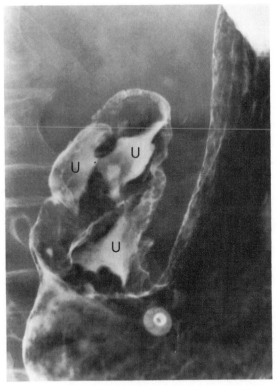

Figure E–178. Diffuse abnormality of the gastric antrum with ulceration (U) and nodular thickening of the rugal folds. This was due to lymphoma, although carcinoma could present similarly.

always warrants a complete examination of the esophagus and the esophago-gastric region.

Gastric lymphoma, like carcinoma, may present in a variety of different morphologic forms, and is usually a differential consideration whenever gastric carcinoma is suspected (Fig. E–178). On the other hand, most gastric leiomyo-sarcomas present as large polypoid masses, often with prominent central ulceration. Other mesenchymal malignancies of the stomach are extremely rare and tend to resemble leiomyosarcoma in appearance.

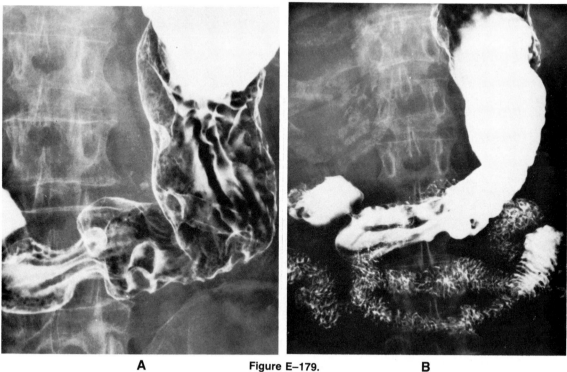

A   **Figure E–179.**   B

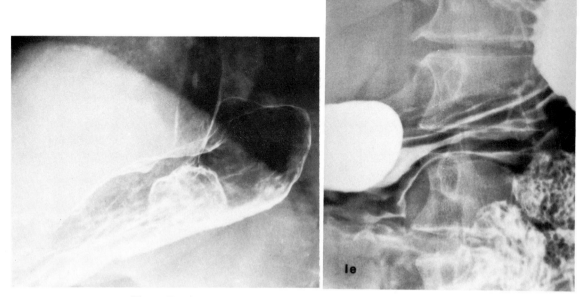

Figure E–180.   **Figure E–181.**

CLINICAL FINDINGS

Case 48–1 (Fig. E–179A and B). Sixty-five-year-old woman with atrophic gastritis, supine (A) and prone (B) films of stomach.

Case 48–2 (Fig. E–180). Fifty-five-year-old woman with epigastric pain.

Case 48–3 (Fig. E–181). Forty-five-year-old man with dyspepsia.

Questions

48–1. In Case 48–1, the MOST likely diagnosis is?
A. Multiple pancreatic rests.
B. Multiple leiomyomas.
C. Multiple neurofibromas.
D. Multiple benign epithelial polyps.
E. Multiple malignant epithelial polyps.

48–2. Which of the following are TRUE?
A. Leiomyomas of the stomach are typically solitary.
B. A pancreatic rest is usually located in the gastric antrum.
C. Most benign gastric polyps are epithelial in origin.
D. Gastric epithelial polyps are hyperplastic or adenomatous.
E. Malignancy is unlikely in a gastric polyp under 2 cm.

48–3. In Cases 48–2 and 48–3, the MOST likely diagnoses respectively are?
A. Leiomyoma–lymphoma.
B. Polypoid carcinoma–leiomyoma.
C. Polypoid carcinoma–pancreatic rest.
D. Lymphoma–leiomyoma.
E. Lymphoma–neurofibroma.

48–4. In differentiating a mucosal from an intramural gastric polypoid lesion, which sign is the LEAST useful?
A. Size of the polypoid lesion.
B. Surface contour of the lesion.
C. Transition with the adjacent gastric wall.
D. Shape of the lesion.
E. Presence of calcification in the lesion.

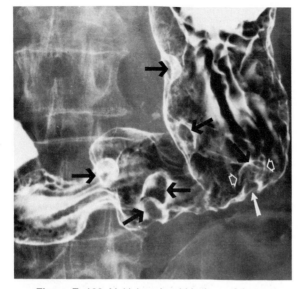

Figure E–182. Multiple polypoid lesions of the stomach (arrows) seen in double-contrast relief. Fewer polyps are evident on the prone film because of obscuration from the dense barium.

Table E–13. CAUSES OF GASTRIC FILLING DEFECTS

Intraluminal filling defects
 Gastric bezoars
 Blood clot*
 Foreign body (e.g., fruit pits)*
Benign polypoid defects
 Hyperplastic polyp*
 Adenomatous polyp*
 Leiomyoma
 Pancreatic ectopia (rest)
 Rarer, polypoid tumors
Malignant polypoid defects
 Polypoid carcinoma
 Lymphoma*
 Leiomyosarcoma
 Metastatic neoplasm**
Miscellaneous defects
 Hypertrophic gastritis**
 Menetrier's disease**
 Gastric varices**
 Esophageal mucosal prolapse
 Postoperative defect
 Jejunogastric intussusception

*May be multiple.
**Typically multiple.

Radiologic Findings. In Case 48–1, multiple filling defects, all measuring less than 2 cm, are present in the body and antrum of the stomach (Fig. E–182). These represented multiple hyperplastic polyps **(D is the correct answer to Question 48–1).** Pancreatic rest, leiomyoma, and neurofibroma are usually solitary gastric lesions **(Question 48–2A is true).** Furthermore, the pancreatic rest occurs typically in the antrum **(Question 48–2B is true).** Benign gastric polyps are usually of epithelial origin **(Question 48–2C is true),** with the hyperplastic and adenomatous types being most common **(Question 48–2D is true).** Size is important in assessing malignant potential. An epithelial polyp of the stomach under 2 cm is rarely malignant **(Question 48–2E is true).**

Cases 48–2 and 48–3 represent relatively large polypoid lesions of the stomach. The radiographic features in Case 48–2 include surface irregularity, abrupt transition with the gastric wall, and near complete intraluminal projection, indicating a lesion of mucosal origin. At surgery, polypoid adenocarcinoma was found. In Case 48–3, the features include a smooth contour, draping of intact rugal folds, gradual transition with the gastric wall, and partial projection into the lumen. This appearance suggests an extramucosal or intramural lesion, and would be most consistent with a leiomyoma **(B is the correct answer to Question 48–3).** This differentiation is least dependent on the size of the lesion **(A is the correct answer to Question 48–4).**

Discussion. Polypoid lesions of the stomach are due to many different causes (Table E–13). Intraluminal defects, such as phytobezoar, are easily distinguished because of their mobility. Hypertrophic gastritis and Menetrier's disease have a characteristic appearance, while gastric varices, esophageal mucosal prolapse, and postoperative defects have a distinctive clinical history. Conversely, fixed and focal polypoid defects of the stomach are more difficult to differentiate from each other. These lesions can be classified according to number, size, and site of origin.

Polypoid lesions of the stomach can be divided into epithelial and nonepithelial types. Those commonly arising from the epithelium include the hyperplastic and adenomatous polyps, and the polypoid adenocarcinoma. The leiomyoma is the most common nonepithelial neoplasm, while other gastric mesenchymal tumors are distinctly rare.

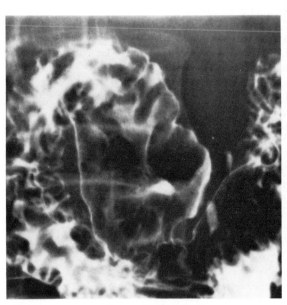

Figure E–183.

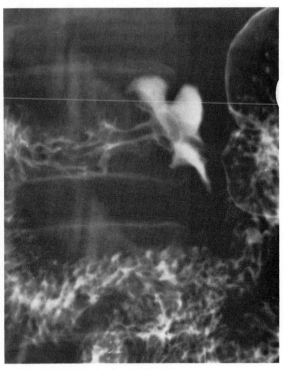

Figure E–184.

CLINICAL FINDINGS

Case 49–1 (Fig. E–183). Forty-five-year-old woman with epigastric pain.
Case 49–2 (Fig. E–184). Fifty-year-old man with dyspepsia.

Questions

49–1. In Case 49–1, what should be the NEXT STEP in this patient's management?
A. Therapeutic trial should be initiated.
B. Gastric analysis to rule out Zollinger-Ellison syndrome.
C. Serum gastrin to rule out Zollinger-Ellison syndrome.
D. Endoscopy to exclude a duodenal carcinoma.
E. Wait and repeat the radiographic examination.

49–2. What is the MOST accurate statement regarding the appearance of the duodenal
bulb in Case 49–2?
A. Deformity facilitates the radiographic diagnosis of acute ulcer.
B. Deformity facilitates the endoscopic diagnosis of acute ulcer.
C. Deformity necessitates the use of endoscopy for accurate diagnosis.
D. Deformity indicates the need for peptic ulcer surgery.
E. Deformity indicates the presence of chronic peptic ulcer disease.

Radiologic Findings. In Case 49–1, a collection of barium is present in the duodenal bulb. This is constant in size and shape on multiple views, and represents an active duodenal ulcer. In contrast to gastric ulceration, the potential for malignancy in duodenal ulcer is nil, whereas Zollinger-Ellison syndrome is a rare entity that does not warrant routine exclusion. The radiographic demonstration of a duodenal ulcer is sufficient evidence for its existence. Thus, the appropriate management in this patient would be a therapeutic trial **(A is the correct answer to Question 49–1).**

In Case 49–2, the duodenal bulb is markedly deformed, an appearance that has been called the "cloverleaf deformity." This configuration invariably indicates chronic peptic ulcer disease. Unfortunately, the radiographic and endoscopic diagnosis of acute duodenal ulcer is less reliable in the presence of deformity. The clinical management of such patients is more dependent on symptomatology than on the radiographic or endoscopic appearance of the duodenal bulb **(E is the correct answer to Question 49–2).**

Discussion. The radiographic diagnosis of duodenal ulcer is accurate when a constant collection of barium is shown on multiple views. It is less reliable if only inconstant collections of varying size and shape are demonstrated. Marked deformity of the duodenal bulb indicates chronic peptic ulcer disease, and adversely affects the ability of radiographic examination to judge acute activity.

Since 95% of all duodenal ulcers occur within the duodenal bulb, this area must be meticulously examined. Prone and supine oblique views are routinely obtained. The prone or barium-filled views assess overall shape of the bulb, while the supine or air-contrast views most accurately demonstrate ulceration, as in Case 49–1.

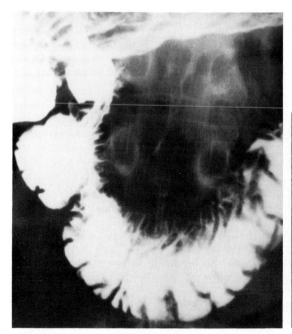

Figure E–185.

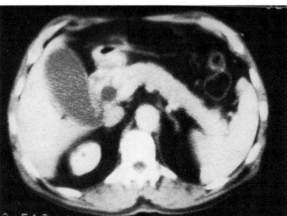

Figure E–186.

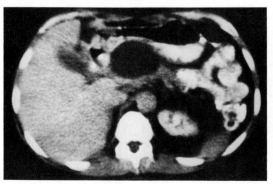

Figure E–187.

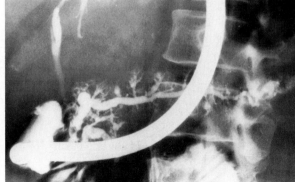

Figure E–188.

CLINICAL FINDINGS

Case 50–1 (Fig. E–185). Fifty-five-year-old man with weight loss.

Case 50–2 (Fig. E–186). Sixty-year-old man with epigastric pain (courtesy of Dr. Neil Wolfman).

Case 50–3 (Fig. E–187). Forty-five-year-old woman with retrogastric mass (courtesy of Dr. Neil Wolfman).

Case 50–4 (Fig. E–188). Fifty-year-old man with chronic alcoholism.

Questions

50–1. In Case 50–1, the spiculation along the medial aspect of the duodenum is LEAST likely due to?

A. Pancreatic pseudocyst.
B. Pancreatic carcinoma.
C. Acute pancreatitis.
D. Chronic pancreatitis.
E. Relapsing pancreatitis.

50–2. In Case 50–2, computed abdominal tomography at the level of the pancreas suggests?

A. Carcinoma of the tail of the pancreas.
B. Carcinoma of the body of the pancreas.
C. Carcinoma of the head of the pancreas.
D. Carcinoma of the common bile duct.
E. Carcinoma of the gallbladder.

50–3. In Case 50–3, computed abdominal tomography shows the cause of the retrogastric mass to be?

A. Pancreatic cystadenoma.
B. Islet cell tumor.
C. Pancreatic carcinoma.
D. Pancreatic pseudocyst.
E. Chronic pancreatitis.

50–4. In Case 50–4, endoscopic pancreatography is MOST consistent with which of the following?

A. Chronic pancreatitis.
B. Acute pancreatitis.
C. Pancreatic carcinoma.
D. Pancreatic pseudocyst.
E. Pancreatic cystadenoma.

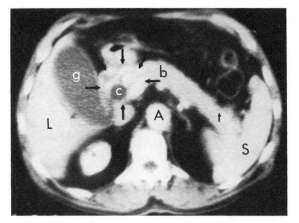

Figure E–189. The body (b) and tail (t) of the pancreas appear normal, while the pancreatic head is enlarged (arrows). The common bile duct (c) and gallbladder (g) are also enlarged, indicating biliary obstruction (A = aorta; L = liver; S = spleen).

Radiologic Findings. In Case 50–1, the medial border of the duodenum shows a spiculated appearance indicative of pancreatic disease secondarily involving the duodenum. These findings on the upper gastrointestinal series are often nonspecific, necessitating correlation with the clinical history and with other imaging methods. Spiculation of the medial duodenum strongly suggests acute pancreatitis or carcinoma of the pancreatic head. Chronic or relapsing pancreatitis would be less likely considerations, while pancreatic pseudocyst, which typically causes a smooth duodenal impression, would be unlikely **(A is the correct answer to Question 50–1).** Pancreatic carcinoma was found at surgery.

In Case 50–2, enlargement of the pancreatic head, dilatation of the common bile duct, and distention of the gallbladder are present (Fig. E–189). This combination of findings is virtually diagnostic of carcinoma of the head of the pancreas **(C is the correct answer to Question 50–2).** Abdominal ultrasound and computed tomography have shown sensitivities averaging 85 to 90% for detecting pancreatic carcinoma, comparable to figures achieved with visceral angiography and endoscopic pancreatography.

In Case 50–3, a large mass is present in the midabdomen, displacing the stomach anteriorly (Fig. E–190). It is homogeneous and radiolucent, suggesting a fluid-filled structure, an impression confirmed by ultrasound. Because of this appearance, pancreatic pseudocyst is the most likely diagnosis **(D is the correct answer to Question 50–3).** The findings of a retrogastric mass on an upper gastrointestinal series is usually a perplexing problem; however, the recent use of abdominal ultrasound and computed tomography have permitted a correct diagnosis in nearly all cases.

In Case 50–4, diffuse dilatation of the main pancreatic duct, along with ectasia of most of its side branches, is evident. A ductal stone is seen as a filling

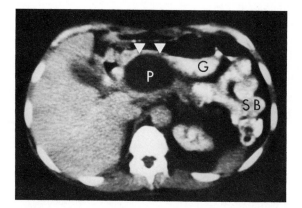

Figure E–190. Large pancreatic pseudocyst (P) displacing the stomach anteriorly (arrowheads) and accounting for the retrogastric mass seen on the upper gastrointestinal series. The opaqueness of the gastric fluid (G) and left upper quadrant small bowel loops (SB) is due to orally ingested contrast media.

Table E-14. RADIOLOGIC EVALUATION OF THE PANCREAS

Poor method of evaluation	Good method of evaluation
Plain abdominal films	Abdominal ultrasound
Barium examinations	Computed tomography
Radionuclide imaging	Visceral angiography
	Endoscopic pancreatography

defect near the papilla of Vater. Abdominal ultrasound was normal. The endoscopic pancreatogram, however, indicates chronic pancreatitis **(A is the correct answer to Question 50-4).**

Discussion. Recently, evaluation of the pancreas has been facilitated by the introduction of newer and more sensitive diagnostic techniques (Table E-14). The traditional methods for examining the pancreas included plain film radiography and the upper gastrointestinal series. The plain abdominal film is often of limited use. It can be of value in acute pancreatitis with focal ileus, chronic pancreatitis with calcification, and pancreatic abscess with gas formation. The upper gastrointestinal series may show secondary changes involving the stomach and medial portion of the duodenum as a result of adjacent pancreatic inflammatory or neoplastic disease. Unfortunately, the sensitivity and specificity of the barium study are poor.

Ultrasound and computed tomography have been largely responsible for the improvements in pancreatic imaging. Alterations in the size and shape of the pancreas are readily demonstrated with either technique. Changes in the internal architecture of the gland, such as ductal dilatation and calcification, may occasionally be seen. Pseudocysts are easily shown, and can be conveniently followed. Furthermore, percutaneous biopsy of suspicious pancreatic masses can be accomplished under ultrasonic or computed tomographic guidance. This has provided the clinician with important information, and has facilitated the management of many patients. As a result, visceral angiography has been largely superseded by these less invasive techniques.

Endoscopic retrograde cholangiopancreatography (ERCP) allows direct visualization of the pancreatic and biliary ductal systems. ERCP is often complementary to abdominal ultrasound and computed tomography. However, in chronic pancreatitis, biliary stricturing, and choledocholithiasis, the endoscopic method usually is a more sensitive and specific means of evaluation.

SMALL BOWEL SERIES
(Fig. 10–7A–D)

Personal experience suggests that the high-density barium employed for double-contrast visualization of the stomach and duodenum (250% weight over volume) is not the ideal agent for examination of the small intestine beyond the duodenum; under these circumstances, a so-called full-column upper gastrointestinal study only is done. The roentgen signs of abnormality of the small intestine are frequently masked by the high-density barium. The full column barium (60 to 85% weight over volume) is carefully followed through the small intestinal loops and each loop of the jejunum and ileum is carefully identified as the barium passes through to the ileocecal junction. Usually, this requires the administration of at least two additional 8-oz doses of the 85% barium sulfate in colloidal suspension. Gastrografin may be added to the barium in small doses to speed up the study. The normal "transit time" (passage time for barium from duodenum to ileocecal junction) varies between one and three hours normally. If delayed beyond six or eight hours, it is abnormal. If increased speed through the small intestine is desired, 2 ml of metoclopramide hydrochloride (Reglan) is administered intravenously. In the presence of malabsorption or other disease, the characteristic mucosal pattern of the small intestine is modified, so that these other abnormalities may be appropriately filmed with spot films and studied thereafter. Apart from malabsorption, regional enteritis is probably the most frequent abnormality we have encountered. Tumors of the small bowel do occur, but are rare by comparison with those involving the upper gastrointestinal tract or colon.

A more selective method for examining the small intestine is obtained by passing the so-called "Bilbao-Dotter" type catheter to the region of the proximal jejunum and the instillation through the tube of a 30% barium sulfate suspension, with about two feet of hydrostatic pressure so that good distention of the small intestine is obtained by this "small bowel enema." This is carried forward from start to finish under fluoroscopic control, with spot films obtained at strategic intervals as the barium is seen to pass through the various loops of jejunum and ileum. The Bilbao-Dotter catheter is particularly suited for this purpose, since it contains a central coiled wire for rigidity, which prevents coiling of the catheter in the stomach and allows easier passage of the catheter through the pyloric sphincter. Approximately 1000 ml of 30% barium sulfate suspension is employed.

BARIUM ENEMA
(Figs. 10–8A, B and 10–9A–D)

As previously indicated, the colon is examined either by full-column or double-contrast technique. Double-contrast technique is preferred whenever feasible, particularly since mucosal abnormalities of the colon reflect extremely important disease and permit the diagnosis of sessile polypoid lesions 5 to 10 mm in size, which in rare instances contain small foci of malignancy. Since 80% of malignant neoplasms of the colon occur in the immediate vicinity of the sigmoid, the detection of early polypoid excrescences is extremely important. Many of these may be removed by endoscopy alone and do not require open laparotomy if discovered early enough. Size is not the only determinant for the presence of malignancy, since very often even a polyp on a long pedicle may contain malignant transformation in the very tip of the polyp. A sessile polyp may be suspect with regard to malignancy, and under these circumstances, the surgeon may prefer to remove this type of lesion by direct visualization and laparotomy, with excision of a segment of the colon. By performing the excision in this manner, the adjoining lymph nodes are examined at the same time.

One must learn to differentiate between diverticula and polypoid excrescences, and for this purpose, films in the erect, supine, and prone positions are often required, employing oblique and horizontal central ray visualization along with prone, supine, and oblique positions of the patient.

Usually, with such diverse positioning, the barium enters a diverticulum, but surrounds a polyp. If the colon is adequately cleansed, the full-column study is probably adequate for polypoid lesions 10 mm or larger and is utilized particularly in patients who have difficulty retaining the gas of a double-contrast enema. In general, the double-contrast enema is preferred whenever feasible, even in the presence of regional

Text continued on page 306

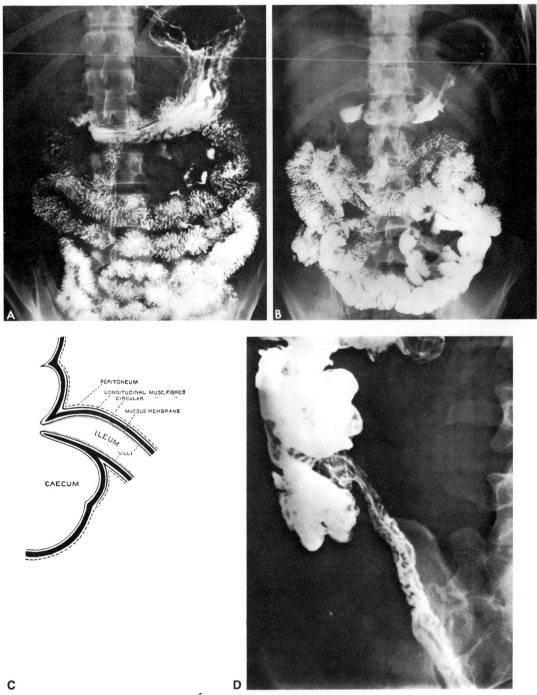

Figure 10–7. Illustrations demonstrating frequent-interval film and fluoroscopy method for examination of small intestine: *A*, At 1 hour following administration of the barium; *B*, at 2 hours. *C*, Schematic diagram of ileocecal junction. *D*, Radiograph of ileocecal junction.

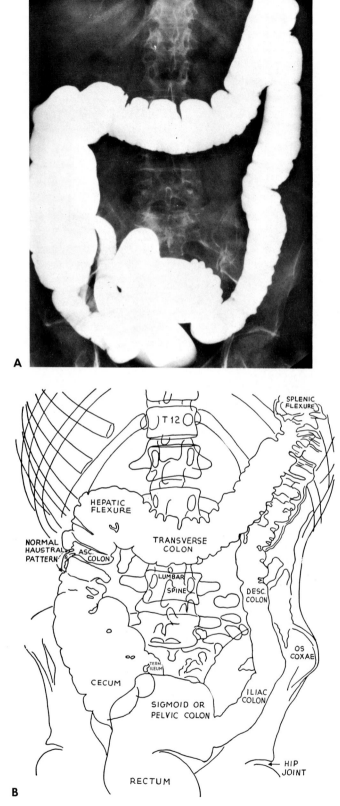

A

B

Figure 10–8. *A*, Radiograph obtained in posteroanterior projection. *B*, Labeled tracing.

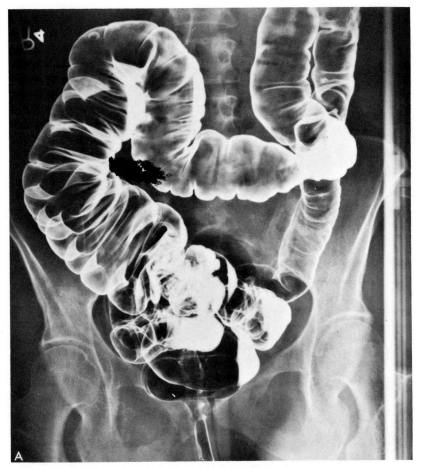

Figure 10–9. Sample radiographs of double-contrast high-density barium-air enemas: *A*, Routine posteroanterior projection.

Illustration continued on following page

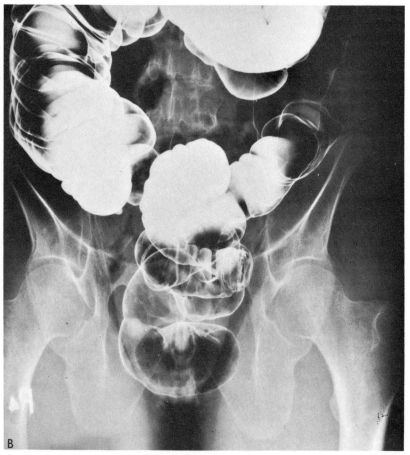

Figure 10–9 *Continued. B,* Special projection with the patient prone, table tilted with head down for better visualization of double contrast of the rectum and sigmoid.

Illustration continued on opposite page

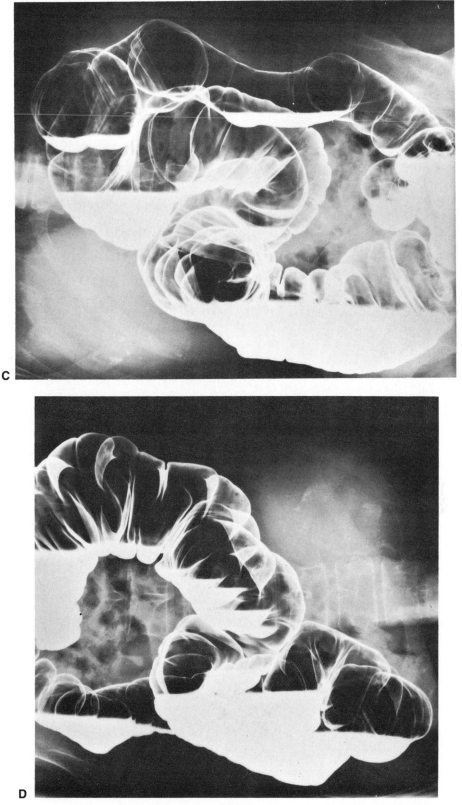

Figure 10–9 *Continued. C,* Horizontal beam study with patient's left side uppermost for best visualization of the descending colon in particular but also for some double contrast visualization of portions of the transverse colon. *D,* Horizontal beam study with the patient's right side uppermost for best visualization of the right half of the colon in double contrast.

enteritis or diverticula of the colon, being careful to regulate the pressure so that perforation of the colon will not occur. With the double-contrast study, protocols may differ somewhat, but the ultimate purpose is the same: Every square centimeter of the colon must be visualized in adequate double-contrast no matter how redundant the colon may be.

In either the full-column or double-contrast study, a postevacuation film may be obtained for further additional examination of any suspicious areas.

Films are studied immediately after they have been obtained, and any suspicious areas are refilmed until a final solution is possible. Lateral decubitus films may also be obtained if a small amount of feces is seen, since the feces often drops by gravity into the barium, leaving a coating of the barium adherent to the mucosa.

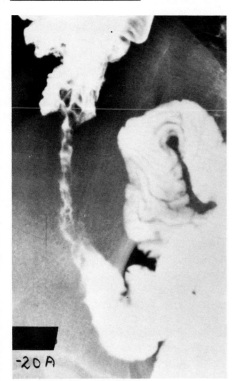

Figure E–191.

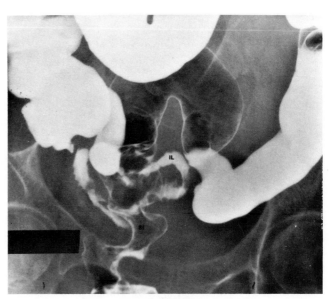

Figure E–192.

CLINICAL FINDINGS
Case 51–1 (Fig. E–191). Thirty-year-old man with intermittent diarrhea.
Case 51–2 (Fig. E–192). Fifty-five-year-old woman with carcinoma of the cervix.

Questions
51–1. In Case 51–1, a coned-down view of the terminal ileum is MOST consistent with?
A. Lymphoma of the ileum.
B. Carcinoma of the ileum.
C. Tuberculous ileitis.
D. Amebic ileitis.
•E. Crohn's ileitis.

51–2. In Case 51–2, double-contrast examination of the colon (SI = sigmoid) with ileal reflux (IL) shows?
A. Cervical carcinoma invading the colon and ileum.
☞B. Radiation proctosigmoiditis and ileitis.
C. Ischemic disease of the colon and ileum.
D. Crohn's disease of rectosigmoid colon and ileum.
E. Ulcerative proctosigmoiditis with backwash ileitis.

Radiologic Findings. In Case 51–1, a peroral small bowel examination shows narrowing and irregularity of the terminal ileum. The appearance and length of involvement would be unusual for a neoplastic process. Although in the past tuberculosis commonly affected this area, it is rarely seen today. Amebiasis typically involves the colon but spares the ileum. Therefore, the most likely cause is Crohn's ileitis (**E is the correct answer to Question 51–1**). Yersinial infection of the ileum may have a similar radiographic appearance. Stool cultures, serologic testing, and sequential small bowel examinations are occasionally needed for differentiation.

Case 51–2 shows irregular narrowing of both the rectosigmoid colon and the ileum. In view of the clinical history, however, neoplastic invasion from cervical carcinoma or radiation injury from its treatment would be the most likely considerations. Cervical carcinoma typically invades the bladder base, causing ureteral obstruction, and, less commonly, involves the bowel. Thus, the extensive involvement of the rectosigmoid colon and ileum in this case is most likely the result of radiation injury (**B is the correct answer to Question 51–2**).

Discussion. Except for duodenal ulcer disease, most primary disorders of the small bowel are uncommon. The major exceptions include obstruction due to adhesion or external hernia and inflammatory disorders, such as Crohn's and radiation enteritis. Secondary involvement of the small bowel by metastatic deposits and intraperitoneal spread of tumor or infection is often seen.

The small intestine can be examined by various methods (Table E–15). The peroral examination is the standard antegrade method, involving ingestion of 16 to 24 ounces of barium and serial filming of the abdomen. Injection of barium through an indwelling small bowel tube or through a special catheter passed into the jejunum (enteroclysis technique) are other antegrade methods. The small bowel can be examined in a retrograde fashion by instilling barium from the opposite direction. This may be accomplished by refluxing the small bowel during a routine barium enema, or by filling it secondarily via a colostomy or directly from an ileostomy.

Table E–15. RADIOGRAPHIC EXAMINATION OF THE SMALL INTESTINE

Antegrade methods	Retrograde methods
Peroral examination	Reflux examination
Enteroclysis technique	Via a colostomy
Indwelling tubes	Via an ileostomy

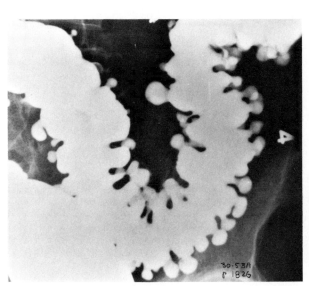

Figure E–193.

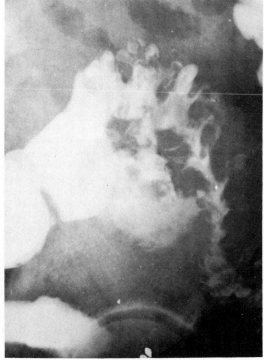

Figure E–194.

CLINICAL FINDINGS

Case 52–1 (Fig. E–193). Sixty-year-old woman with left lower quadrant pain.
Case 52–2 (Fig. E–194). Fifty-year-old man with fever and left lower quadrant mass.

Questions

52–1. Which of the following are TRUE concerning the disease shown in Case 52–1?
A. It is the most common structural disease of the colon.
B. It is acquired rather than congenital.
C. The pathogenesis may relate to a dietary deficiency.
D. The sigmoid colon is the least common site of involvement.
E. It is rarely symptomatic with few complications.

52–2. Which of the following are TRUE concerning the complication of diverticular disease shown in Case 52–2?
A. It is the most frequent complication of diverticular disease.
B. It is often associated with gross rectal bleeding.
C. It results from perforation of multiple diverticula.
D. It most commonly involves the sigmoid colon.
E. It commonly leads to generalized peritonitis.

309

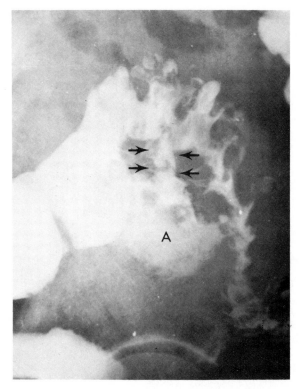

Figure E–195. The sigmoid colon is affected by diverticular disease, and partially narrowed by the adjacent inflammatory process. Extravasation from a perforated diverticulum (arrows) into a diverticular abscess (A) is well shown.

Radiologic Findings. Case 52–1 illustrates the typical appearance of uncomplicated diverticular disease involving the sigmoid colon. The multiple sacculations represent diverticula protruding between bands of thickened colon musculature.

Case 52–2 shows severe diverticular disease of the sigmoid colon. The paracolic extravasation represents diverticulitis with abscess formation (Fig. E–195).

Discussion. Diverticular disease is the most common structural disorder of the colon (**Question 52–1 A is true**), and is felt to be an acquired disease, rarely seen in individuals under 40 years (**Question 52–1 B is true**). The diverticula represent mucosal protrusions that herniate through the vascular clefts of the colonic musculature. Abnormal pulsion forces within the colon presumably promote the formation of diverticula. The pathogenesis of this disorder is not completely understood but has been related to long term fiber deficiency in the diet (**Question 52–1 C is true**).

Although diverticula may occur anywhere in the colon, the sigmoid area is the most common site (**Question 52–1 D is false**). The pathologic findings include prominent thickening of the circular muscle and the presence of diverticula. In some patients, these components, particularly muscle thickening, may be seen separately (Fig. E–196). Diverticular disease is a frequent cause of lower gastrointestinal symptomatology, and significant complications are not uncommon (**Question 52–1 E is false**).

Diverticulitis is the most common complication of diverticular disease of the colon (**Question 52–2 A is true**). Indeed, most of the complications from this disease begin as focal diverticulitis (Table E–16). The main exception is gross rectal bleeding, which usually occurs in the absence of overt diverticulitis (**Question 52–2 B is false**). Diverticulitis is nearly always due to perforation of a single diverticulum with fecal leakage initiating abscess formation (**Question 52–2 C is false**). The sigmoid colon is most commonly involved (**Question 52–2 D is true**).

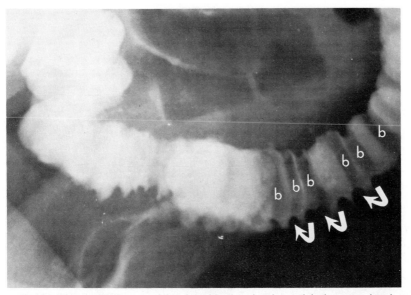

Figure E–196. Diverticular disease of the sigmoid colon showing mainly the muscular abnormality. Muscle thickening is seen as transverse bands crossing the lumen (b), and as corrugation along the edge of the colon (arrows).

Diverticulitis usually remains confined as a paracolic abscess. Colonic obstruction may occur acutely if significant inflammatory narrowing and spasm are present. Chronic stricturing may also occur and cause obstruction. Occasionally, diverticulitis does not remain confined, and is then an important cause of pelvic fistulization. Focal peritonitis usually accompanies diverticulitis; however, generalized peritonitis due to free communication of the abscess with the peritoneal cavity is rare (**Question 52–2 E is false**). When proper precautions are followed, little risk is involved in doing a barium enema. If contrast extravasation is seen radiographically, the procedure should be terminated, since the diagnosis is evident. Water soluble contrast media may be used instead of barium sulfate.

Table E–16. COMPLICATIONS OF DIVERTICULAR DISEASE OF THE COLON

Diverticulitis
Obstruction
Fistulization
Peritonitis
Hemorrhage

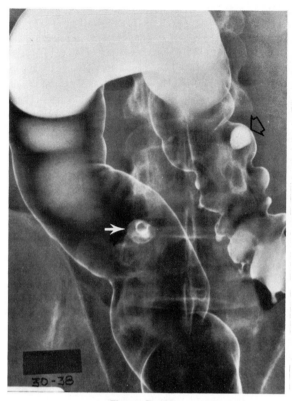

Figure E–197.

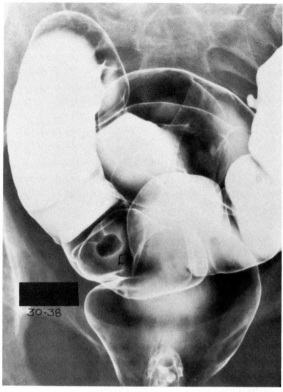

Figure E–198.

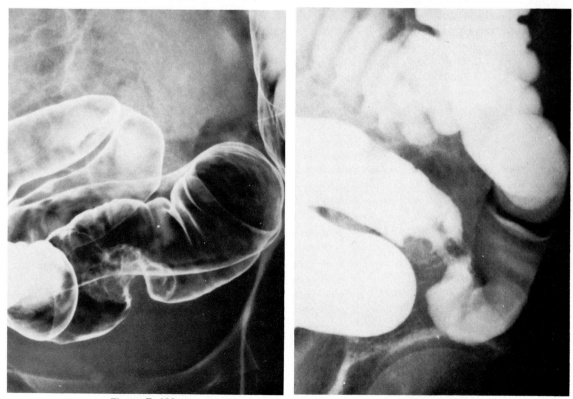

Figure E–199.

Figure E–200.

CLINICAL FINDINGS
Case 53–1 (Fig. E–197). Forty-five-year-old man with constipation.
Case 53–2 (Fig. E–198). Fifty-year-old woman with occult rectal bleeding.
Case 53–3 (Fig. E–199). Sixty-year-old woman with gross rectal bleeding.
Case 53–4 (Fig. E–200). Seventy-year-old woman with obstipation.

Questions
53–1. In case 53–1, two sigmoid lesions (arrows) shown MOST likely represent?
A. Diverticulum (lower arrow) – polyp (upper arrow).
B. Diverticulum (lower arrow) – stool (upper arrow).
C. Diverticula for both sigmoid lesions.
D. Polyps for both sigmoid lesions.
E. Polyp (lower arrow) – diverticulum (upper arrow).

53–2. In Case 53–2, the MOST LIKELY conclusion regarding the appearance of the
    sigmoid polyp (arrow) is?
A. A hyperplastic polyp.
B. A villous adenoma.
C. An adenomatous polyp.
D. A polypoid carcinoma.
E. An annular carcinoma.

53–3. In Case 53–3, which feature of the polypoid sigmoid lesion is LEAST reliable
    for malignancy?
A. Absence of an associated pedicle.
B. Size of the polypoid lesion.
C. Shape of the polypoid lesion.
D. Indentation at the base of the lesion.
E. Irregular surface of the lesion.

53–4. In Case 53–4, the MOST likely diagnosis is?
A. Endometriosis involving the colon.
B. Leiomyosarcoma of the colon.
C. Lymphoma of the colon.
D. Adenocarcinoma of the colon.
E. Squamous carcinoma of the colon.

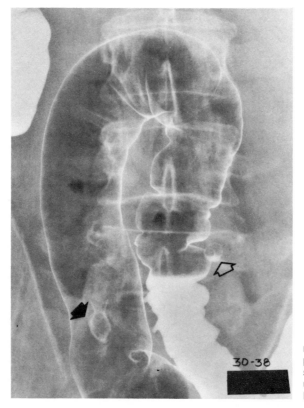

30-38

Figure E–201. Upright view of the rectosigmoid colon. A pedunculated polyp (closed arrow) is near the rectosigmoid junction. A projecting diverticulum (open arrows) with an air-barium level is easily distinguished.

Figure E–202. Large polypoid carcinoma of the sigmoid colon (arrowheads). The surface is markedly irregular and the base of the lesion is indented (arrow).

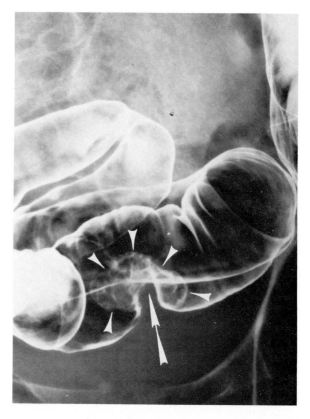

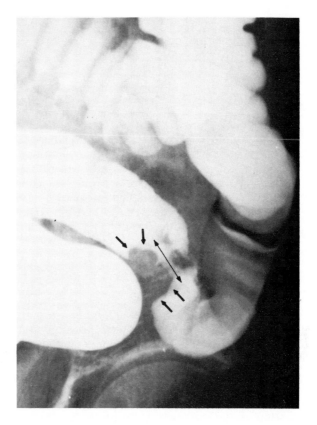

Figure E–203. Single-contrast barium enema showing an annular carcinoma with overhanging edges (arrows). The lumen (connected arrows) is markedly narrowed by the encircling tumor.

Radiologic Findings. In Case 53–1, two lesions are seen in the sigmoid colon on a double-contrast barium enema. The more proximal one fills with barium and is a diverticulum. The lesion near the rectosigmoid junction is less dense because of barium coating and represents a polyp (**E is the correct answer to Question 53–1**). Differentiation of colonic polyp from diverticulum may be difficult. However, if a lesion fills with barium or projects off the colonic lumen, the diagnosis of diverticulum is easily made (Fig. E–201).

Case 53–2 represents a pedunculated polyp in the sigmoid colon. The size of the lesion and the presence of a stalk argue against this being a hyperplastic polyp. The villous adenoma is uncommon and is usually sessile with an irregular surface. The presence of a pedicle is an important finding, indicating that the polyp is most likely benign. Although pedunculated polyps may habor focal carcinoma, neoplastic invasion into the adjacent colonic wall is rare. As expected, this lesion proved to be a benign adenomatous polyp (**C is the correct answer to Question 53–2**).

In Case 53–3, a lobulated polypoid lesion of the sigmoid colon is present. It measures 3 by 4 cm and shows indentation at its base (Fig. E–202), suggesting malignant infiltration of the colonic wall. Size and, to a lesser extent, surface lobulation are important criteria for estimating malignant potential. A sessile polyp less than 1 cm has only about a 1% chance of malignancy, while a lesion over 2 cm has nearly a 50% chance. Conversely, the absence of a pedicle, particularly with smaller polyps, is of little value in estimating malignant risk (**A is the correct answer to Question 53–3**).

Case 53–4 represents an annular or "apple-core" carcinoma of the colon (Fig. E–203). This appearance is almost pathognomonic for adenocarcinoma (**D is the correct answer to Question 53–4**). All other primary malignancies of the colon are extremely rare. Although endometriosis may affect the colon, the age of the patient and configuration of the lesion are atypical.

Table E–17. EPITHELIAL POLYPS OF THE COLON

Hyperplastic polyp	Inflammatory polyp
Neoplastic polyp	Hamartomatous polyp
Benign adenoma	Juvenile polyp
Adenoma with carcinoma	
Polypoid carcinoma	

Discussion. Primary colonic neoplasms almost always arise from the epithelium. The polypoid type is the most common morphologic form. Not all epithelial lesions of the colon, however, are true neoplasms (Table E–17). Hyperplastic polyps are found in most adults over 40 years of age. They are smooth and sessile protuberances, usually measuring less than 5 mm, and make up the bulk of all colon polyps in this size range. Pathologically, neoplastic polyps range from the benign adenoma to the polypoid carcinoma. Intermediate types include the villous adenoma and the adenoma containing focal carcinoma. Adenomas are estimated to occur in 8 to 12 per cent of the adult population, with higher incidences in the later decades of life. Inflammatory, hamartomatous, and juvenile polyps are much less common, and occur typically within a specific clinical setting.

Adenomas may be sessile or pedunculated, with a smooth or lobulated surface. In general, smaller adenomas are usually sessile and smooth, while larger ones tend to be stalked and lobulated (Fig. E–204). Size is the most important radiographic criterion for estimating the risk of invasive carcinoma within an otherwise benign adenoma. Lesions over 1 cm have an increasing risk of malignancy, and should be appropriately removed.

Adenocarcinoma of the colon is the most common gastrointestinal malignancy. A variety of morphologic types exist, ranging from the small polypoid carcinoma to the obstructing, annular type. The presence of a focal, annular lesion in the colon is almost diagnostic of carcinoma. Unfortunately, this appearance indicates advanced disease and portends a poorer prognosis. Carcinoma of the colon and sigmoid diverticulitis are the two most common causes of colonic obstruction in adults.

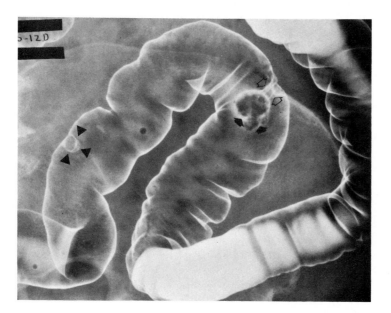

Figure E–204. Sigmoid colon containing two polyps. The smaller polyp (arrowheads) is smooth and sessile, while the larger polyp is pedunculated (open arrows) and has a lobulated or irregular surface (closed arrows).

Exercise 54: Inflammatory Disease of the Colon

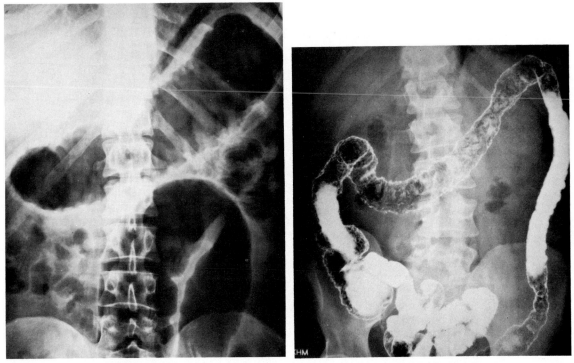

Figure E–205.   **Figure E–206.**

CLINICAL FINDINGS

Case 54–1 (Fig. E–205). Thirty-two-year-old man with abdominal pain and diarrhea.
Case 54–2 (Fig. E–206). Twenty-eight-year-old man with fever and bloody diarrhea.

Questions

54–1. What is the MOST appropriate radiographic management in Case 54–1?
A. Serial plain films of the abdomen.
B. Upper gastrointestinal series.
C. Small bowel series.
D. Water-soluble contrast enema.
E. Barium contrast enema.

54–2. In Case 54–2, what is the MOST likely diagnosis?
A. Ulcerative colitis.
B. Crohn's colitis.
C. Bacterial colitis.
D. Amebic colitis.
E. Tuberculous colitis.

Table E–18. INFLAMMATORY DISEASE OF THE COLON

Idiopathic causes	Drug related causes
Ulcerative colitis	Antibiotic colitis
Crohn's colitis	Cathartic abuse
Infectious causes	Radiation induced colitis
Bacterial agents	Miscellaneous causes
Parasitic agents	Ischemic colitis
Viral agents	Pseudomembranous colitis
Fungal agents	Obstruction related

Radiologic Findings. In Case 54–1, the abdominal plain film shows dilatation of the colon with loss of the normal haustral contour of the transverse portion. This represents toxic megacolon related to fulminant ulcerative colitis. Because of the risk of perforation, radiographic contrast studies are contraindicated. These patients must be followed clinically and with serial abdominal films to assess progressive colonic dilatation (**A is the correct answer to Question 54–1**). Surgical intervention is often necessary.

In Case 54–2, a supine film from a double-contrast examination of the colon shows pancolitis with ileal sparing. The colon lacks haustration, has a coarse surface granularity, and is diffusely ulcerated. These features are most consistent with ulcerative colitis (**A is the correct answer to Question 54–2**). Crohn's disease and amebic colitis would be the major differential considerations, but would rarely cause a symmetrically diffuse pancolitis.

Discussion. Inflammatory disease of the colon is due to many different causes (Table E–18). A number of these disorders may clinically and radiographically simulate ulcerative colitis and Crohn's disease. Radiation proctitis, for example, is often indistinguishable from ulcerative colitis, and certain infectious causes may occasionally mimic the idiopathic diseases. Therefore, it is important to exclude these more specific causes through clinical correlation and by appropriate laboratory testing.

Radiographic differentiation between ulcerative colitis and Crohn's disease is possible in most cases (Table E–19). The features that most suggest ulcerative colitis are continuous disease with rectal involvement, ahaustral shortening of the colon, and a finely ulcerated or granular mucosal pattern (Fig. E–207). On the other hand, the characteristic features of Crohn's colitis include discontinuous disease with ileal involvement, eccentric wall involvement (Fig. E–208), discrete or deep ulceration, intramural fissuring, and fistulization (Fig. E–209).

Table E–19. SUMMARY OF THE MORE SPECIFIC DIFFERENTIAL FEATURES OF ULCERATIVE AND CROHN'S COLITIS

Ulcerative colitis	Crohn's colitis
Continuous, circumferential disease	Discontinuous, eccentric disease
Rectal and left-sided involvement	Right-sided colitis with rectal sparing
Pancolitis with ileal sparing	Frequent, typical ileal involvement
Smooth, ahaustral colon	Discrete "aphthoid" ulceration
Granular mucosal pattern	Criss-crossing, deep ulceration
Finely serrated ulceration	Fissure formation and fistulization

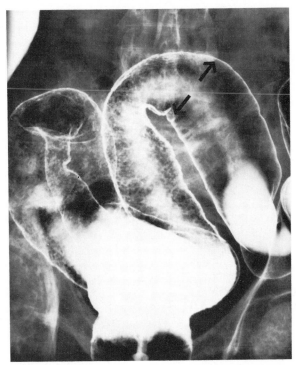

Figure E–207. Double-contrast barium enema showing diffuse granularity due to ulcerative proctosigmoiditis. The uninvolved sigmoid colon is smoothly and homogeneously coated with barium (proximal to arrows).

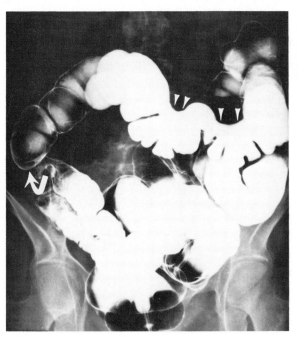

Figure E–208. Crohn's ileocolitis with cecal contraction and ileal narrowing (curved arrow). Eccentric involvement of the superior wall of the mid-transverse colon (arrowheads) is also seen.

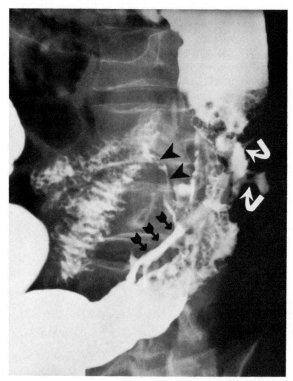

Figure E–209. Segmental Crohn's disease of the descending colon. Deep transverse ulceration and fissuring (curved arrows) are present, along with longitudinal (arrows) and small bowel (arrowheads) fistulization.

Toxic megacolon results from a variety of different causes; however, ulcerative colitis is the most common (Table E–20). In the acutely dilated colon in ulcerative colitis, the bowel wall is weakened and prone to perforation. Radiographic contrast studies, particularly the barium enema, are contraindicated.

Table E–20. CAUSES OF TOXIC MEGACOLON

Ulcerative colitis
Crohn's colitis
Ischemic colitis
Infectious colitides
Hirschsprung's disease
Drug-induced dilation

11

Biliary System

ORAL CHOLECYSTOGRAPHY
(Fig. 11–1A, B)

Of the various commonly employed cholecystographic oral agents, the most frequently used agent in Telepaque, or iopanoic acid. The usual dose for a single examination is 3 gm contrast agent, so that when Telepaque, for example, is utilized, six tablets are administered to the patient.

Clinically, any suspicion of biliary tract disease is sufficient indication for cholecystography, provided: (1) jaundice is not too severe, since a total failure of opacification will occur, and (2) renal failure is not present, since the contrast agent is ultimately excreted *via* the urinary tract. Usually, a bilirubin level greater than 1.5 mg/dl precludes oral cholecystography (4 mg/dl precludes *intravenous* cholangiography). Side reactions, such as nausea and vomiting, are common in patients undergoing oral cholecystography.

Wherever possible a plain film of the abdomen should be taken prior to the administration of any contrast study, including oral cholecystography, but unfortunately, since the examination is conducted over a 14-hour period, many x-ray laboratories omit a plain film of the abdomen prior to the procedure. However, most patients will have had a KUB film in the course of other studies, particularly of the gastrointestinal tract, which will suffice.

The patient is given the iodinated con-

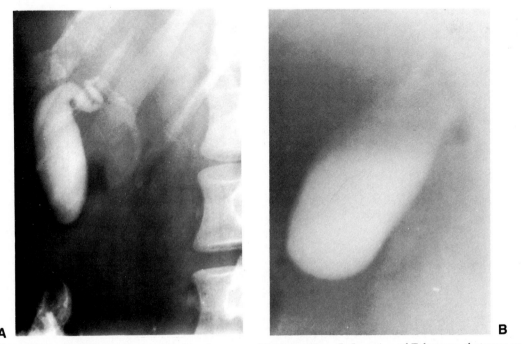

A **B**

Figure 11–1. A, Radiograph of gallbladder in prone oblique position. B, Layering of Telepaque that may occur normally in the gallbladder.

trast agent in the 3-gm dosage and is instructed generally to remain on a fat-free diet after the dinner meal, after which the contrast agent is administered. The noon meal should have contained sufficient fat for evacuation of the gallbladder prior to the examination, so that bile salts will appear in the small intestine.

The optimum concentration of the contrast agent is obtained approximately 14 hours after its oral administration, so that if it is administered at 6:00 PM the night prior to the procedure, the examination is conducted at 8:00 AM the following day.

The examination is conducted first with spot film studies of the gallbladder area obtained in the erect position, and thereafter in the right posterior oblique, or left anterior oblique projections in the supine and prone. Every effort is made to obtain a clear visualization of the gallbladder with no interference by gaseous shadows. If it is impossible to obtain a clear visualization of the gallbladder, tomograms are indicated.

It is important to combine the upright examination with the recumbent in order to obtain the "layering out" or gravity effect of gallstones, which allows visualization in many instances when they otherwise may not be seen.

Unfortunately, carcinoma of the gallbladder usually leads to nonfunction of the organ and requires an examination of the gallbladder other than oral cholecystography for visualization (i.e., ultrasonography or computed tomography).

If the gallbladder is not visualized following the first dose of six tablets of Telepaque, which may be the case in 15 to 25% of patients, a second dose of six tablets is administered that evening and the examination repeated the following morning. Sometimes this is erroneously referred to as a double-dose procedure. Within a 7-day period, it is ordinarily required that no further Telepaque be administered, since it is especially contraindicated on the basis of its nephrotoxicity.

With the advent of ultrasonography (as will be detailed in the description of ultrasonography [Fig. 11–2]), at times the patient is referred directly to the ultrasonographer, since this method of examination has become very accurate for the detection of very small filling defects within the gallbladder, whether they be due to stones, papillomas, or cholesterol plaques. However, this is a morphologic demonstration rather than a physiologic study, as is oral cholecystography.

It is important to note that for oral cholecystography to be successful, bile salts must be present in the small intestine at the time the water-insoluble contrast agent, such as

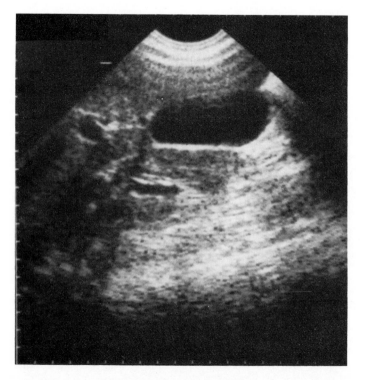

Figure 11–2. Normal longitudinal ultrasonogram of the gallbladder. (Courtesy of Dr. Nat Watson.)

Telepaque, is administered. Only under this circumstance is the agent absorbed by the small intestine, transported by the blood stream to the liver parenchyma (usually attached to albumin), and conjugated in the liver with glucuronic acid to an ester of glucuronide. This conjugation provides a more water-soluble molecule of increased molecular weight for excretion into bile that cannot diffuse back into the liver across the lipid membrane of its canaliculi. It must therefore be understood that bile salts per se, independent of their choleretic effect, are the important determinants of iopanoate excretion.

In the absence of circulating bile salts, biliary excretion rate of iopanoate is markedly reduced. Thus, when a low-protein diet has been administered to the patient, there is a reduction of biliary excretion rate of bile salts. This, in turn, impairs the intestinal solubility and absorption of iopanoate, limits its rate of excretion, and probably causes poor visualization of the gallbladder.

Similar impairment results from fasting. Within the gallbladder there is a reabsorption of water, which does not occur in the bile duct proper. Thus, visualization of the bile ducts is determined by the rate of excretion solely of the contrast agent, and the basal bile flow. Upon leaving the liver, although a small portion of the biliary contrast material flows directly into the duodenum, when the cystic duct is patent the flow is primarily into the gallbladder. Here it is concentrated by the reabsorption of water. The peak radiographic opacification of the gallbladder then occurs 14 to 19 hours after ingestion of the contrast material. It is important to recognize that nonvisualization cannot be attributed to failure of the gallbladder to reabsorb water, but rather that the conjugated iopanoate is too readily reabsorbed from the inflamed gallbladder.

Most of the contrast material, after conjugation in the liver and storage in the biliary tree, is excreted into the gastrointestinal tract. In the colon it may be deconjugated and permit reabsorption of the unconjugated compound, but generally about 65% of the administered dose may be recovered in the stool. Renal excretion is the other major route of elimination of the biliary contrast agents, and this in turn is directly related to the concentration of the conjugated form of contrast agent in plasma. It is of clinical importance that the iopanoate glucuronide in the urine may produce a false-positive protein-precipitation test for albumin, and positive

reactions for the latter should be verified by a colorimetric dipstick method. Failure of visualization of two doses of the Telepaque usually indicates disease of the gallbladder or gallstones with approximately 95% accuracy. For visualization of the cystic and common bile duct, it is sometimes desirable to administer a fatty meal or other gallbladder stimulant (cholecystokinin), and films are obtained at 10, 20, 30, and 45 minute intervals in the right posterior olbique supine projection. At times tomography is employed for best visualization. Often, however, if there is a diseased gallbladder, it will fail to contract, and a failure of visualization of the ductal system will also ensue.

INTRAVENOUS CHOLANGIOGRAPHY (IVC)

With the advent of newer procedures, such as percutaneous cholangiography, ultrasonography, endoscopic retrograde cholangiopancreatography (ERCP), and computed tomography, intravenous cholangiography has seldom been employed. It is usually performed when the common bile duct is of prime interest rather than the gallbladder. It is contraindicated when the bilirubin exceeds 4 mg/dl.

In this procedure a scout film is first performed with a scout tomogram at the approximate level of the common bile duct in the right posterior oblique projection. Thereafter, a slow injection of 20 ml of Cholegrafin is performed, and the common bile duct is visualized moderately well, particularly with the aid of tomography, within 20 to 30 minutes. Films taken later at 2 and 4 hours are required for visualization of the gallbladder proper. For optimal visualization of the common bile duct, tomograms are essential for detail.

Radionuclide imaging of the liver and biliary system is particularly useful when obstructive disease of the biliary system or acute cholecystitis is suspected (see section on "Nuclear Medicine").

ENDOSCOPIC RETROGRADE CHOLANGIOPANCREATOGRAPHY (ERCP)
(Fig. 11–3)

With the aid of an endoscope in the duodenum, the ampulla of Vater is cannulated and iodinated water-soluble contrast agent injected first for visualization of the

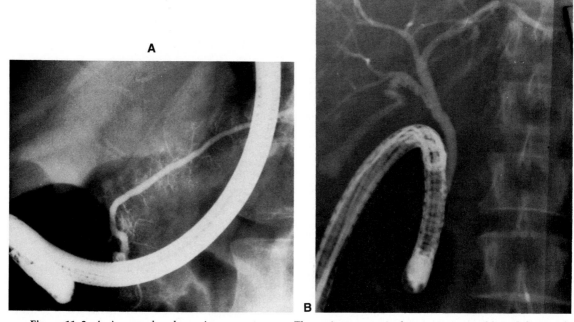

Figure 11–3. *A*, A normal endoscopic pancreatogram. The main pancreatic duct tapers smoothly, while its side branches are fine and uniform in size. *B*, Biliary ductal system by ERCP.

pancreatic duct and thereafter into the common bile duct for visualization of the common bile duct, right and left hepatic ducts, and biliary radicles. If the gallbladder is intact, it too will be visualized at this time by passage of the contrast agent through the cystic duct into the gallbladder.

Whenever possible, the complete procedure should be performed for visualization of both of these areas. It is particularly accurate for visualization of pancreatic ductal abnormalities, such as may occur with pancreatitis and carcinoma of the pancreas; for visualization of the gallbladder when it is nonvisualized by oral cholecystography and occupied by neoplasm or stones; or for visualization of common bile duct or hepatic ductal stones.

DIRECT PERCUTANEOUS TRANSHEPATIC CHOLANGIOGRAPHY

In this procedure, a fine-gauge needle is inserted into the right lobe of the liver until a bile duct is encountered. The water-soluble iodinated contrast agent is injected and films obtained in sequence thereafter until the main biliary radicles are visualized as well as the common hepatic and common bile duct.

The procedure is particularly indicated when obstruction of the biliary tree is anticipated, and it is desired that the cause of the obstruction be elucidated. Usually, in these patients, the bilirubin level is too high for either intravenous or oral cholangiography, and an ERCP examination either is noncommital in its results or cannot be performed. The small-gauge rather flexible needle is well tolerated by the patient without serious complications in practically all instances.

INTRAOPERATIVE CHOLANGIOGRAPHY

This procedure is performed on the operating table at the time of cholecystectomy, after the surgeon has removed the gallbladder, and a small catheter is placed into the common hepatic duct, near the cystic duct. Its main purpose is to visualize any residual stones or abnormalities that might otherwise have been missed during the surgical procedure. If visualized at this time, the surgeon is equipped to remove these stones. Contrast agent is injected under direct visualization and a film obtained immediately of the entire common hepatic duct and common bile duct, and the flow of the contrast agent into the duodenum is visualized.

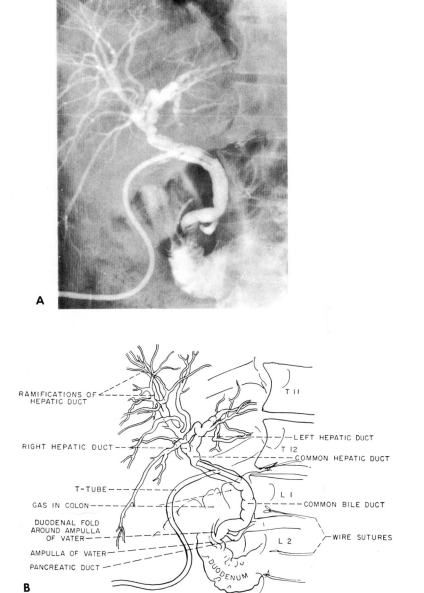

A

RAMIFICATIONS OF
HEPATIC DUCT

RIGHT HEPATIC DUCT

T-TUBE

GAS IN COLON

DUODENAL FOLD
AROUND AMPULLA
OF VATER

AMPULLA OF VATER

PANCREATIC DUCT

T 11

LEFT HEPATIC DUCT

T 12

COMMON HEPATIC DUCT

L 1

COMMON BILE DUCT

WIRE SUTURES

L 2

DUODENUM

B

Figure 11–4. Thirty-five per cent Renografin T-tube cholangiogram (A) and its tracing (B). This contrast medium gives a more complete visualization of all hepatic radicles. This is extremely important because stones may be concealed in the hepatic radicles only to descend later and cause recurrence of symptoms.

T-TUBE CHOLANGIOGRAPHY
(Fig. 11–4)

Following cholecystectomy, particularly in the presence of a stone in the common bile duct, a T-tube is placed in the common bile duct by the surgeon and exteriorized. Usually one week or 10 days after the operation, retrograde injection of water-soluble iodinated contrast agent is performed into this tube after all air bubbles have been evacuated from the system. The contrast agent first outlines the right hepatic duct with its radicles; then the left hepatic duct by tilting the patient toward the left side; and finally, the common hepatic and common bile duct in their entirety. The ideal examination allows one to visualize the entire biliary tree, including the left hepatic duct particularly, since this is often a reservoir for stones that have formed since the operative procedure, or may be residual following the cholecystectomy. The examination is never considered complete unless the left hepatic duct is well visualized, since this structure is notorious as a reservoir for residual stones.

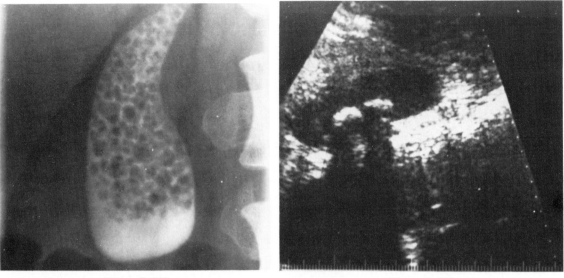

Figure E–210.

Figure E–211.

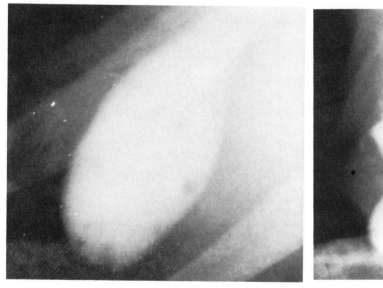
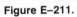

Figure E–212.

Figure E–213.

326

CLINICAL FINDINGS
Case 55–1 (Fig. E–210). Forty-five-year-old woman with dyspepsia.
Case 55–2 (Fig. E–211). Fifty-year-old man with right upper quadrant pain (courtesy of Dr. Neil Wolfman).
Case 55–3 (Fig. E–212). Fifty-five-year-old man with fatty food intolerance.
Case 55–4 (Fig. E–213). Sixty-year-old woman with epigastric pain.

Questions
55–1. In Case 55–1, the oral cholecystogram shows?
A. Acute cholecystitis.
B. Emphysematous cholecystitis.
C. Gallbladder carcinoma.
D. Cholesterol polyps.
E. Multiple gallstones.

55–2. In Case 55–2, longitudinal ultrasound of the gallbladder indicates?
A. Solitary gallstone.
B. Multiple gallstones.
C. Cholesterol polyps.
D. Multiple papillomas.
E. Gallbladder carcinoma.

55–3. In Case 55–3, UPRIGHT film of the gallbladder is MOST suggestive of?
A. Multiple papillomas.
B. Multiple gallstones.
C. Cholesterol polyps.
D. Adenomyomatosis.
E. Carcinomatosis.

55–4. In Case 55–4, the proposed cause of the gallbladder appearance is?
A. Congenital origin.
B. Neoplastic origin.
C. Inflammatory origin.
D. Degenerative origin.
E. Traumatic origin.

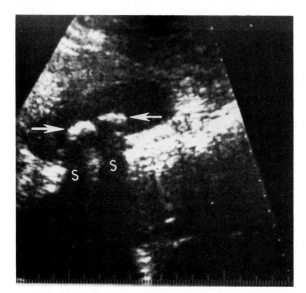

Figure E–214. Two stones (arrows) are seen as echogenic foci within the gallbladder. Prominent acoustic shadowing (S) is produced by both stones.

Radiologic Findings. In Case 55–1, multiple defects are present within the gallbladder. Many have a faceted appearance, which is characteristic of cholelithiasis (**E is the correct answer to Question 55–1**). In acute or emphysematous cholecystitis and in carcinoma, the gallbladder typically fails to visualize. Cholesterol polyps are round in shape and much fewer in number.

In Case 55–2, ultrasonic examination of the gallbladder shows several echogenic structures associated with acoustic shadowing (Fig. E–214). The latter is produced by the poor sound transmission, and is typically seen with gallstones (**B is the correct answer to Question 55–2**). Noncalculous defects in the gallbladder generally cause focal echogenicity, but without prominent acoustic shadowing.

In Case 55–3, multiple defects are present within the gallbladder on an upright film. Because of their movability, gallstones would be expected to layer inferiorly (Fig. E–215). Consequently, these are more likely fixed defects, with the most common cause being multiple cholesterol polyps (**C is the correct answer to Question 56–3**).

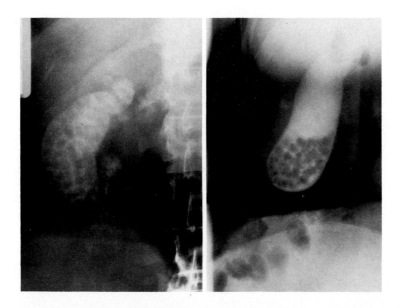

Figure E–215. Multiple lucencies are present within the gallbladder on the supine film (left). On the upright film (right), the defects layer in the dependent portion of the organ and are therefore gallstones. Cholesterol polyps would not change their position.

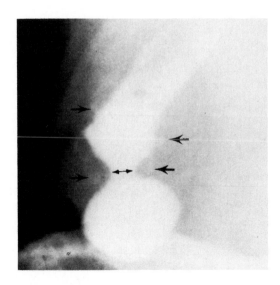

Figure E–216. Segmental narrowing (connected arrows) of the gallbladder with diverticula-like outpouchings known as Rokitansky-Aschoff sinuses (arrows).

In Case 55–4, the gallbladder is segmentally narrowed with multiple out-pouchings resembling diverticula (Fig. E–216). This represents adenomyomatosis of the gallbladder, a benign degenerative disorder **(D is the correct answer to Question 55–4).**

Discussion. The two primary methods for imaging the gallbladder are oral cholecystography and ultrasound. The oral cholecystogram has been traditionally used but involves the ingestion of an iodinated contrast medium on the day preceding the examination and exposure to ionizing radiation. Its major disadvantage is that 15 to 35% of patients will have a nondiagnostic study following the first dose. Up to 20% of those with initial nonvisualization and 65 to 75% with poor visualization will have normal gallbladders after a second additional dose. Thus, "nonvisualization" of the gallbladder as a valid diagnosis necessitates two consecutive doses. In some institutions, ultrasound has replaced the oral cholecystogram as the initial examination. The main advantages of ultrasound are avoidance of ionizing radiation, elimination of the risk of a contrast reaction, and reliable evaluation of the gallbladder poorly seen or nonvisualized on oral cholecystography.

Figure E–217. The supine film of the gallbladder was normal; however, a string of minute stones is evident on the upright view.

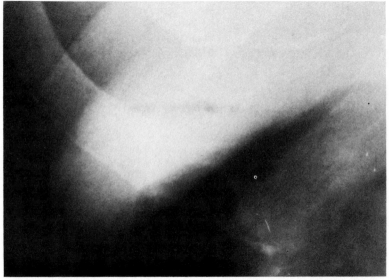

Table E–21. CAUSES OF FIXED DEFECTS WITHIN THE GALLBLADDER

Common causes	Uncommon causes
Cholesterol polyp*	Congenital septum
Adenomyoma	Inflammatory polyp*
Adherent calculus*	Benign neoplasms
Adenoma (papilloma)	Malignant neoplasms
	Postoperative defect

*May be multiple.

When defects are seen within the gallbladder, comparison of horizontal and upright films is crucial to ascertain their movability. Cholelithiasis is certain if the defects are movable. Furthermore, small calculi in the gallbladder may be seen only in the upright position (Fig. E–217). On the other hand, fixed defects in the gallbladder are rarely due to stones (Table E–21). Nearly all fixed defects appearing in a well opacified gallbladder are caused by benign processes. Most importantly, carcinoma of the gallbladder is invariably associated with a non-visualized oral cholecystogram.

Cholesterolosis and adenomyomatosis are the two most common types of an unusual group of gallbladder disorders called the cholecystoses. These are felt to be degenerative, noninflammatory processes, which may be associated occasionally with gallstones. Their clinical significance is often uncertain. Cholesterolosis is seen as either single or multiple cholesterol polyps or as a diffuse process called the "strawberry gallbladder," while adenomyomatosis may be seen as a focal, segmental, or diffuse process (Fig. E–218).

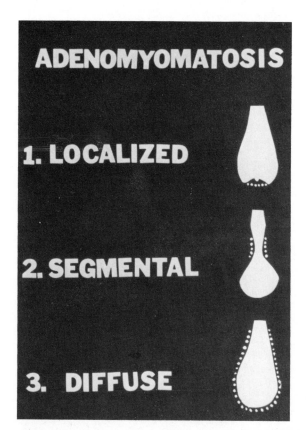

Figure E–218. The three general types of adenomyomatosis of the gallbladder shown schematically. The localized form occurs in the fundus and is usually called the adenomyoma. Rokitansky-Aschoff sinuses are commonly seen in all types.

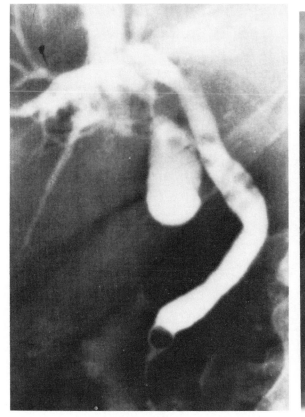

Figure E–219.

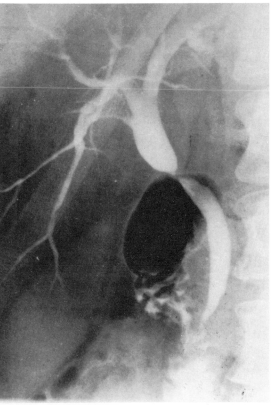

Figure E–220.

CLINICAL FINDINGS

Case 56–1 (Fig. E–219). Forty-five-year-old woman with right upper quadrant pain and jaundice.

Case 56–2 (Fig. E–220). Fifty-year-old man with right upper quadrant pain following cholecystectomy.

Questions

56–1. In Case 56–1, a transhepatic cholangiogram shows all EXCEPT which of the following?

A. Stricture of the common bile duct.
B. Several stones within the gallbladder.
C. Multiple extrahepatic ductal stones.
D. Impacted stone in lower common bile duct.
E. Extravasation into the liver parenchyma.

56–2. In Case 56–2, the MOST likely cause of the biliary ductal abnormality is?

A. Cholangiocarcinoma.
B. Gallbladder carcinoma.
C. Pancreatic carcinoma.
D. Sclerosing cholangitis.
E. Iatrogenic stricture.

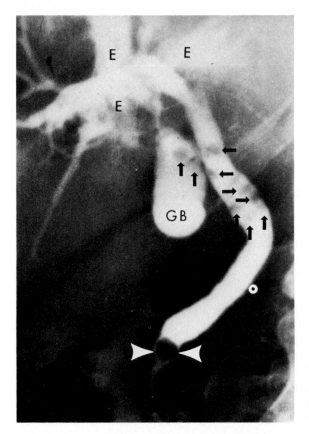

Figure E–221. Multiple stones (arrows) are present in the extrahepatic ductal system and in the gallbladder (GB). A larger stone (arrowheads) is impacted at the lower end of the common duct. Extravasation (E) into the liver is evident, a common occurrence with transhepatic cholangiography.

Radiologic Findings. Case 56–1 shows multiple lucencies within the extrahepatic biliary tree, several within the gallbladder, and a single filling defect impacted at the lower end of the common bile duct (Fig. E–221). These represent ductal and gallbladder stones. Stricture of the common duct, however, is not present (**A is the correct answer to Question 56–1**).

In Case 56–2, focal narrowing involves the midportion of the extrahepatic ductal system. The most common cause of this appearance·following cholecystectomy is an iatrogenic stricture (**E is the correct answer to Question 56–2**). Vigorous dissection of the cystic duct or traction at this level during surgery contributes to this complication.

Discussion. Evaluation of the biliary tract has been greatly facilitated in recent years through the introduction of newer and improved imaging modalities.

Table E–22. METHODS OF DIRECT CHOLANGIOGRAPHY

Commonly used methods
Percutaneous transhepatic cholangiography
Endoscopic retrograde cholangiography
Operative cholangiography
T-tube cholangiography
Less common methods
Barium cholangiography
Transjugular cholangiography
Cholecystostomy cholangiography
Laparoscopic cholangiography

Table E-23. CAUSES OF BILIARY NARROWING

Benign stricture	Malignant stricture
Postoperative	Cholangiocarcinoma
Cholangitis	Gallbladder carcinoma*
Stone related	Pancreatic carcinoma*
Chronic pancreatitis*	Porta hepatis metastases*

*Represent extrinsic involvement.

Ultrasound and computed tomography of the abdomen have revolutionized the study of the jaundiced patient, usually providing a specific preoperative diagnosis. In addition, a variety of methods are available for direct visualization of the biliary tree (Table E-22). Endoscopic retrograde cholangiopancreatography permits evaluation of both the biliary and pancreatic ductal systems. The recent use of thinner (22-23 gauge) and flexible percutaneous needles has revived an interest in transhepatic cholangiography. When properly performed, these techniques are safe, with serious complications occurring in less than 5% of cases, and with a mortality rate under 0.2%.

In the United States, choledocholithiasis is nearly always secondary to passage of stones from the gallbladder into the biliary tree. Up to 10 to 15% of patients with cholelithiasis will also have ductal stones. Operative cholangiography is available at the time of cholecystectomy to accurately assess the status of the biliary system. Most ductal stones are extrahepatic in location, while those situated intrahepatically are usually found in or near the right and left hepatic ducts. T-tube cholangiography is used to evaluate the biliary tree postoperatively, and occasionally detects stones that were inadvertently left at surgery. These retained stones can often be retrieved radiologically via the T-tube sinus tract, through the use of special instruments.

Focal narrowing of the biliary tract can result from many causes (Table E-23). Separation of benign from malignant biliary stricturing is not always easy. Clinical correlation with the appearance and location of the ductal narrowing is important.

Recurrent symptoms following cholecystectomy are not uncommon. The causes of the so-called "postcholecystectomy syndrome" are numerous and varied (Table E-24). Occasionally, the gallbladder was not at fault and disease outside the biliary tract is eventually discovered. More commonly, however, complications related to surgery or stone disease are found.

Table E-24. CAUSES FOR THE POSTCHOLECYSTECTOMY SYNDROME

Unrelated, undiagnosed problem
Surgical complications
Retained or recurrent stones
Benign ductal stricture
Diseased cystic duct remnant
Papillary stenosis/dysfunction

12

Special Studies

ANGIOGRAPHY

Angiography is utilized for visualization of arteries or veins at a site of physiologic or clinical interest. The blood supply on images so obtained, very often in rapid sequence, allows us a most accurate method for diagnostic imaging of congenital aberrations, trauma, inflammations, and neoplasms. Bleeding areas may be thereby detected and treated with appropriate pharmacologic agents, and angioplasties performed on stenotic blood vessels. Similarly, an effort may be made to obliterate the vasculature of a neoplasm.

The vessel most frequently employed for catheterization is the femoral artery. This is done by the Seldinger method, which requires that a needle first be inserted directly into the vessel and a flexible guidewire thereafter passed through it into the vessel in question. A catheter is passed over the guidewire, and the guidewire is removed when it is determined by fluoroscopic control that the catheter is in good position in the major vessel desired. The contrast agent is rapidly injected, either by a mechanical device, which allows for the rapid injection of a sufficient volume of the contrast agent, or manually, depending on the blood vessels being investigated.

Highly selective catheterization may be performed under fluoroscopic control. Serial film studies following the injection are obtained by special devices that allow as many as 12 films per second, in rapid sequence, or in any preordained fashion; or cineradiography in the 16-mm or 35-mm format of the image on the output phosphor of the fluoroscopic image amplifier. This method is especially preferred in coronary angiography, and in children and infants, since less radiation of the patient is thereby sustained.

Injection of the contrast agent into the arteries leading to the brain constitutes neurologic angiography; that which requires the injection of the blood vessels of the heart, coronary angiography; the viscera, visceral angiography. The latter include the direct injections into the celiac artery, its branches, the superior mesenteric, or the inferior mesenteric arteries. Injection of peripheral arteries is similarly performed. The method is ideal for study of the anatomic position of these major vessels as well as the neovasculature that forms with primary or metastatic tumors. Aneurysms and arteriovenous malformations may be visualized in the same manner.

Thoracic angiograms are at times performed for visualization of the entire aorta, including its major blood vessels, or for visualization of traumatic dissection.

The sequential films are obtained through the venous phase if the latter will be helpful in analysis of the anatomy or to confirm thrombosis or invasion by inflammation or tumor.

Pulmonary angiograms are at times performed when pulmonary thromboses are suspected and surgical removal of these is contemplated, or when arteriovenous malformations are suspected.

At times venography itself is employed without the aid of arteriography preceding it. This is true not only for peripheral veins but also for sampling of blood, as in the case of angiotensin determinations in the two renal veins if renovascular hypertension is suspected.

Cerebral angiography has to a great extent been replaced by computed tomography (to be described subsequently), but there is still considerable employment of this procedure when the computed tomogram does not yield sufficient data. Fortunately, the central nervous system can be examined adequately in many ways—with nuclear medicine, angiography, the injection of air into the ventricles of the brain either directly (ventriculography) or through the lumbar subarachnoid space (pneumoencephalography); or computed tomography. With the advent of computed tomography, pneumoencephalography and ventriculography have almost disappeared from radiologic practice. Nuclear magnetic resonance imaging of the brain has already proved to be eminently successful and helpful.

MYELOGRAPHY

Myelography is performed by direct percutaneous injection of a suitable radiopaque material into the subarachnoid space for visualization of this space, surrounding the spinal cord, in its entirety. The primary clinical indications are back pain, or neurologic findings that point to the spinal cord or the neural canal as the site of disease.

The radiopaque agents most frequently employed are: (1) Pantopaque, and (2) metrizamide (Amipaque, Winthrop). The former is an iodinated oil of sufficiently low viscosity to allow its almost complete removal from the subarachnoid space following the fluoroscopic and radiographic procedure. The latter is a nonionic water-soluble contrast medium in a 20-ml vial of sterile aqueous diluent containing 0.05 mg/ml of sodium bicarbonate in water for injection and pH adjusted with carbon dioxide if necessary. In the lowest recommended concentration (170 mg of iodine per ml), it has a specific gravity of 1.184 at 37°C, is isotonic with cerebrospinal fluid, and has a pH of approximately 7.4. Amipaque solution and powder are sensitive to heat or light and must be protected from this exposure. Unlike Pantopaque, which is not absorbed, Amipaque is absorbed from cerebrospinal fluid into the blood stream. Approximately 60% of the administered dose is excreted unchanged through the kidneys within 48 hours. Following spinal subarachnoid injection, conventional radiography and fluoroscopy will continue to provide diagnostic imaging for approximately an hour. At 4 to 5 hours the contrast is hazy and it is no longer detectable at 24 hours. Irrespective of the position of the patient, Amipaque diffuses upward and contrast enhancement is achieved in the thoracic region in about one hour, in the cervical region in about 2 hours,

and in the basal cisterns in 3 to 4 hours. However, during the radiographic and fluoroscopic procedure, it moves cephalad under gravity control. Even the lateral, third and fourth ventricles may also be visualized by computed tomography. The contrast in these latter areas is markedly diminished at 6 hours and disappears by 24 hours. The cerebrospinal fluid will be enhanced in the region of the cortical sulci and interhemispheric fissures at 6 hours. Between 12 and 24 hours, the surfaces of the cerebrum and cerebellum, in contact with the subarachnoid space, will develop a "blush" effect on the computed tomographic scan, which normally disappears at 36 to 48 hours. It is probable that less irritating contrast agents will soon be available (Iopamidol-Squibb).

If grossly bloody cerebrospinal fluid is encountered, the utilization of either contrast agent must be considered with great caution. Specific administration of Amipaque before the age of 12 years is as yet not recommended.

Caution is advised in the use of Amipaque in patients with a history of epilepsy, severe cardiovascular disease, chronic alcoholism, multiple sclerosis, or bronchial asthma or other allergic manifestations. It is true, however, that no conclusive relationship between severe reactions and antigen-antibody reactions or other manifestations of allergy have been established. Prophylactic anticonvulsant treatment with barbiturates or Diazepam orally for 24 to 48 hours should be considered when there has been an inadvertent intracranial entry of a large or concentrated bolus of Amipaque. Phenothiazine derivatives which lower the seizure threshold or MAO inhibitors, tricyclic antidepressants, antihistamines, central nervous system stimulants, psychoactive drugs, and major tranquilizers should not be administered coincident with examination with Amipaque. There should be a discontinuation for at least 24 hours before myelography. In patients with severe renal insufficiency or failure, Amipaque is excreted from the liver into the bile at a much slower rate. Patients with hepatorenal insufficiency should not be examined unless the possibility of benefit clearly outweighs the additional risk, and any re-examination should be delayed for 5 to 7 days. With regard to Amipaque, a relatively recently introduced contrast agent, the most frequently occurring adverse reactions are headache, nausea, and vomiting, which occur 3 to 8 hours after injection, but sometimes even as late as 24 hours. Backache, neck stiffness, numbness and paresthesia, and leg or sciatic pain occur less frequently, often in the form of transient exacerbation of pre-existing symptomatology. Temperature elevations and dizziness have also been reported. Rarely, muscle spasm or generalized convulsions have occurred 4 to 8 hours following injection, or in some cases have been attributed to a history of epilepsy. Central nervous system irritation has been described, of a mild and transitory nature with hallucinations, depersonalization, anxiety, depression, hyperesthesia, visual and auditory or speech disturbances, confusion, and disorientation. Malaise, weakness, electroencephalogram changes, and meningismus have occurred. Certain cardiovascular alterations have also occurred, such as chest pain, tachycardia, bradycardia, and arrhythmia.

With regard to Pantopaque, occasional droplets may remain after virtually complete removal of the iodized oil from the subarachnoid space, which may cause minimal adhesions but are considered clinically tolerable. Occasionally air myelography is employed, although rarely. With myelograms it is possible to demonstrate extradural, intradural, and intramedullary spinal lesions. A cervical approach for the injection of the contrast agent may be employed, and with gravity the Pantopaque passes down the subarachnoid space to a possible level of obstruction or other abnormality.

Cisternomyelography may be employed for visualization of the area around the internal acoustic meatus in the head, although this procedure has been virtually replaced with the aid of computed tomography and the much simpler injection of a small amount of air allowed to accumulate around the cerebellopontine angle. This allows optimum visualization of the structures in this immediate vicinity (for tumors, abscesses, or other abnormalities).

Exploratory studies of the vertebrae, intervertebral discs, and spinal canal would indicate excellent anatomic detail feasible without contrast enhancement with nuclear magnetic resonance imaging.

ARTHROGRAPHY

In this procedure, a small amount of air, or air intermixed with a water-soluble opaque contrast agent of the diatrizoate group, is injected directly into a joint and the joint surfaces studied fluoroscopically and radio-graphically. Almost any joint of the body may be examined in this manner, but the most common are the knee, the shoulders, and the hip. In the case of the knee, a very small amount of the contrast agent is injected in the suprapatellar bursa followed by the injection of air. The knee joint is spread so that the cartilaginous menisci and the internal structures of the knee are portrayed in various obliquities. Tears or fractures of the menisci, as well as ligamentous structure tears, may be visualized. Injections of the shoulder and hip are usually carried out with the water-soluble iodinated opaque contrast media alone for visualization of tears in the joint capsule or its adjoining sheaths.

HYSTEROSALPINGOGRAPHY

Hysterosalpingography is primarily used in the study of infertility and its many causes. A water-soluble diatrizoate or iothalamate agent, thickened somewhat for special visualization of the uterine cavity and oviducts, is used optimally for this procedure. Under direct vaginal visualization of the uterine cervix with a speculum, the uterine cervix is held taut with an appropriate instrument, and a radiolucent plastic cone at the end of a syringe is inserted into the cervical canal. The vaginal speculum is withdrawn into the vagina, and the contrast agent is injected under fluoroscopic control in approximately 3-cc fractions, with films obtained intermittently to demonstrate the uterine carity, uterine horns, oviduct, fimbriated end of the oviduct, and spillage into the pelvic peritoneal space, bilaterally. If abnormalities are encountered, such as sacculation or retention of the contrast agent, a delayed film is obtained in approximately 30 minutes, since reabsorption of the water-soluble agent ordinarily does not occur if hydrosalpinx or pelvic abscess is encountered. Likewise, blockage of one or both of the tubes, caused by prior infection, may prevent complete visualization of the oviducts. The visualization of the uterine cavity is important from the standpoint of demonstrating filling defects from small neoplasms, synechiae resulting from previous operations, or masses of other origin which might prevent implantation of a fertilized ovum.

BRONCHOGRAPHY

This procedure involves the injection of appropriate opaque media into the trachea and bronchial tree either under fluoroscopic control or in fractional doses, obtaining overhead radiography of each lobe or segment of the lung. This can be accomplished by intratracheal intubation through the nose or mouth or by needle puncture of the trachea. The purpose of this procedure is to demonstrate bronchiectasis, bronchial obstruction, chronic bronchitis, and any other processes that may be envisioned to damage or distort the bronchi. Although in times past bronchography was also utilized to a great extent to obtain histologic smears and microscopic sections by fiberoptic endoscopy or helicon (wire) brush biopsy techniques, direct needle puncture of the appropriate portion of the lung under fluoroscopic guidance has largely replaced this technology. Computed tomography has also proved to be helpful in determining the nature of a nodule in the lung and has, to some extent, replaced bronchography.

LARYNGOGRAPHY

Laryngography is closely related technically to bronchography in that the larynx is studied before and after phonation and before and after distention of the larynx, the pyriform sinuses, and contiguous structures, all under fluoroscopic control. The soft palate may be studied in respect to its motion during phonation. This procedure, like bronchography, is performed after topical anesthesia of the mucous membrane and spot films are obtained. A laryngogram provides an excellent visualization of the false cords, true cords, laryngeal ventricle, valleculae, laryngeal tumors, pyriform sinuses, epiglottis, nodules on the cords, and any other abnormality that might be suspected of producing gross morphologic change in this region. It should be noted, however, that since the advent of computed tomography, which is obviously less invasive than either bronchography or laryngography, this procedure is favored to replace these examinations whenever possible.

Special algorithms may reconstruct the vocal cords and areas around the larynx by computed tomography, and this format is particularly useful.

SIALOGRAPHY

Although Stensen's duct leading to the parotid gland is probably the most frequent

duct injected for this purpose, the submaxillary and sublingual glands are similarly studied. A thickened iodized oil or somewhat thickened water-soluble medium can be utilized through a very fine catheter inserted into the ostium of the duct in the mouth. Masses, invaded areas of the gland or contiguous structures, calculi, inflammations, and dilatations of the ductal structures of the gland as occur in Sjögren's syndrome may be demonstrated with considerable accuracy.

LYMPHOGRAPHY (LYMPHANGIOGRAPHY AND LYMPHADENOGRAPHY)

Classically, lymphangiograms as well as lymphadenograms are most frequently employed to investigate the lymphatics of the legs, thighs, and groins, and the paraortic, pericaval, and supraclavicular lymph nodes. This is accomplished by subcutaneous enhancement of the lymphatics, usually in the web space between the great toe and the second toe, and cannulation of this lymphatic thereafter. The iodized oil (Ethiodol) is slowly pumped with a special pumping mechanism, usually over a period of approximately 2 hours, through the lymphatics on both sides. A film is obtained, at 2 to 4 hours, of the leg, thigh, and abdomen in the anteroposterior, oblique, and lateral projections. In 24 hours the patient is returned when the Ethiodol or equivalent substance contained within the lymph nodes draining the areas is visualized in conjunction with intravenous urography to ascertain the relationship of the lymphatics to the upper urinary tract. Although size has conventionally been considered very important in respect to abnormality of lymph nodes (greater than 3 cm in any dimension), it is actually the filling defects contained within the nodes, obstruction, or the actual architecture of the lymph nodes that is studied most carefully. Occasionally, a rupture of a lymphatic may be detected, demonstrating a lymphocele, especially in the pelvis minor.

INTERVENTIONAL RADIOGRAPHY

Interventional radiography employs the expertise of the diagnostic radiologist in the introduction of appropriate catheters or fiberoptic endoscopes for therapeutic problems. Special catheters have been developed for this purpose, for example, to dilate constricted arteries (Grünzig catheter). Usually these catheters have a balloon on their end that can be blown up to a specific volume, and this distention then cracks the thickened endothelial lining of an artery just enough to permit an ischemic organ beyond this artery to receive a more adequate blood supply. At times "scraping" techniques have been employed, although these are significantly more dangerous.

The removal of gallstones through T-tubes has likewise been accomplished in this fashion. Liver puncture, first performed to enable transhepatic cholangiography for biopsy purposes, is now being performed with a fine gauge needle ("skinny needle" technique) to inject the bile ducts and fill them with contrast agents, in order to identify and analyze an obstruction to the common hepatic or one of the major ductal systems. These "skinny needle" techniques are quite safe with little morbidity, and have even permitted pancreatic and renal biopsies to be done. This, in turn, provides microscopic information in relation to masses visualized by other diagnostic methods. The procedures are performed under fluoroscopic, ultrasonic, or computed tomographic control. Bone biopsies may be similarly performed with fluoroscopic guidance so that a major surgical procedure may be avoided.

DIGITAL VIDEO SUBTRACTION

In older methods of x-ray subtraction, a film of an anatomic part was obtained prior to injection of a contrast agent, and a series of films was taken immediately thereafter, with no movement of the anatomic part being x-rayed. The noncontrast radiograph may be called a "mask" (M) and the contrast-containing radiograph a "contrast-enhanced image" (CEI). The CEI is superimposed over the M exactly, and the two films are transilluminated; a third film is obtained in which only the blood vessels will be visualized, since the remaining structures are "subtracted."

Computerization of the mask initially, and thereafter the contrast-enhanced image, permits a computer to achieve this subtraction—giving rise now to **computerized digital subtraction.** If a video image is obtained with a signal-to-"noise" ratio of 1000:1 or better (to avoid degradation of the image), and if several masks are taken initially to obtain one that would best compensate for the slightest motion in the anatomic part being contrast-enhanced, a digital video subtraction with high resolution is thereby obtained. The contrast enhancement may be obtained by transvenous or intra-arterial injection, or by introduction of the contrast through a catheter closer to the blood vessels to be visualized.

Both the multiple masks and digitalized contrast-enhanced images may be stored in the computer and remanipulated to achieve the following: (1) linear subtraction; (2) log subtraction; (3) edge enhancement; (4) a smoothing effect mathematically; (5) signal averaging; (6) image addition; (7) compensatory manipulations to overcome noise or movement artifacts; or (8) flow measurements. The signal images may be studied at any time after the completion of the computerization.

Hand or power injections may be employed as desired.

The applications are manifold: (1) diagnosis (and treatment thereafter) of atherosclerosis in virtually any desired blood vessel; (2) a screening test for patients with audible bruit over blood vessels; (3) avoidance of catheterization of a blood vessel where this might be contraindicated; and (4) wherever contrast injections are employed intravenously for other purposes, such as urography, allowing for supplemental information regarding feeder arteries and draining veins.

The full scope of this new computerized technique is still being realized, but it is envisaged that this technique may ultimately substitute for more hazardous methods of angiography now requiring catheterization.

13

Xeroradiography and Mammography

In xeroradiography, the x-ray beam emerging from the patient strikes an electrostatically charged plate instead of an x-ray film. The charge imparted to the plate is directly proportional to the number of photons in the x-ray beam. The plate is then placed in a special processor, and a blue powder is blown on the plate so that it adheres to the parts still containing a charge. The amount of powder that adheres is in direct proportion to the amount of charge in the plate.

A photograph is then made of the plate reproduced ordinarily on photographic paper. Usually the image is seen as either blue on white or white on blue. In the positive mode, the air appears blue and the bone white.

Xeroradiography has been particularly useful in that at each change of tissue environment there is an "edge enhancement," which serves as a useful tool in delineating the fat planes within an anatomic part. The paper containing the image is treated to produce a permanent image. The xeroradiographic plate may thereafter be discharged and reused.

This method has been particularly useful in mammography, but also has been applied successfully in the study of cadaveric slices particularly because of this "edge enhancement" technique. The technology is also useful in the visualization of bones with another modality, since edge enhancement allows for a more detailed visualization of the trabeculae and bone marrow, and for evaluation of many of the soft tissues, such as the larynx.

Despite the development of special films, screens, and cassettes for mammography, and despite the fact that xeroradiography requires slightly greater dosage to the breast by ionizing radiation than does conventional radiography, there are many who still prefer xeroradiographs of the breast for mammography because of the clearer image of the stroma, the vessels, and the subcutaneous tissues.

Although the first report concerning mammography dates back to 1913, it did not achieve its optimum utilization until an x-ray tube with a molybdenum target, beryllium window, and 30 mμ added molybdenum filtration became available. It was also apparent that with this tube the optimum kilovoltage would be 25 to 30 Kvp. With present day tubes and equipment, xeroradiography may be utilized for the average breast with an average skin entry dose of approximately 0.4 rads. With special film and screen applications, newer mammographic equipment has reduced the dosage to the skin tenfold.

Prior to radiography, the patient's breast should be carefully inspected and palpated, in both the recumbent and erect positions. During the mammographic procedure it is important that a craniocaudal projection, with the patient sitting, a lateral projection (mediolateral projection) with the patient sitting or supine, and a special axillary projection of the breast be obtained. If a nonscreen film technique other than xeroradiography is used, there are a number of specially made films and screens for this purpose available. When the study is obtained the films are examined with a magnifying glass for discernment of detail. Interpretation of the mammogram requires familiarity with the structural anatomy of the breast, its normal appearance in the vicinity of the nipple, the appearance of its fatty tissue, arteries, and veins, and the lymphatics and lymph flow to the axillary and parasternal and regional lymph nodes. The overlying skin of the breast is readily recognized in a mammogram with suitable lighting and varies in thickness from 0.5 to 2 mm. Skinfolds should be recognized, since they may readily be misinterpreted as representing intramammary pathology.

Variations of normal should be readily understood, such as: polymastia, which indicates an extranumerary nipple in association with underlying parenchymal tissue, and accessory breast parenchyma which may be recognized beneath the anterior axillary fold most frequently. Moreover, hormonal influences produce certain physiological changes in the mature breast throughout the menstrual cycle. Following ovulation the breast is generally enlarged due to progesterone, and this should not be misinterpreted as fibrocystic disease. During the premenstrual phase the breast may appear increased in size and greater in density, with a greater prominence of the venous system. When menses appears, there is a generalized involution of the parenchyma with lesser density of the breast.

Moreover, during pregnancy there are gestational changes in the female breast which must be understood. The density of the parenchyma is increased; the glandular lobules enlarge, and the total mass becomes coarser and denser radiographically. It may be very difficult during gestation to recognize pathological processes.

When lactation ceases, the breast becomes somewhat involuted and the lactiferous ducts become smaller. The parenchyma may be replaced by fatty tissue, which is readily recognized by xeroradiography. The trabeculae of the breast become smaller and less distinct.

Senile involution of the breast occurs during and after the menopause. Parenchymal acini become atrophic, and fat may become the dominant tissue of the breast.

There are still many controversies in the diagnosis and management of breast disease. It must be recognized, however, that despite improved therapeutic modalities involving surgery, radiation therapy, and chemotherapy, there has been no decrease in the mortality rate in breast cancer in the last 50 years. Breast cancer in 1978 was the leading cause of cancer death in women between the ages of 15 and 34; and in 1982 it has been estimated that breast cancer will continue to lead all other cancers, with 112,000 new cases and

37,000 deaths. It accounts for approximately 26 per cent of all malignant disease in women and 19 per cent of their deaths from cancer. There are regional or distant metastases in over 50 per cent of patients at the time of initial diagnosis.

It is probable that the major benefit will come from early detection. Early detection will probably require a screening method better than self-examination or physician examination. There is a lower frequency of lymph node involvement when the lesion is detected by screening techniques other than palpation. Also the cancer is smaller upon first detection by a screening method other than physical examination.

Apart from realizing that screening for breast cancer may discover it at an earlier stage, understanding certain *risk factors in relation to breast cancer* is also important. The National Cancer Institute, influenced by concern for the cumulative risks of ionizing radiation to the breast, has recommended annual mammographic screening of women over the age of 50, but not those between the ages of 39 to 49, unless they or their immediate family have a history of breast cancer. Unfortunately data from the Breast Cancer Detection Demonstration Projects show that 25% of cancers occur in women under the age of 50.

Mammography is also indicated in women under 50 who complain of painful nodularity in the breast, or in whom a malignancy is at all suspected. The radiographic findings include those of thickening of the skin, indentation, amorphous fine pulverization of calcification or irregular nodularity within the breast proper. A mass with a loss of its margination, even though it does not contain pulverized calcification, may be regarded as suspect for biopsy. Mammography has been particularly useful in patients with fibrocystic disease when the cysts themselves feel nodular and malignancy is difficult to establish. Careful follow-up of these patients is certainly indicated because their rate of malignant disease is known to be higher than the rate for the general female population.

In our experience, ultrasonography has had its main usefulness in this area of differentiating cystic from solid structures; and to assist in accurate needle biopsy of a lesion identified by any imaging technique.

Transillumination of the breast has also been used as a screening procedure (diaphanography), but remains an investigational approach that warrants further controlled study before its clinical application. Also, thermography has been proposed as a screening procedure to be utilized prior to mammography, despite a false-negative ratio of greater than 50 per cent.

The risk factor regarding ionizing radiation is often quoted as the greatest deterrent to the use of mammography. At the present time, however, doses are extremely low, making it difficult to implicate mammography as the cause of an increased incidence of breast cancer. It is generally accepted that breast carcinoma will not result from ionizing radiation under the following conditions: a total lifetime dose of under 50 rads; exposure over the age of 30; periods of years between exposures and the use of 25 to 45 KvP (Brenner). *In a special breast cancer detection project conducted by the American Cancer Society in 1973, approximately one half of all the histologically proven cancers were detected by mammography alone.* These, then, were clinically occult malignancies. Moreover, one third of all breast cancers occur between the ages of 35 and 50.

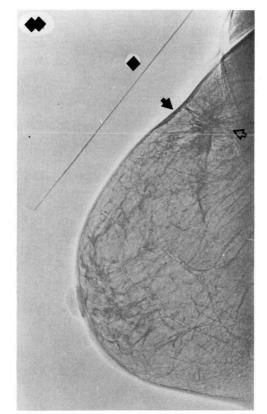

Figure 13–2. Occult xeroradiographic mammogram demonstrating stellate radiations around a very small lesion with microcalcifications. (Courtesy of American College of Radiology Mammogram File.)

Thus as a general rule, every female 35 years of age or older should have at least a baseline mammogram. She may thereafter have a mammogram, if she is not in the greater risk factor group, on alternate years until the age of 50. Every female older than 50 years of age may by present radiologic low dose techniques be examined probably as often as twice a year and the 50 rad maximum would not be exceeded in the usual lifetime.

The accompanying illustrations of xeroradiography of the breast demonstrate: (1) a normal xeroradiograph mammogram; (2) a small, occult, non-palpable carcinoma of the breast detected by xeroradiography; (3) the thickening of the skin overlying a carcinoma of the breast—a very important sign apart from the microcalcifications; and (4) a fibrocystic breast disease with the increased density making it somewhat difficult to detect the carcinoma of the breast partially concealed by this underlying condition (Fig. 13–1 to 13–4).

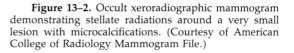

Figure 13–1. Normal xeroradiographic mammogram of the breast.

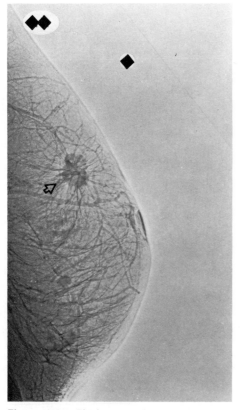

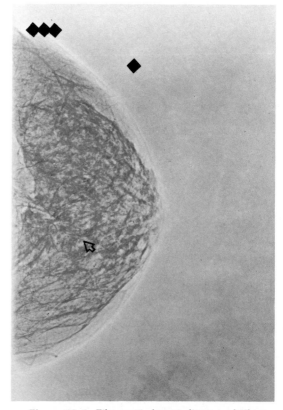

Figure 13–3. Thickening of the skin overlying a small carcinoma of the breast demonstrated by xeroradiography. (Courtesy of American College of Radiology Mammogram File.)

Figure 13–4. Fibrocystic breast disease which may conceal a carcinoma of the breast, particularly at a depth, if one is not thoroughly familiar with recognition of this disorder under these circumstances. (Courtesy of American College of Radiology Mammogram File.)

14

Nuclear Medicine

Following the development of the atomic bomb, it became readily apparent that many radionuclides could be obtained for peaceful use in diagnostic imaging, either from the decay products of the split uranium and plutonium or by atomic particulate bombardment with the aid of a cyclotron. A further source for radionuclides virtually revolutionized the procurement of these substances for diagnostic imaging: It was discovered that the radioactive decay of some substances (called metastable), when washed with an appropriate diluent, would yield decay products of appropriate kilovoltage and short half-lives, so that these in turn could be produced in virtually any laboratory. The development of these latter generators allowed the further production radiopharmaceutically of special radionuclide complexes shown in Tables 14–1 and 14–2 for visualization of many organs of the body. It is now possible, for example, to evaluate the liver, spleen, bones, urinary tract, lungs, heart, thyroid, and brain most accurately. Tumor and abscess imaging with radionuclides is often achieved before radiographic images are altered visibly with the aid of thallium citrate. Likewise, it is possible to instill into the body radionuclides that emit x-rays, and these are captured on a device very similar to the computed tomograph machine, although in this instance the detectors are capturing emitted radiation rather than transmitted radiation. It is anticipated by some that these emission type detector machines may ultimately be even more valuable than the transmission machines, particularly in relation to tracing physiologic rather than morphologic changes. The further development of special camera devices for phosphorescence, as they are struck by the photons of energy emitted from the patient, have allowed for "camera" development of imaging as well as translation of the photons by computerization into numeric data. The gamma camera, coupled with a computer, has become an extremely useful and important device for the investigation of dynamic functions in the body, such as blood flow in arteries in the brain; the passage of a radionuclide through the liver, bile duct system, common bile duct, and into the gastrointestinal tract; and the passage of radionuclides through the kidney into the collecting system, ureters, and urinary bladder. With appropriate use of radionuclides, not only can the passage of the radionuclide be detected, but by means of the computerization, such special physiologic functions as glomerular filtration, tubular excretion, clearance ratio, and filtration fraction may all be accomplished. Indeed it is anticipated that nuclear medicine in the long run may play just as important a role in physiologic analysis of body function as does the transmission computed tomograph in its morphologic depiction.

THYROID IMAGING

The major uses of radionuclide thyroid imaging are as follows: (1) recording of the activity of the thyroid gland in respect to the patient being euthyroid, hyperthyroid, or hypothyroid; (2) depiction of the gland and its content when it is enlarged, to determine whether nodules contained therein are either functional or nonfunctional—whether they are toxic or nontoxic. Generally, the thyroid nodule that is not toxic is much more apt to be malignant than are the others. Likewise, metastases from thyroid tumors or ectopic thyroid tissue may appear months or years after resection of a primary malignancy of the thyroid gland, and for this purpose these radionuclides are ideal.

Table 14–1 CURRENT RADIOPHARMACEUTICALS FOR SELECTED NUCLEAR MEDICINE IMAGING

Imaging Study and Uptake Pattern	Radiopharmaceutical	Activity Administered	Time to Image Post-Injection	Gonads Testes	Gonads Ovaries	Kidneys	Liver	Total Body	Other
Brain. Agent "crosses" disruptions in blood brain barrier	Tc-99m sodium pertechnetate	15–25 mCi	2 hours	0.012	0.017		0.015		0.20 (thyroid) 0.53 (bladder wall) 0.20 (lower large intestine)
	Tc-99m gluceptate	15–20 mCi	1 hour	0.004	0.007	0.3		0.01	
	Tc-99m DTPA*	15–20 mCi	1 hour	0.005	0.007	0.09		0.02	0.45 (bladder wall)
Skeleton. Localizes in areas of increased osteogenesis	Tc-99m methylene diphosphonate (MDP medronate) Tc-99m Hydroxydiphosphonate (HDP-oxidronate)	15–20 mCi	2–3 hours	0.034	0.046	0.03	0.01	0.013	0.05 (bone)
Liver/Spleen/Bone Marrow. Agent is phagocytized by reticuloendothelial cells, plasma T½ = 3 minutes	Tc-99m sulfur colloid	2–5 mCi	15 minutes	0.019	0.023		0.34	0.019	0.21 (spleen)
Liver. Removed by hepatocytes and excreted via biliary pathway (patient preparation may include high protein, low fat meal)	I-131 Rose Bengal	200–300 μCi	10 minutes	0.14	1.6		0.8	0.01	35 (lower large intestine)
	Tc-99m HIDA (imminodiacetic acid derivatives)	2–5 mCi	5 minutes	0.025	0.05		0.09		0.55 (upper large intestine)
Lungs. Macroaggregates of human serum albumin (15–35 μ) are "filtered" in smaller pulmonary vessels, depict regional blood flow	Tc-99m albumin macroaggregates	2–5 mCi	15 minutes	0.007	0.009	0.16	0.017	0.008	0.2 (lungs)

Study / Mechanism	Radiopharmaceutical	Dose	Imaging Time					Critical Organ (rads)
Lungs. Radiogas ventilation with inert element	Xe-133 Xenon gas	10–20 mCi	Immediately	0.26	0.26	0.0062		39 (lungs— breathing 3 min. in closed system 1 mCi/l)
Heart. Depicts myocardial infarction, uptake in damaged tissues	Tc-99m pyrophosphate	15–20 mCi	90 minutes	0.034	0.046	0.03	0.13	0.05 (bone)
Heart. Potassium-like analog	Tl-201 Thallous chloride	2 mCi	Immediately after exercise; then 4 hours	0.55	0.50	1.25	0.23	0.6 (liver) 0.55 (heart wall)
Thyroid. Iodide uptake mechanism	I-123 sodium iodide	300 μCi	24 hours	0.025	0.034		0.03	2.4 (5% uptake) 7.5 (15% uptake) 13.0 (25% uptake)
Tumor/Abscess Imaging. (patient preparation— cathartic PM prior to imaging)	Ga-67 citrate	3–5 mCi	24–48 hours	0.26	0.26	0.41	0.45 0.16	0.6 (spleen) 0.9 (lower large intestine)
Renal Imaging. Passing filtration of nonprotein-bound fraction	Tc-99m sodium pertechnetate	5–10 mCi	Immediately	0.012	0.017		0.015	0.20 (thyroid) 0.53 (bladder wall)
	Tc-99m DTPA	5–15 mCi	Immediately	0.005	0.007	0.09	0.02	0.20 (lower large intestine) 0.45 (bladder wall)
Tubular secretion with some filtration	I-131 orthoiodohippuric acid (OIHA)	150–300 mCi	Immediately through 30 mins	0.040	0.064	0.10	0.10	12 (bladder wall)
Concentrated renal cortex static imaging agent	Tc-99m DMSA (dimercapto-succinic acid-succimer)	1–5 mCi	2–3 hours	0.014	0.023	0.75		48 (kidney)

*Diethylenetriamine pentaacetic acid

Compiled by: Henry M. Chilton, Pharm.D., Bowman Gray School of Medicine, Winston-Salem, N.C.

[131]I was developed early following World War II, but thereafter many other isotopes of iodine and other radionuclides have been demonstrated to have superior physical qualities for these several purposes. Even [99m]technetium, extracted from a generator as a pertechnetate, has been utilized for thyroid visualization. [131]I has become significantly less popular for routine clinical use because of its long physical half-life and emission of beta radiation. Generally, the gamma emissions of ^{123}I and technetium pertechnetate are ideally suited for the Anger type camera in common usage today, particularly when the collimator is a pinhole type.

BRAIN IMAGING

Computed tomography has in great measure replaced radionuclide brain imaging, but there are still a number of instances in which nuclear medicine is the method of choice. These are in particular brain abscesses, in which a "doughnut" sign is shown; encephalitis or meningitis, in which there have been alterations in the blood/brain barrier; and specific lesions especially in the posterior fossa, such as medulloblastomas and cystic atrocytomas in children. There are some conditions in which a patient is unable to flex the neck adequately for posterior study with computed tomography, and the radionuclide brain scan affords an excellent opportunity for visualization of this region. Moreover, brain scanning is valuable in the detection of dynamic cerebral flow through the carotid artery as well as the intracerebral arteries if views of the brain and neck are obtained in rapid sequence. The bolus of contrast agent is injected intravenously.

The overall sensitivity of radionuclide brain imaging for brain tumors is about 85%; however, lesions situated near the sella turcica and brain stem are best visualized with computed tomography. The overall sensitivity of radionuclide imaging for metastatic tumor lesions of the brain is approximately 90%.

LIVER-SPLEEN IMAGING

Apart from investigating diffuse parenchymal disease and looking for possible space-occupying lesions within the liver or spleen, radionuclide scanning of this area makes it possible, with rapid sequencing, to demonstrate certain functional aspects of the liver parenchyma and the secretion of bile from the liver into the biliary ductal system, and thereafter into the gastrointestinal tract. This procedure therefore is particularly valuable in the differential diagnosis of complete *versus* incomplete biliary obstruction (Fig. 14–1A–D), as well as for the evaluation of acute cholecystitis. One of the great advantages of [99m]technetium-labeled agents indicated in Table 14–1 is that it allows visualization of the biliary tree when the serum bilirubin is greater than 1.5 mg/dl when oral cholecystography is not helpful. The sensitivity of true positivity in a liver/spleen scan is in the order of 85%, and hence this study would rank high among those ordered for detection of hepatic disorders. If a defect is detected, the ultrasound study is valuable in determining whether a lesion is cystic or solid before percutaneous biopsy is performed. The radionuclide study may show multiple focus defects and demonstrate diffuse parenchymal disease, which does not necessarily require confirmation.

BONE SCANNING

Bone scans reveal abnormality long before such lesions can be detected by conventional radiography, especially such lesions as metastases (Fig. 14–2), osteomyelitis, or changes related to stress fractures. In only about 5% of patients will the radiography show an abnormality in which the scan is normal. Basically, bone scanning depends on active bone turnover with osteoblastic activity, and lytic lesions may not be evident if they are relatively static. Apart from those indications already mentioned, bone scans are done (1) for evaluation of delayed union of fractures; (2) in a child complaining of hip pain when routine radiographs are normal and avascularity of femoral head is suspected; (3) in adults with suspected avascular necrosis; and (4) for evaluation of hip prostheses, particularly when total hip replacement has occurred. Persistent radionuclide activity around the acetabulum and upper femur 6 months after surgery is abnormal and is often associated with infection or loosening of the prosthetic device. In every instance it is advisable to correlate the bone scan with the radiographic image.

Table 14–2 NUCLEAR PROPERTIES OF RADIONUCLIDES COMMONLY USED
IN NUCLEAR MEDICINE

Radionuclide	Physical Half-Life	Decay Mode	Principal Gamma Emissions (KeV)	Mean % Disintegration
Gallium-67	78 hours	Electron capture	93	40
			184	24
			296	22
Technetium-99m	6.0 hours	Isomeric transition	140	88
Iodine-123	13.3 hours	Electron capture	159	83
Iodine-131	8.1 days	Beta emission	364	82
Xenon-133	5.3 days	Beta emission	81	35
Thallium-201	73.1 hours	Electron capture	68–80	95
			(mercury x-rays)	

Prepared by: Henry M. Chilton, Pharm.D., The Bowman Gray School of Medicine, Winston-Salem, N.C.

RENAL IMAGING

Renal imaging with radionuclides has proved to be particularly useful in (1) assessing renal blood flow; (2) evaluating renal function, with respect to both glomerular and tubular excretion; (3) assessing filtration fraction; and (4) determining the presence of vesicoureteral reflux.

Renal function studies may be performed either with radioactive iodinated hippuran, which is to a great extent handled by the renal tubule physiologically, or radioactive diatrizoates, iothalamates, or ^{99m}technetium compounds, more specifically handled by glomerular filtration. Comparison studies between the right and left kidneys are valuable. Function studies may also be performed to evaluate renal transplant rejection.

Although vesicoureteral reflux can be readily detected by conventional radiography and voiding cystourethrography, the radionuclide technique may be performed by in-

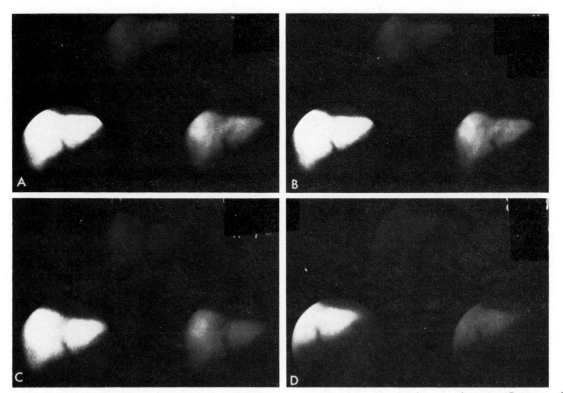

Figure 14–1. Tc-99m HIDA hepatobiliary scan showing complete obstruction at the porta hepatis. (Courtesy of Dr. Nat Watson.)

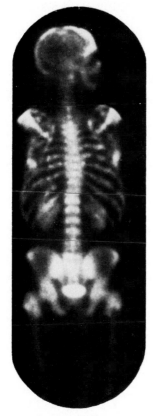

Figure 14–2. Tc-99m diphosphonate bone scan showing a lymphoma involving the skeleton in numerous areas. (Courtesy of Dr. Nat Watson.)

troducing [99m]technetium as a pertechnetate solution into the urinary bladder through a catheter. The radionuclide study allows monitoring both the filling and voiding phases, so that rapid and transient reflux can be detected.

LUNG SCANNING

Lung scanning is particularly useful in (1) the detection of perfusion defects by injection of a radionuclide into the vascular systems, and (2) the detection of ventilatory defects by the use of a radioactive gas such as [133]xenon. The most common indication for perfusion lung scanning is the suspicion of pulmonary emboli or infarction. The ventilatory studies are performed by assaying the patient after he has inhaled a single breath of radioxenon gas. Normal perfusion and ventilation lung scans exclude the possibility of significant pulmonary embolus. In either instance, it is important to make comparison with the conventional chest radiograph. Un-

fortunately, the lung scan is not specific and abnormalities may be seen with pneumonia, chronic lung disease, asthma, and tumor.

Quantification may be obtained by computerization of the counts as they appear in the Anger camera and hence the pulmonary perfusion can be assessed in a very accurate mode.

CARDIAC STUDIES

Radionuclide studies of the heart at present include (1) assessment of myocardial perfusion, (2) evaluation of blood flow through the cardiac chambers and great vessels, (3) blood pool studies of ventricular anatomy and function, and (4) imaging of myocardial infarction.

Myocardial perfusion is best assessed with the utilization of [201]thallium, administered intravenously. An abnormal study shows a focal area of decreased or absent uptake. Usually strenuous exercise or a "stress test," immediately preceding the administration of the tracer, is employed to accentuate the myocardial perfusion abnormality. This test is accurate in over 80% of patients with significant coronary artery impairment.

If one assesses the passage of [99m]technetium-labeled radionuclide as it passes through the great vessels of the heart, an evaluation of blood pool can thereby be derived, particularly if the counts are computerized as they are "visualized" by the Anger camera and recorded graphically. Blood pool tracers used are particularly [99m]technetium-labeled albumin or [99m]technetium-labeled red blood cells. Actually, parameters such as ejection fractions, cardiac output, and ventricular asynchrony, as well as dyskinesis and akinesis, can be well defined. Unfortunately, differentiation between acute and nonacute myocardial infarction cannot be made. [99m]Technetium pyrophosphate, a bone scanning agent, has been found to indicate an acute myocardial infarction within 4 to 8 hours of the insult, with a peak activity at 24 hours; a scan taken 2 weeks after the infarct is usually normal.

GALLIUM SCANNING

The main purpose of [67]gallium scanning is the detection of neoplastic and inflammatory tissue throughout the body. Ordinarily, abscesses as young as 4 hours, or as old as 5 to 10 days may sequester this radionuclide, but the optimum time for imaging abscesses is 24 to 48 hours after the administration of the ^{67}gallium. The gallium deposits itself in the wall of the abscess predominantly.

The tumors that are most frequently and selectively visualized by ^{67}gallium are (1) malignant lymphomas, (2) bronchogenic carcinomas, and (3) inadequately treated or recurrent tumors. In an initial study of patients with malignant lymphoma, the accuracy approaches 85%; the actual demonstration of abnormal uptake is indicative of probable tumor presence in all but about 5%.

With bronchogenic carcinoma the positive accuracy approaches 90%. Normal bronchogenic tissues usually do not sequester ^{67}gallium.

Unfortunately, positive ^{67}gallium uptakes may be obtained with pneumonia, sarcoidosis, active tuberculosis, and radiation pneumonitis; hence, the pulmonary process is nonspecific. Correlation with a chest radiograph is essential.

As noted, ^{67}gallium scans are also particularly useful in following patients who are undergoing radiotherapy or chemotherapy, since a decrease of uptake within the neoplastic tissue indicates improvement, whereas the recurrence of uptake indicates recurrence of tumor.

15

Clinical Ultrasonography

Ultrasonography is the visualization of the deep structures of the body by recording the reflections of ultrasonic impulses directed into the tissues. Sound waves of about 20,000 cycles per second are employed (or 20 kilohertz, where hertz refers to the number of cycles per second). Although earlier devices required immersion of the organ or patient in a tank of water for optimum results, further development of ultrasonic equipment has made this no longer necessary, and now only the skin of the patient is appropriately moistened at the site of sound introduction and a device known as a "transducer" (Fig. 15–1) sends forth the sound and receives the echo for recording purposes. Actually, the sound is produced by the "ringing" of a ceramic material (called piezoelectric) inside the housing of the transducer probe. The natural frequency of the sound waves pro-

duced by the piezoelectric element is determined by its thickness and constitution.

Thus, a sound wave is produced that is of a known velocity until it meets a barrier from which it is reflected; this reflected surface is called the "acoustic interface." The product of the density of the substance encountered and the velocity of the sound wave is called "acoustic impedance." The greater the acoustic impedance between two substances, the greater is the amount of sound reflected back from a boundary between these two substances toward the source of production of the sound waves. The transducer is connected with an appropriate screen, so that the distance between the vibrating piezoelectric substance and the return interface is displayed on the screen, producing the so-called "A-mode" method of scanning (Fig. 15–2).

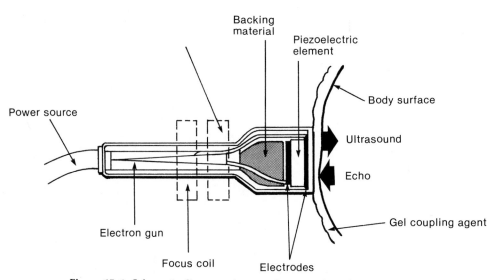

Figure 15–1. Schematic diagram of a transducer used in ultrasonography.

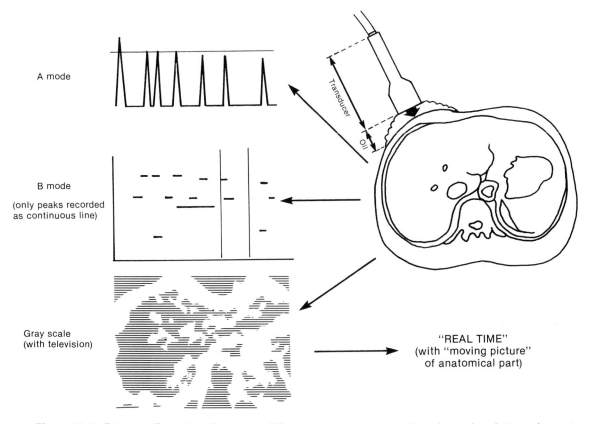

A mode

B mode
(only peaks recorded
as continuous line)

Gray scale
(with television)

"REAL TIME"
(with "moving picture"
of anatomical part)

Figure 15–2. Diagram illustrating the major differences among A-mode, B-mode, and real time ultrasonic techniques.

Figure 15–3. Longitudinal ultrasonogram of the abdominal aorta. (Courtesy of Dr. Nat Watson.) (A = aorta)

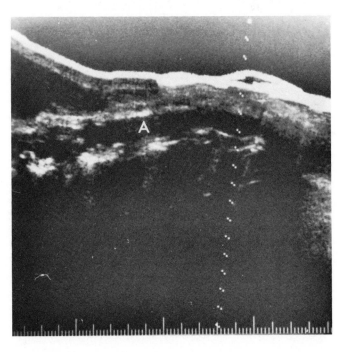

In B-mode scanning the brightness of the reflection or its intensity is recorded on the screen. These brightness spots are compounded together to produce a two-dimensional representation spoken of as a "compound-scan."

There is a third form of ultrasonography employed called the M-mode—or motion scanning. In this mode, one particular dot is selected and watched over a period of time, and one of its greatest applications is in echocardiography, in which the reflecting surface might be the mitral valve or some such structure. The M-mode is also particularly useful for almost any reflecting surface of the heart from one side to the other, evaluating chamber size, and discovering such abnormalities as pericardial effusions.

There are two additional or recent refinements of ultrasonography clinically: (1) the so-called "gray scale," and (2) "real time." The gray scale provides us with a mechanism for recording a spectrum of echoes arising within the substance of the organ—not just from its various surfaces, displaying textures in varying shades of gray—especially on a television screen. Real time imaging is just like fluoroscopy in that instantaneous images are rapidly evaluated in sequence. Although B-mode scanning utilizes a pencil-like sound beam, real time employs a much larger sound beam in one

of three ways: (1) with a linear array of sound-producing crystals in a rectangular configuration; (2) by the utilization of a group of crystals in "phased array"; and (3) by a beam oscillating in such a fashion as to produce a fanlike distribution of the sound waves, "mechanical sector scanning."

CLINICAL APPLICATIONS OF ULTRASOUND

Differentiation of Solid from Cystic Structures

Solid structures contain internal echoes; cystic structures do not. This has very wide application in many organs of the body.

Heart

Echocardiography with the M-mode has already been mentioned. Various parameters of study include the speed of closure of such valves as the mitral valve, ejection fraction, stroke volume, and septal and leaflet motion within the heart.

Breast

Well-circumscribed solitary masses within the breast 1 cm or greater in size may be recognized as being solid or cystic.

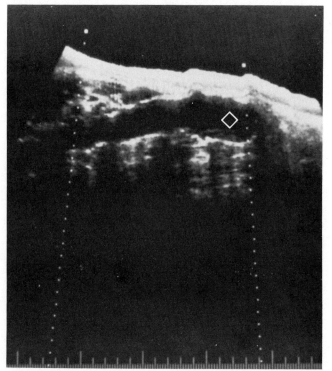

Figure 15–4. Sonogram showing a small aneurysm at the bifurcation of the aorta into the two common iliac arteries. (Courtesy Dr. Nat Watson.) (◇ = aneurysm)

Abdomen

In the abdomen there is wide usage of ultrasound so long as the sound wave is not required to traverse a gaseous medium. To overcome this, a liquid substance may be introduced within the gaseous medium such as the stomach. One of the greatest areas of utilization is the liver, where not only may solid or cystic mass lesions be appreciated but the ductal and vascular system recognized and depicted quite accurately. Interventional radiography may likewise be guided by ultrasonic evaluation employing the "skinny-needle" technique.

The spleen may be evaluated for solid or cystic content.

In recent years, the gallbladder has become an important area for evaluation. Gallstones 3 to 5 mm in size may be detected. This technique may be adjunctive to oral cholecystography, which is a function study as well, or even during cholecystography.

The pancreas also has become accessible to this modality, by which pancreatic masses

Figure 15–5. *A,* Sonogram of a simple ovarian cyst with smooth contours and no internal echoes. *B,* Sonogram of a "complicated" ovarian cyst due to hemorrhage or infection. (Courtesy of Dr. Nat Watson.)

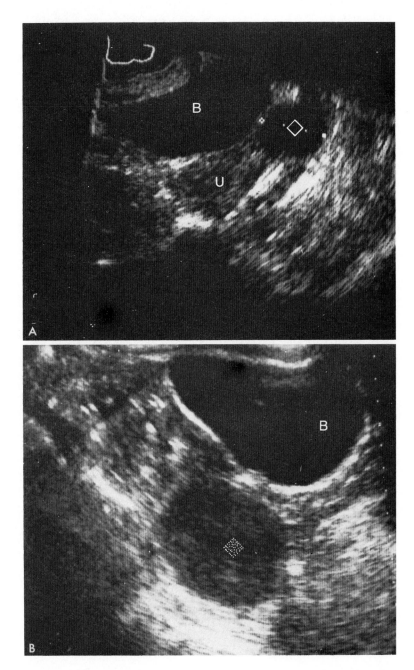

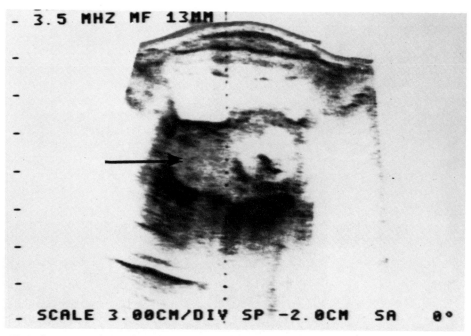

Figure 15–6. Sonogram of a pedunculated uterine fibroid mistaken for a pregnancy. (Courtesy of Dr. Lewis Nelson.)

and the guidance of biopsy needles can be visualized.

The abdominal aorta is readily recognized and aneurysms and branches of the aorta accurately depicted (Fig. 15–3). The aorta can be measured as can the size of the aneurysm (Fig. 15–4).

In the retroperitoneum, information can be gathered regarding the following: (1) renal size and content as well as location, (2) renal mass evaluation, and (3) renal biopsy. The urinary bladder can be evaluated if it is filled with fluid or water.

Pelvis

Ultrasonic evaluation of the pelvis has opened up an entire sphere of investigation for gynecologic (Fig. 15–5) and obstetric utilization (Fig. 15–6). Generally, the patient's urinary bladder is full, and the patient is placed supine, with longitudinal sonograms being the first ones to be employed from the umbilicus downward. Thereafter, cross-sec-

tional evaluation at 90 degrees to the midline is obtained. In evaluation of the cross-section, the urinary bladder is first visualized; behind it the uterus; and the ovaries may be seen lateral to the uterus (although variably identified). If a pelvic mass is identified, its texture can be further studied and differentiated, particularly in view of the great value of the ultrasonic beam in differentiating cystic from solid masses. Loculated fluid accumulations in the female pelvis can be detected and even aspirated by percutaneous guidance and biopsy.

In the study of obstetric problems, the placenta and uterus are readily identified. Moreover, the age of the fetus can be documented by measuring the biparietal diameter of the fetal skull and by such other measurements as the crown-rump length. Fetal death can be diagnosed by the appearance of the fetal head, even as it is suggested in conventional radiography, and the absence of fetal heart beat or movements of the fetus with M-mode evaluation.

16

Computed Tomography

Computed tomography, first developed in 1969 by Ambrose, a neuroradiologist, and Hounsfield, a physicist, has virtually revolutionized radiologic diagnostic imaging. In this technique, organs are viewed in cross-section rather than with the traditional *en face* approach. The initial device developed by these investigators required that a pencil-like beam of x-rays pass through the body, which contains tissues of different densities—called x-ray absorption coefficients. The beam of x-rays is attenuated in accordance with the absorption of the photons by the tissues. The original device required that this fine pencil-like beam move 1 degree each interval in a 180 degree arc around the individual, with a detector phosphorescent crystal receiving the photons emanating from the patient at each of these intervals. The width of the beam was 1.3 cm. The body was theoretically divided into small cubes measuring $1.3 \times 1.3 \times 0.5$ cm; and by an algorithm applied to the remnant radiation derived at each 1 degree interval, the transmitted radiation was calculated in relation to the absorption of the photons from the originating beam into each of the volume elements composing the cross-section. These volume elements are called "voxels." By means of this backward type of calculation and transmission of this information through a computer, the information was translated into an image displayed on either a cathode ray oscilloscope or television screen. Thus, the computer reconstructs a cross-sectional image of the patient (Fig. 16–1), depending on the size of the voxel employed.

Initially, this highly collimated x-ray beam scanned the patient in one direction and was indexed to move 1 degree at a time, but in later developments, the x-ray beam was allowed to fan out through the patient so that a number of detectors were struck simultaneously by this fan beam and related back to the voxels contained within the cross-section of the patient. By utilizing a fan beam rather than a slit beam, the x-ray beam could move 10 or 15 degrees in a very short interval of time, and thus the time of the procedure was significantly diminished, so that now as many as 2400 detectors may be utilized around the patient and a fan beam may scan an entire cross-section of the patient in as short a time interval as one second. The detector devices that have been used are either phosphorescent crystals or small xenon gas tubes. Not only can a picture of the cross-section be thereby derived, but by appropriate application of algorithms, coronal and sagittal sections may be recreated on the television screen. Moreover, the content of the tissue may be in part predicted from the absorption coefficients, so that an approach to histologic content of the tissue is thereby obtained. Small nodules of the lung have been analyzed; the fan beam, although scanning the patient more rapidly and allowing a better resolution type image, has unfortunately permitted a scatter of photons from one voxel to another, so that analysis of absorption coefficients in relation to histologic structure has become somewhat less accurate. It may be predicted that in the future histologic accuracy might be anticipated with appropriate development of machinery. However, even as of this writing, gray matter in the brain may be differentiated from white matter, white matter from cerebrospinal fluid (Fig. 16–2A–C), nuclear tissues of the brain differentiated from all other tissue, and hemorrhage differentiated from edema. Additionally, in the spine, the intravertebral disc may be clearly seen as different from the bony structures and the subarachnoid space, and spinal cord as well as nerve roots are clearly delineated.

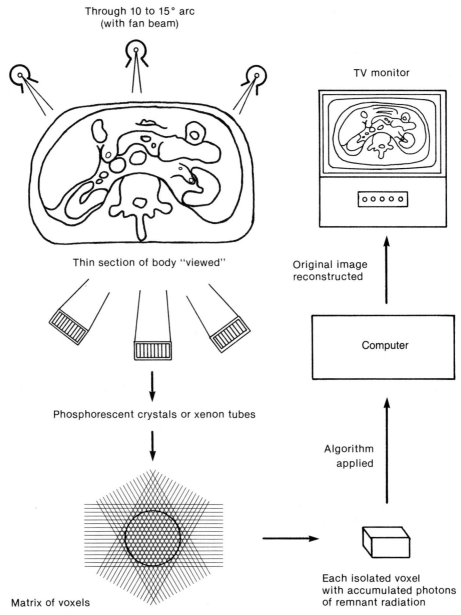

Figure 16–1. Diagrammatic representation of the basis for computed tomography.

By the intravenous injection of water-iodinated contrast media, blood vessels contained within the cross-section may be visualized—in which case this technique is "contrast enhancement." In similar fashion, contrast in low dilution may be injected into the gastrointestinal tract or any orifice of the body to enhance the visualization of contiguous anatomic structures.

The control mechanism for the device is equipped with a "window, width," which permits the selection of the range of absorption coefficients or units between the black and the white peaks displayed on the cathode ray tube or television screen. There is also a "window level" control to determine the center of the range selected by the window width control. Although in most machines this range is now from -1000 to $+1000$ with 0 being water, and -1000 being air and $+1000$ being bone, in one machine the $+1000$ has now been called $+2000$ for bone.

Computed tomography has already found wide application in studies of the brain, for which it was originally developed,

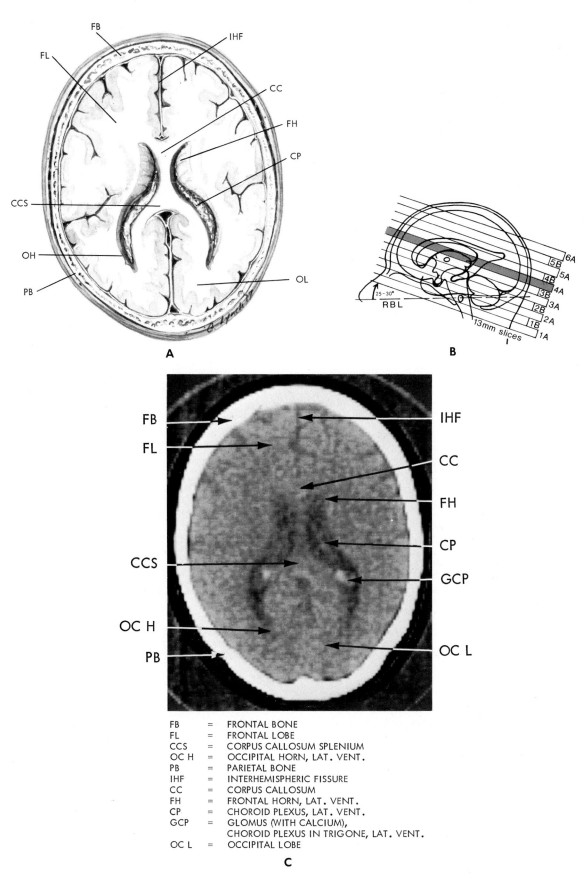

FB	=	FRONTAL BONE
FL	=	FRONTAL LOBE
CCS	=	CORPUS CALLOSUM SPLENIUM
OC H	=	OCCIPITAL HORN, LAT. VENT.
PB	=	PARIETAL BONE
IHF	=	INTERHEMISPHERIC FISSURE
CC	=	CORPUS CALLOSUM
FH	=	FRONTAL HORN, LAT. VENT.
CP	=	CHOROID PLEXUS, LAT. VENT.
GCP	=	GLOMUS (WITH CALCIUM), CHOROID PLEXUS IN TRIGONE, LAT. VENT.
OC L	=	OCCIPITAL LOBE

C

Figure 16–2. *A,* Diagram of brain through 4A level. *B,* Orientation for usual tomographic slices obtained (25–30 degrees to RBL). *C,* Tomographic slice at 4A level.

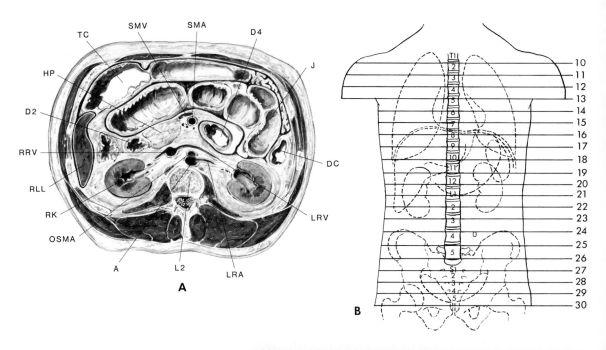

A

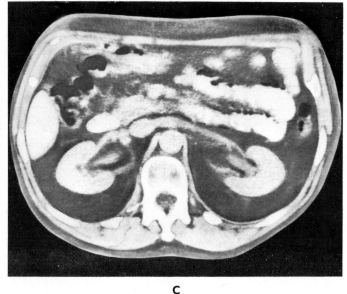

C

Figure 16–3. *A,* Diagram at upper abdomen level (L2) at cut No. 21, showing anatomic parts encountered in this slice. *B,* Line drawing showing the position of the computed tomographic cuts of the thorax and abdomen. *C,* Computed tomograph obtained approximately at this level. (Courtesy of Dr. Neil Wolfman.) A = aorta; OSMA = origin of superior mesenteric artery; RK = right kidney; RLL = right lower lobe; RRV = right renal vein; D2 = 2nd part of duodenum; HP = head of pancreas; TC = transverse colon; SMV = superior mesenteric vein; SMA = superior mesenteric artery; D4 = fourth part of duodenum; J = jejunum; DC = descending colon; LRV = left renal vein; LRA = left renal artery.

whereby such lesions as infarctions, epidural hematomas, subdural hematomas, brain tumors, and contusions of the brain could be readily identified. In addition, by application of this technique to cross-sections of the body, minute lesions in the tracheobronchial tree, the lung, the pleura, and throughout the abdomen may also be visualized. Retroperitoneal lesions (Fig. 16–3*A–C*) may be evaluated in respect to extent and organs of involvement, so that to a great extent the etiology of a disease may be predicted. The kidneys and suprarenals may be visualized. The pancreas, which hitherto has escaped

radiologic imaging, is clearly defined, and mediastinal lesions may be evaluated with an accuracy hitherto unanticipated. This method may also be utilized for examination of even orbital structures in which the oculus, the lens, the oribital muscles, the periorbital fat, the lacrimal gland, and the lacrimal duct may all be seen in extensive detail. These structures, which have hitherto defied radiographic imaging, can now be accurately depicted. Fractures that might have defied ordinary radiography might likewise be detected in the spine or elsewhere in the body.

Index

Note: Page numbers in *italic* type refer to illustrations; page numbers followed by (t) refer to tables.

Chest *Continued)*
oblique studies of, 21
PA view of, in staphylococcal pneumonia, *58*
pediatric problems of, 221–224
plain film examination of, apical lordotic view in, 23
chest walls and supraclavicular area in, 16
costophrenic angles in, 15, *15*
decubitus views in, 23
expiration views in, 23
in cardiac hypertrophy and dilatation, with pulmonary infarction, 33–34, *33*
in pleural effusion, 34–35, *35*
in pneumothorax, 31–32, *31*
inspiration views in, 23
lateral projection in, for definition of heart and left ventricle, *21, 22*
left PA oblique projection in, *19*
lung fields in, 15, 16, 21
oblique studies in, 23
PA projection in, 16, *17*
with barium in esophagus, *20*
position of heart in, 16
positions of pulmonary arteries in, 16
routine for study of, 15, *15, 16*
special views of ribs in, 23
trachea and mediastinal area in, 16
Children, abdominal problems in, 225
acute gastric dilatation in, 225
acute mastoiditis in, 225
acute osteomyelitis in, 232
air distention in upper abdomen of, 225
anomalies of base of first cervical vertebra in, 235
anomalies of base of skull in, 235
asthma in, 223, *224*
body surface area of, nomogram for determination of, 75(t)
brachial plexus injuries in, 235
cellulitis of knee in, 232
central cord syndrome in, 235
cervical cord and nerve root injuries in, 235
chest problems in, 221–224
congenital ureteropelvic obstruction in, *228,* 229–231, *230*
emergency conditions in, involving extremities, 232–234
Salter-Harris classification of, 233
enlarged lymph nodes in, 221
epistaxis in, 225
extension injuries of lower cervical spine in, 234
extraluminal gas patterns in, 226
head injury in, 234
hernias in, 227
ileus in, paralytic vs. mechanical, 225
ingestion of corrosive fluids by, 232
ingestion of foreign bodies by, 232
injuries of atlas in, 234–235
injuries of axis in, 234–235
intestinal volvulus in, 227
intravenous urography in, 238
intussusception in, 226
lateral flexion injuries of spine in, 235
multicystic kidney in, *228,* 229–231
neuroblastoma in, *228,* 229–231
pancreatic trauma in, 227
perforated appendicitis in, 226, *226*

Children *(Continued)*
pneumomediastinal air collections in, 223
pneumonia in, PA and lateral views in, *222, 223*
problems related to, 221
pulmonary edema in, 223
retropharyngeal abscess in, 225
rotation injuries of cervical spine in, 235
sentinel loop in, 225
septic arthritis in, 232
sinusitis in, 225
spinal problems in, 235
splenic torsion in, 227
tear-drop fracture in, 234
torus fracture in, 232
toxic synovitis in, 232
trauma to thoracolumbar spine in, 235
Wilms' tumor in, *228,* 229–231, *230*
Cholangiography, direct, methods of, 332(t)
percutaneous transhepatic, 324
intraoperative, 324
T-tube, 325, *325*
Cholangiopancreatography, endoscopic retrograde, 299, 323–324, *324*
Cholecystectomy, symptoms following, 333, 333(t)
Cholecystography, oral, of biliary system, 321–323, *321, 322*
Cholecystosis, 330
Choledocholithiasis, causes of, 333
Cholelithiasis. See *Gallstones.*
Cholesterol polyps, *326,* 327–328
Cholesterolosis, 330
Chondrosarcoma, plain film examination in, 53, *54*
Chordoma, plain film examination in, 53, *54*
Chronic obstructive lung disease, diagnostic studies for, 45–46
plain film examination in, 43–44, *43*
Clavicle, fracture of, *158,* 166
"Clay shoveler's" fracture, 162, 182
Coarctation of aorta, aortic knob in, 94, *95, 96*
rib notching in, *95, 96*
Coccyx, injuries of, 165
Colitis, ulcerative, 317–318, *317*
versus Crohn's colitis, 318(t)
Colles' fracture of wrist, 189, *190*
Colon. See also under *Intestine(s).*
adenocarcinoma of, 313, 315, *315,* 316
"apple-core" carcinoma of, 313–315, *315*
architecture of, analysis of, 11
diverticular disease of, 309–311, *309–311,* 311(t)
double-contrast, high-density barium air enema radiographs of, horizontal beam, *305*
routine PA studies, *303*
with patient prone and table tilted, *304*
epithelial polyps of, 316(t)
inflammatory disease of, 317–320, *317, 319–320,* 318(t)
neoplasms of, 300, *312,* 313–316, *314–316*
PA projection of, 302
polyps of, differentiation between types of, 300
rectosigmoid, annular carcinoma of, *315*
diverticular disease of, 309–310, *309, 310, 311,* 311(t)
polypoid carcinoma of, *314*